Operative Hip Arthroscopy

Second Edition

J.W. Thomas Byrd, MD

Assistant Clinical Professor, Department of Orthopaedics and Rehabilitation, Vanderbilt University School of Medicine, Nashville, Tennessee; Orthopaedic Center, Baptist Medical Plaza, Nashville Sports Medicine and Orthopaedic Center, Nashville, Tennessee

Editor

Operative Hip Arthroscopy

Second Edition

With 581 Illustrations in 814 Parts, 292 in Full Color

Forewords by Lanny L. Johnson, MD, and James R. Andrews, MD

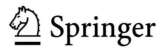 Springer

J.W. Thomas Byrd, MD
Assistant Clinical Professor
Department of Orthopaedics and Rehabilitation
Vanderbilt University School of Medicine
Nashville, TN
and
Orthopaedic Center
Baptist Medical Plaza
Nashville Sports Medicine and Orthopaedic Center
Nashville, TN 37203
USA

Library of Congress Cataloging-in-Publication Data
Byrd, J.W. Thomas (John Wilson Thomas), 1957–
    Operative hip arthroscopy / J.W. Thomas Byrd,—2nd ed.
        p. ; cm.
    Includes bibliographical references and index.
    ISBN 0-387-21011-3 (hc : alk. paper)
    1. Hip joint Examination.—2. Arthroscopy.   I. Title.
    [DNLM: 1. Arthroscopy methods.—2. Hip Joint—surgery.   3. Hip Joint—pathology. WE
860 B995o 2004]
    RD772.B97 2004
    617.5'810597—dc22   2004045358

First edition © Thieme, New York, Stuttgart

ISBN 0-387-21011-3   Printed on acid-free paper.

Printed in China.   (MP/EVB)

9 8 7 6 5 4 3 2 1   SPIN 10939703

springeronline.com

This second edition remains dedicated to my family, Donna, Allison, and Ellen, and to the two finest surgeons that I have known, Benjamin Franklin Byrd, Jr., and James Reuben Andrews.

My father, B.F. Byrd, Jr., has dedicated his entire life to fighting cancer, a much more admirable pursuit than anything I will do. He detoured only briefly from this battle to champion another cause, as a highly decorated medial officer overseeing the care of wounded from Normandy Beach through the fields of Europe. Through his lifelong example, he has shown me what being a physician is all about. As he put it, "a surgeon is just a regular doctor, with a few special skills."

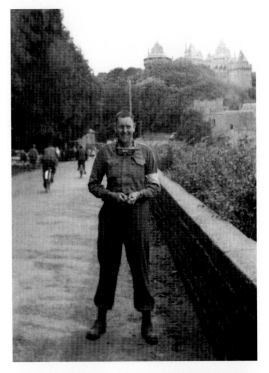

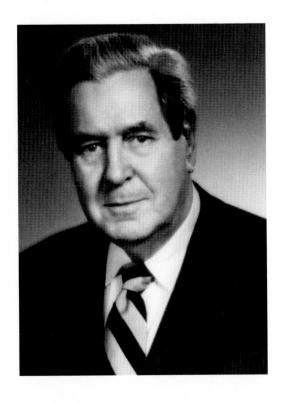

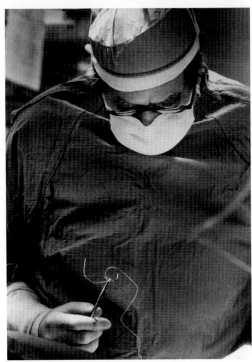

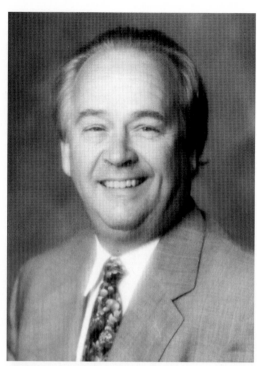

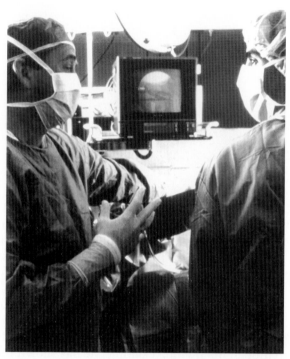

Dr. Andrews taught me the art and the philosophy of sports medicine. He also taught me much about how to treat patients as people and, fortunately, he shared with me a few of his remarkable surgical skills. Per- haps more importantly, through his example, he in- stilled in me the burning desire to make the most of my abilities.

J.W.T.B.

Preface

The fundamental principles for effectively performing hip arthroscopy remain unchanged from the first edition of this text. These include proper patient selection, attention to patient positioning for the procedure, careful orientation to the anatomy, meticulous technique in portal placement and instrumentation of the joint, and thoughtful guidance through the postoperative recovery.

However, the indications continue to expand and the available interventional technology is growing at an accelerated rate. This second edition attempts to capture these state-of-the art advancements and provides outcomes data now available with many of these methods.

Our knowledge of the normal arthroscopic anatomy is more complete. Interpretation of pathological anatomy is much improved, and we are now beginning to understand the pathomechanics involved in the development of many of these conditions. We have met with success in reducing the symptoms associated with a variety of painful conditions, improving the quality of life for many patients. However, it is through better understanding of the pathomechanics and pathophysiology that we can now start to influence the natural history and progression of many of these pathological states.

There are unique challenges to hip arthroscopy that should discourage the casual consideration of this procedure without clear indication and purpose. The dos and don'ts are clearly emphasized in this text. If you prepare to embark on a case of arthroscopic surgery of the hip, be sure of your indications, be versed in the technique, but read about the complications twice. As my father's chief, Barney Brooks, MD, Chief of Surgery Vanderbilt University, 1925–1952, was quoted as saying to one of his residents "Son, you don't have to learn about all the complications for yourself; you can read about a few of them."

The title *Operative Hip Arthroscopy* reflects a de-emphasis on the role of simply diagnostic procedures. In the chapter, Physical Examination, the diagnosis of intraarticular hip lesions may still be elusive. Arthroscopy may be considered without clear knowledge of the nature of the pathology, but usually with at least a good degree of predictability that there is something that can be addressed. If in doubt, most hip problems amenable to arthroscopy declare themselves over time.

In many respects, the distinction between diagnostic arthroscopy and operative arthroscopy is analogous to what Lewis Grizzard, the colorful journalist from Atlanta, said about the difference between naked and nekkid. "*Naked* means you ain't got no clothes on, and *nekkid* means you ain't got no clothes on and you're up to something." In this respect, with arthroscopy, we prefer to go "nekkid."

J.W. Thomas Byrd, MD

Contents

Contributors

Keith R. Berend, MD
Chief Resident, Division of Orthopedics, Duke University Medical Center, Durham, NC 27713, USA

J.W. Thomas Byrd, MD
Assistant Clinical Professor, Department of Orthopaedics and Rehabilitation, Vanderbilt University School of Medicine, Nashville, TN; Orthopaedic Center, Baptist Medical Plaza, Nashville Sports Medicine and Orthopaedic Center, Nashville, TN 37203, USA

Michael Dienst, MD
Assistant Professor, Department of Orthopedic Surgery, University Hospital, 66421 Homburg/Saar, Germany

Roy E. Erb, MD
Western Colorado Radiology Associates, Grand Junction, CO 81501, USA

Karen M. Griffin, PT, ATC
Physical Therapist/Athletic Trainer, STAR Physical Therapy, Nashville, TN 37115, USA

Kay S. Jones, MSN, RN
Clinical Nurse Specialist, Nashville Sports Medicine and Orthopaedic Center, Nashville, TN 37203, USA

Bert R. Mandelbaum, MD
Santa Monica Orthopaedic and Sports Medicine Group, Santa Monica, CA 90404, USA

William C. Meyers, MD
Professor and Chairman, Department of Surgery, Assistant Dean, Interdisciplinary Studies, Drexel University College of Medicine, Philadelphia, PA 19102, USA

Steve A. Mora, MD
Santa Monica Orthopaedic and Sports Medicine Group, Santa Monica, CA 90404, USA

Archit Naik
Medical Student, Department of Surgery, Drexel University College of Medicine, Philadelphia, PA 19102, USA

Nicholas D. Potter, DPT, ATC
Physical Therapist, Department of Orthopaedics, Duke University Medical Center, Durham, NC 27710, USA

T. Kevin Robinson, PT, DSc OCS
Associate Professor, School of Physical Therapy, Belmont University; Physical Therapist, STAR Physical Therapy, Nashville, TN 37115, USA

Jeff Ryan, PT
Physical Therapist, Department of Orthopedics, Drexel University College of Medicine, Philadelphia, PA 19102, USA

Thomas G. Sampson, MD
Associate Clinical Professor, Department of Orthopaedic Surgery, University of California, San Francisco, CA, Orthopaedic Surgeon, San Francisco, CA 94109, USA

Nicola Santori, MD, PhD
Centro Diagnostico, 00154 Rome, Italy

Levente J. Szalai, MD
Resident, Department of Surgery, Drexel University College of Medicine, Philadelphia, PA 19102, USA

Thomas Parker Vail, MD
Associate Professor, Director of Adult Reconstructive Surgery, Division of Orthopaedic Surgery, Duke University Medical Center, Durham, North Carolina 27710, USA

Richard N. Villar, MS, FRCS
Cambridge Hip and Knee Unit, BUPA Cambridge Lea Hospital, Impington, Cambridge CB4 4EL, UK

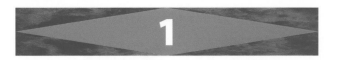

Overview and History of Hip Arthroscopy

J.W. Thomas Byrd

The history of endoscopic in vivo examination of the human body is well known to students of arthroscopic techniques.[1] This history dates back almost 200 years to the Austrian, Philipp Bozzini, who in 1806 devised the *Lichtleiter* (Austrian for light conductor). This instrument, designed for inspection of the rectum and vagina, actually gained clinical record for its use in inspection of the larynx and vocal cords.[2]

Instruments for viewing human anatomy were heralded as providing indisputable evidence of disease. Previously, only indirect evidence of various disorders was usually available. It is worthy to note that, at the time of Bozzini's invention, auscultation was the principal method of examining the human body. However, when auscultation skills and instruments were initially introduced, they were not without their detractors. Many physicians believed that it would necessitate that they abandon other examination methods that they had spent years developing and feared they might not possess the necessary skills for performing effective auscultation.[2] Centuries later, these same barriers existed in the acceptance of modern arthroscopic techniques.

Following Bozzini's initial design, crude cystoscopes of various constructs were developed over the ensuing 100 years. All of these were limited by lack of an adequate light source. However, by the early 1900s, electricity was discovered and Edison had invented the incandescent light bulb. This accomplishment opened new horizons in the development of endoscopic instruments. In 1918, Kenji Takagi[3] visualized the interior of a cadaveric knee joint with a cystoscope. The first recorded attempt at arthroscopic visualization of the hip is attributed to Michael S. Burman[4] in 1931 (Figures 1.1, 1.2). For his purposes, an arthroscope was constructed by Reinhold Wappler with a diameter of 4 mm, not dissimilar to the dimensions of our current arthroscopes (Figure 1.3). Burman used fluid distension for visualization, examining the interior of more than 90 various joints in cadaver specimens, correlating the arthroscopic anatomy with the gross anatomy on subsequent dissection. Twenty of these were hip joints.

Burman made several pertinent and prudent observations that still hold true today, more than over 60 years later. His examination of the hip did not use distraction, and the structures that he successfully visualized correspond with the structures that currently are discernible via arthroscopy without distraction (Figure 1.4). These aspects include much of the articular surface of the femoral head, seen by placing the hip through range of motion, and the intracapsular portion of the femoral neck. With this approach, the acetabulum, fossa, and ligamentum teres could not be visualized.

Burman noted that "visualization of the hip joint is limited to the intracapsular part of the joint." This statement still has much bearing in current applications of hip arthroscopy. Although arthroscopy has been used for release of a snapping iliopsoas tendon and for extracapsular bone fragments that impinge on the joint, intraarticular sources of pathology are most amenable to arthroscopic intervention.

Burman further stated:

"We experimented with a number of punctures and the anterior paratrochanteric puncture proved the best. . . . The anterior paratrochanteric puncture is undoubtedly the best and is made slightly anterior to the greater trochanter along the course of the neck of the femur. . . . The puncture is not hard to do and one can visualize the hip with it in almost every case. Originally we were skeptical as to whether anything could be seen in the hip joint, but we have had unusual success with this puncture."

The anterior paratrochanteric (or anterolateral; see Chapter 7) portal is clearly the workhorse portal for modern arthroscopy. Although there is some variation of the other portals described by numerous authors, this is the one position common to all and, according to an anatomic study, it is the safest.[5]

Burman continued:

"We have been careful to choose cadavers of slender build since our trochar is not long enough to puncture the hip of a well muscled person. . . . A special long trochar with a correspondingly long telescope should thus be used for the hip joint. The line of the femoral artery and the position of the head of the fe-

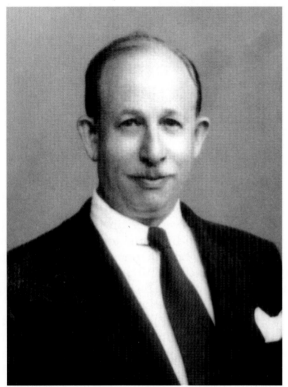

FIGURE 1.1. Dr. Michael Samuel Burman (1901–1975). (Reprinted with permission of New York Academy of Medicine.)

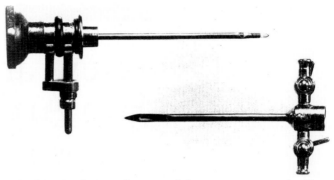

FIGURE 1.3. Photograph reprinted from Burman's article illustrates the arthroscopic instruments devised by Reinhold Wappler and used by Dr. Burman in his investigative studies. The upper portion is the telescope (measuring 3 mm in diameter); the lower portion is the trochar sheath (measuring 4 mm in diameter.) (From Burman,[4] with permission.)

mur should be marked beforehand to avoid possible damage to the vessels. This should only be a theoretical accident."

For the surgeon who only occasionally is challenged by the role of arthroscopic surgery of the hip, size may be a relative contraindication, and even for an experienced arthroscopist it may preclude the ability to enter the hip joint. Indeed, as recommended by Burman, extra-length cannulas and instruments are used but, in some cases, even these may not be adequate. Also, a careful appreciation of the orientation

of the major neurovascular structures is always critical. There are anecdotal accounts such as a case of irreparable damage to the femoral nerve. This type of catastrophic scenario should be unlikely with basic understanding and orientation of the extraarticular anatomy.

The first clinical application of the arthroscope in the hip of a patient was reported by Takagi[3] in 1939 (Figure 1.5). This report consisted of four hips, including two cases of Charcot joints, one tuberculous arthritis, and one suppurative arthritis.

The clinical implications of arthroscopic techniques, especially about the knee, began to flourish following the publication of the second edition of *Atlas of Arthroscopy* by Masaki Watanabe et al.[6] in 1965 (Figure 1.6). Watanabe was a student of Takagi's. He also visited with Michael Burman in the evolution of his techniques.

However, following Takagi's report in 1939, the clinical applications of arthroscopy about the hip went unmentioned until the 1970s with Aignan's[7] report of attempted diagnostic arthroscopy and biopsy of 51 hips. This study was presented at the 1975 meeting of the International Arthroscopy Association in Copenhagen. In 1977, Richard Gross described 32 diagnostic arthroscopic procedures in 27 children for a variety of pediatric hip disorders including congenital dislocation, Legg–Calvé–Perthes disease, neuropathic subluxation, prior sepsis, and slipped capital femoral epiphysis.[8] A second clinical series appeared in the pediatric literature in 1981 when Svante Holgersson et al.[9] reported on the role of arthroscopy in assessing 15 hips in 13 children with juvenile chronic arthritis. Between these two series, there were two case reports on removal of entrapped cement fragments following total hip arthroplasty, one from the New York City Hospital for Special Surgery and one from Israel.[10,11]

The 1980s brought several important advancements that contributed to the applications of opera-

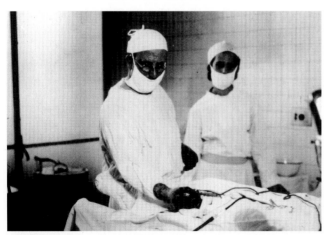

FIGURE 1.2. Dr. Burman performing an arthroscopic procedure at the Hospital for Joint Diseases in 1935. (Courtesy of Serge Parisien, MD; from Parisien,[26] with permission.)

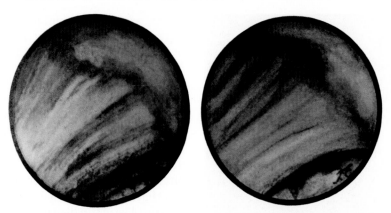

FIGURE 1.4. Burman's illustration of the arthroscopic view of a hip visualizing the ridging of the neck of the femur, the junction of the neck and the femoral head, and a portion of the articular surface of the femoral head. (From Burman,[4] with permission.)

tive hip arthroscopy. In 1981 Lanny Johnson[12] addressed the role of arthroscopy of the hip joint in the second edition of his textbook, *Diagnostic and Surgical Arthroscopy* (Figure 1.7). In 1985, Watanabe[13] also described the technique for carrying out the procedure in *Arthroscopy of Small Joints*. In 1986 Ejnar Eriksson et al.[14] from Sweden described the forces necessary for adequate hip distraction. This was an in vivo study of patients undergoing arthroscopy as well as a study of unanesthetized volunteers, which included Professor Eriksson himself.

James Glick from San Francisco has been recognized as the single greatest influence on the development of hip arthroscopy in North America (Figure 1.8).

Motivated by the creative ideas of Lanny Johnson, Glick began performing the procedure in 1977. He recognized limitations of the technique in obese patients. Influenced by his partner, Thomas Sampson, in 1985 they modified the procedure and began placing the patient in the lateral decubitus position. Their preliminary experiences were reported in 1987.[15] This and subsequent works have been the cornerstones on which other surgeons have founded their approach.[16–18] Arthroscopy by the lateral approach has been found to be accessible and reproducible. Additionally, a custom distractor has been developed that greatly facilitates arthroscopy in this position.

In the mid-1980s, Richard Villar from Cambridge,

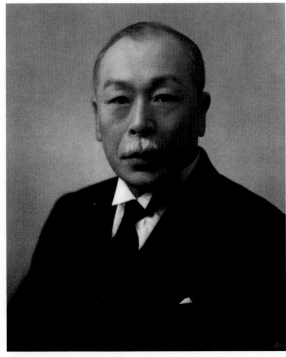

FIGURE 1.5. Dr. Kenji Takagi (1888–1963). (Courtesy of Tokyo Teishin Hospital.)

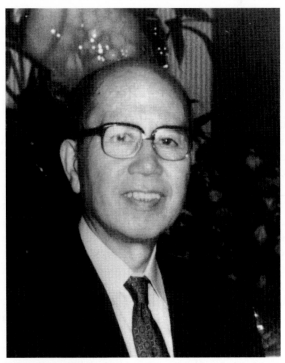

FIGURE 1.6. Dr. Masaki Watanabe (1911–1994). (Courtesy of Tokyo Teishin Hospital.)

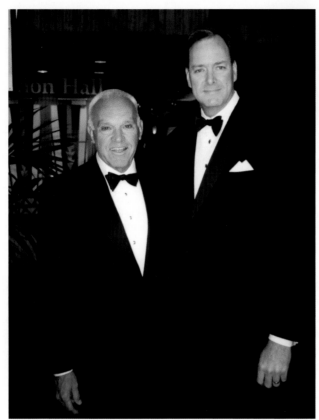

FIGURE 1.7. The author (right) with Lanny Johnson (left), a pioneer of arthroscopy as a clinician, scientist, and inventor. (Courtesy of Dr. J.W. Thomas Byrd.)

England, envisioned several useful roles for arthroscopy of the hip. He corresponded with James Glick and Richard Hawkins, who had published some of the few articles available on the topic at the time.[15–19] Villar subsequently pioneered the technique in England and has taught the procedure to others now beginning to perform it in the United Kingdom. He has reported in detail his extensive experience with arthroscopic anatomy and operative arthroscopy.[20,21]

Brian Day from Toronto accurately envisioned the expanding role for operative hip arthroscopy and has written on the anatomy, indications, and nomenclature for this technique.[22,23] Gary Poehling and Dave Ruch from Winston-Salem, NC, have explored the role of arthroscopy as a supplemental technique in the management of avascular necrosis of the femoral head.[24] Down the road in Durham, Tad Vail has published his experience, useful in selecting potential candidates for hip arthroscopy.[25] Serge Parisien from the Hospital for Joint Diseases in New York City authored several pertinent publications in the 1980s, and Joe McCarthy from Boston has been active reporting his experience in numerous aspects of hip arthroscopy.[23,26,27]

In the United States, little attention has been given to the prospect of performing hip arthroscopy without distraction.[28] However, Henri Dorfmann and Thierry Boyer, a pair of rheumatologists from Paris, France, have accumulated a large number of cases performed by this method.[29,30] Dr. Dorfmann learned the techniques of arthroscopy training under Dr. Watanabe in Japan and pioneered his own method of hip arthroscopy, especially important for viewing the peripheral compartment. As rheumatologists, Drs. Dorfmann and Boyer especially focus on the role of synovial pathology as a source of hip disease. Their method is unsurpassed in being able to address the synovium and often complements the traditional distraction methods that have otherwise been most popular.

Dysplastic hip disease is quite prevalent in Japan.[31] The association of labral lesions with dysplasia may explain why there have been several significant studies regarding labral lesions reported from Japanese centers.[32–34] In 1991, Ide et al.[35] reported what, at the time, was the largest clinical series of arthroscopic procedures.

In Nashville, the author has redefined the application of the supine position and has gained increasing experience in the use of this approach in operative hip arthroscopy.[36,37] Minor modifications to a standard fracture table facilitate many of the advantages attributed to the lateral position.

The progression and application of arthroscopic techniques for the hip have lagged behind those for other joints because of the unique challenges imposed by its anatomy. Although slower, the evolution of hip arthroscopy has paralleled that of other joints. Early clinical applications were followed by a hiatus of four decades. The reemergence of case reports and small clinical series was surrounded by uncertainty regarding the merits of the procedure. Arthroscopic investigation of the joint has subsequently expanded our

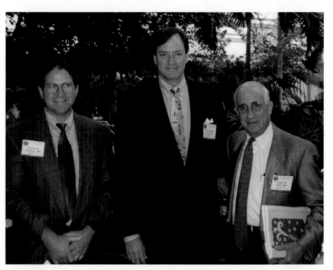

FIGURE 1.8. The author (center) with James Glick (right) and Thomas Sampson (left). Jim Glick, the single greatest figure in modern hip arthroscopy, was motivated by Lanny Johnson and influenced in his techniques by his younger partner, Tom Sampson. (Courtesy of Dr. J.W. Thomas Byrd.)

knowledge of hip disease and injury. This investigative phase has been followed with a clearer understanding of the indications and technique. The evolution is not complete, but the foundation laid by many of these pioneers has provided the basis for the fundamentals of operative hip arthroscopy.

The maturation of arthroscopic methods has begun a transformation to endoscopic techniques for areas surrounding the hip. Already surgeons are able to address bone fragments outside the joint and to address lesions of the iliopsoas tendon. The incentive is to make surgical procedures less invasive. This category will undoubtedly soon include procedures in which the scope is used as an adjunct to arthroscopic and endoscopic assisted techniques. This development will be driven exponentially by the next generation of surgeons and scientists. Each clinician brings a unique perspective and experience that will benefit all those who struggle on the continually changing horizon of technology with which to battle hip disease.

References

1. Joyce JJ, Jackson OR: Historical Perspectives: History of Arthroscopy. American Academy of Orthopaedic Surgeons Symposium on Arthroscopy and Arthrography of the Knee. St. Louis: Mosby, 1978.
2. Reiser SJ: Medicine and the Reign of Technology. Cambridge, UK: Cambridge University Press, 1978.
3. Takagi K: The arthroscope: the second report. J Jpn Orthop Assoc 1939;14:441–466.
4. Burman M: Arthroscopy or the direct visualization of joints. J Bone Joint Surg 1931;13:669–694.
5. Byrd JWT, Pappas JN, Pedley MJ: Hip arthroscopy: an anatomic study of portal placement and relationship to the extraarticular structures. Arthroscopy 1994;11:418–423.
6. Watanabe M, Takeda S, Ikeuchi H: Atlas of Arthroscopy, 2nd ed. Tokyo: Igaku-Shoin, 1970.
7. Aignan M: Arthroscopy of the hip. In: Proceedings of the International Association of Arthroscopy. Rev Int Rheumatol 1976;33:458.
8. Gross R: Arthroscopy in hip disorders in children. Orthop Rev 1977;6:43–49.
9. Holgersson S, Brattström H, Mogensen B, Lidgren L: Arthroscopy of the hip in juvenile chronic arthritis. J Pediatr Orthop 1981;1:273–278.
10. Shifrin L, Reis N: Arthroscopy of a dislocated hip replacement: a case report. Clin Orthop 1980;146:213–214.
11. Vakili F, Salvati EA, Warren RF: Entrapped foreign body within the acetabular cup in total hip replacement. Clin Orthop 1980;150:159–162.
12. Johnson LL: Hip joint. In: Johnson LL (ed). Diagnostic and Surgical Arthroscopy: The Knee and Other Joints, 2nd ed. St. Louis: Mosby, 1981:405–411.
13. Watanabe M: Arthroscopy of Small Joints. Tokyo: Igaku-Shoin, 1985.
14. Eriksson E, Arvidsson I, Arvidsson H: Diagnostic and operative arthroscopy of the hip. Orthopaedics 1986;9:169–176.
15. Glick JM, Sampson TG, Gordon BB, Behr JT, Schmidt E: Hip arthroscopy by the lateral approach. Arthroscopy 1987;3:4–12.
16. Glick JM: Hip arthroscopy using the lateral approach. Instr Course Lect 1988;37:223–231.
17. Glick JM, Sampson TG: Hip arthroscopy by the lateral approach. In: McGinty J, Caspari R, Jackson R, Poehling G (eds). Operative Arthroscopy, 2nd ed. New York: Raven Press, 1995: 1079–1090.
18. Glick JM: Complications of hip arthroscopy by the lateral approach. In: Sherman OH, Minkoff J (eds). Current Management of Complications in Orthopaedics: Arthroscopic Surgery. Baltimore: Williams & Wilkins, 1990:193–201.
19. Hawkins RB: Arthroscopy of the hip. Clin Orthop 1989;249: 44–47.
20. Villar RN: Hip Arthroscopy. Oxford: Butterworth-Heinemann, 1992.
21. Keene GS, Villar RN: Arthroscopic anatomy of the hip: an in vivo study. Arthroscopy 1994;10:392–399.
22. Dvorak M, Duncan CP, Day B: Arthroscopic anatomy of the hip. Arthroscopy 1990;6:264–273.
23. McCarthy JC, Day B, Busconi B: Hip arthroscopy: applications and technique. J Am Acad Orthop Surg 1995;3:115–122.
24. Ruch DS, Sekiya J, Dickson Schaefer W, Koman LA, Pope TL, Poehling GG: The role of hip arthroscopy in the evaluation of avascular necrosis. Orthopedics 2001;24:339–343.
25. O'Leary JA, Berend K, Vail TP: The relationship between diagnosis and outcome in arthroscopy of the hip. Arthroscopy 2001;17:181–188.
26. Parisien JS: Arthroscopy of the hip, present status. Bull Hosp Joint Dis Orthop Inst 1985;45:127–132.
27. Parisien JS: Arthroscopy surgery of the hip. In: Parisien JS (ed). Arthroscopic Surgery. New York: McGraw-Hill, 1988:283–291.
28. Klapper RC, Silver DM: Hip arthroscopy without distraction. Contemp Orthop 1989;18:687–693.
29. Dorfmann H, Boyer T, Henry P, de Bie B: A simple approach to hip arthroscopy. Arthroscopy 1988;4:141–142.
30. Dorfmann H, Boyer T: Arthroscopy of the hip: 12 years of experience. Arthroscopy 1999;15:67–72.
31. Yoshimura N, Campbell L, Hashimoto T, et al: Acetabular dysplasia in Britain and Japan. British Society for Rheumatology, Brighton, 1994, Abstract. Br J Rheumatol 1994;33(suppl 1):102.
32. Ikeda T, Awaya G, Suzuki S, Okada Y, Tada H: Torn acetabular labrum in young patients. J Bone Joint Surg 1988;70B: 13–16.
33. Ueo T, Suzuki S, Iwasaki R, Yosikawa J: Rupture of the labra acetabularis as a cause of hip pain detected arthroscopically, and partial limbectomy for successful pain relief. Arthroscopy 1990;6:48–51.
34. Suzuki S, Awaya G, Okada Y, Maekawa M, Ikeda T, Tada H: Arthroscopic diagnosis of ruptured acetabular labrum. Acta Orthop Scand 1986;57:513–515.
35. Ide T, Akamatsu N, Nakajima I: Arthroscopic surgery of the hip joint. Arthroscopy 1991;7:204–211.
36. Byrd JWT: Hip arthroscopy utilizing the supine position. Arthroscopy 1994;10(3):275–280.
37. Byrd JWT: Operative Hip Arthroscopy. New York: Thieme, 1998.

2

Indications and Contraindications

J.W. Thomas Byrd

The indications for hip arthroscopy continue to evolve (Table 2.1). Even in this evolutionary process, the key to successful results most clearly is proper patient selection. A well-performed procedure fails when performed for the wrong reasons. Proper patient selection includes not only selecting lesions amenable to arthroscopic intervention but also assessing the patient as a whole. The patient must have reasonable expectations of what may be accomplished with arthroscopy. Again, a procedure successfully performed by the surgeon will be deemed a failure if it does not fulfill the patient's expectations.

LOOSE BODIES

Symptomatic loose bodies represent the clearest indication for arthroscopic intervention. The most common source is probably posttraumatic intraarticular fragments.[1] Synovial chondromatosis is another source that has been variously reported.[2,3] The hip is the third most common site of involvement of this disease, and the diagnosis can be elusive, with at least half of the cases unrecognized before arthroscopy, according to McCarthy et al.[4] Fragments may occur in association with Legg–Calvé–Perthes disease due to accompanying osteochondritis dissecans, and excision of these loose articular or osteoarticular fragments may result in remarkable improvement, even in the presence of a severely misshapen femoral head.[5,6] Loose bodies can lead to secondary degenerative arthritis, but sometimes loose bodies simply occur secondary to degenerative disease. In either case, the extent of degeneration may be the limiting factor in the response to arthroscopy and, with advanced deterioration, removing the loose bodies may not be of any benefit. There have also been reports of removal of foreign objects such as bullets.[7–9]

Removal of symptomatic loose bodies represents the clearest indication for hip arthroscopy for three reasons:

1. The diagnosis is usually easy to determine. Radiodense loose bodies may be apparent on plain radiographs and can be substantiated by computer-ized tomography (CT). Radiolucent cartilaginous loose bodies can be better visualized by gadolinium arthrography with magnetic resonance imaging (MRA) or iodinated contrast with CT (Arthro-CT).

2. The importance of loose body removal from the hip has been well documented in the literature, largely based on the work of Epstein,[10,11] who defined the poor prognosis associated with retained intraarticular fragments. In fact, without the alternative of the arthroscopic approach, arthrotomy with dislocation of the hip for adequate debridement would be required.

3. Compared with an arthrotomy, arthroscopy is significantly less invasive and offers numerous advantages. These benefits include fewer and less serious surgical complications, lower associated morbidity, no hospitalization, less postoperative pain, and quicker recovery with return to normal activities.

Three case examples highlight the merits of the arthroscopic approach in addressing symptomatic hips with radiographic evidence of loose bodies.

Case 1

A 17-year-old boy presented 2 years following closed treatment of a posterior column fracture of the right acetabulum. He had developed progressive mechanical hip joint symptoms including pain, catching, and a sensation of giving way, with discomfort localized to the groin area. Radiographs revealed changes consistent with his previous fracture and areas suggestive of intraarticular loose bodies (Figure 2.1A). Multiple cartilaginous and osseous loose bodies were confirmed by double-contrast arthrography followed by CT scan (Figure 2.1B). At arthroscopy, multiple loose bodies were identified (Figure 2.1C). Many were too large to be retrieved through large-diameter cannulas but could be removed free-hand and with extra-length pituitary rongeurs.

Case 2

A 28-year-old man presented 5 years following closed treatment of a posterior wall fracture of the left ac-

Table 2.1. Indications

Loose bodies	Avascular necrosis
Labral lesions	Instability
Chondral injuries	Adhesive capsulitis
Ruptured ligamentum teres	Sepsis
Degenerative arthritis	Status post total hip arthroplasty
Synovial disease	Unresolved hip pain
Impinging osteophytes	Associated with open procedures

etabulum. He described progressively debilitating symptoms of mechanical groin and hip pain, worsened with activities. Radiographs revealed mild changes consistent with his old injury as well as apparent intraarticular bony fragments (Figure 2.2A); this was confirmed by double-contrast arthrography followed by CT scan (Figure 2.2B). At arthroscopy, grade III articular sur-

face wear was debrided with significant symptomatic improvement (Figure 2.2C). The bone fragments were found to be firmly fixed within the acetabular fossa and not involving the weight-bearing portion of the joint. Arthroscopy was beneficial with regard to the chondroplasty and helped define the status of the bone fragments, avoiding the potential alternative consideration of a more extensive operative procedure such as arthrotomy to address these fragments.

Case 3

A 20-year-old man presented with a 3-month history of acute left hip pain that occurred while playing basketball. His history was remarkable for Legg–Calvé–Perthes disease treated conservatively at age 8. He related no recent symptoms until this acute episode. Ra-

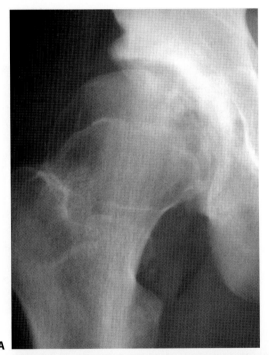

FIGURE 2.1. A 17-year-old man with mechanical right hip pain 2 years following closed treatment of a posterior column fracture of the acetabulum. (A) Anteroposterior (AP) radiograph shows evidence of posttraumatic degenerative changes with mild deformation of the femoral head. (B) A double-contrast iodinated contrast with computed tomography (Arthro-CT) scan confirms the presence of multiple loose bodies represented by the numerous filling defects (arrows) posteriorly on this image through the joint. (C) Arthroscopic view reveals several of the representative loose bodies between the femoral head and acetabulum. (C, from Byrd,[34] with permission of Arthroscopy.)

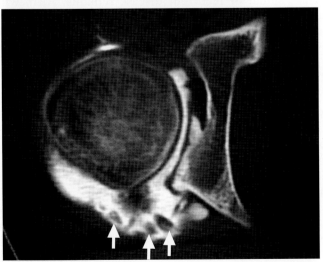

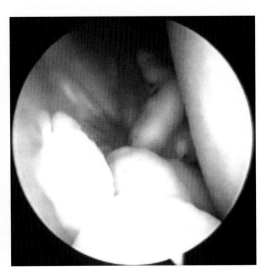

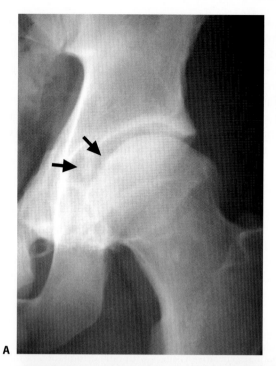

FIGURE 2.2. A 28-year-old man with mechanical left hip pain 5 years following closed treatment of a posterior wall fracture of the acetabulum. (A) AP radiograph reveals changes consistent with an old acetabular fracture and suggests the presence of bony fragments (arrows). (B) A double-contrast Arthro-CT scan shows further evidence of fragments within the joint (arrow). (C) Arthroscopy revealed grade III articular surface damage present in the femoral head (F) and degeneration of the labrum (L) but no free-floating fragments.

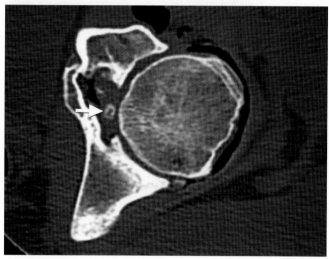

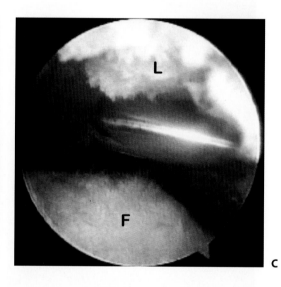

diographs revealed changes consistent with his previous Perthes disease as well as evidence of an intraarticular fragment (Figure 2.3A,B). A CT scan further demonstrated evidence of an intraarticular fragment (Figure 2.3C). Arthroscopy revealed numerous free-floating fragments (Figure 2.3D). Enlarging the anterior portal allowed retrieval of these fragments (Figure 2.3E–G).

Although removal of symptomatic loose bodies represents the clearest indication for hip arthroscopy, there are still potential pitfalls. The premise that loose fragments should be removed is based on Epstein's long-term follow-up of posterior fracture dislocations of the hip. Loose bodies or free fragments associated with disease may have other influencing factors. For example, removal of loose bodies associated with synovial osteochondromatosis may result in significant symptomatic improvement, but the possibility of re-

sidual or recurrent disease remains. Also, when intraarticular fragments are accompanied by degenerative disease, it is the extent of degeneration that is often the limiting factor in the response to surgery. Last, removal of free fragments associated with osteonecrosis can result in significant alleviation of mechanical joint symptoms, but the long-term prognosis will be dependent on the natural history of the underlying area of infarct.

LABRAL LESIONS

Labral tears are the most common indication for hip arthroscopy.[12] Despite the frequency with which these lesions are addressed, there is still much that is not fully understood regarding the pathomechanics

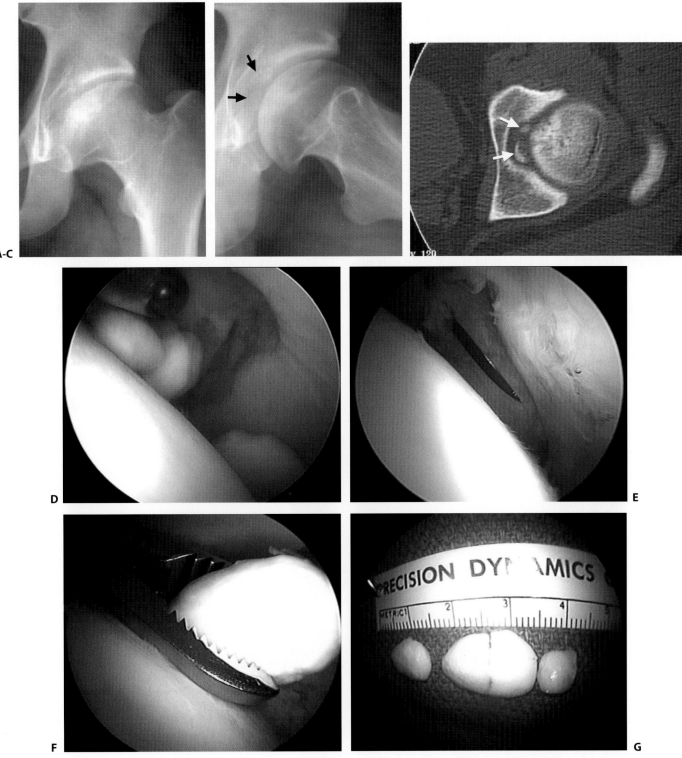

FIGURE 2.3. A 20-year-old man with a 3-month history of acute left hip pain. (A) AP radiograph demonstrates findings consistent with old Legg–Calvé–Perthes disease. (B) Lateral view defines the presence of intraarticular loose bodies (arrows). (C) CT scan substantiates the intraarticular location of the fragments (arrows). (D) Arthroscopic view medially demonstrates the loose bodies.

(E) Viewing anteriorly, the anterior capsular incision is enlarged with an arthroscopic knife to facilitate removal of the fragments. (F) One of the fragments is being retrieved. (G) Loose bodies can be removed whole. (E and F, JWT Byrd. Arthroscopy, December 2003, with permission.)

and natural history. This may partly explain why the results of surgical intervention, although often good, are not uniformly successful.

Labral tears were first reported in the literature as

a detachment associated with posterior dislocation of the hip, serving as a block to reduction or source of recurrent instability.[13–15] Altenberg, in 1977, was the first to report on labral pathology as a cause of hip pain in absence of a dislocation episode.[16] He described two cases treated with open debridement.

The labrum is a fibrocartilaginous rim that encompasses the circumference of the acetabulum, effectively deepening the socket (Figure 2.4). The ring is incomplete inferiorly where the labrum ends at the anterior and posterior margins of the inferior aspect of the acetabular fossa, becoming confluent with the transverse acetabular ligament. The acetabular labrum has not been studied as extensively as has its counterpart, the glenoid labrum of the shoulder. Functionally, it may not be quite as complex, but it is susceptible to acute tearing and degeneration.[17,18]

The constrained ball-and-socket bony architecture of the hip provides much more inherent stability than the glenohumeral joint. Although the acetabular labrum may not be as critical to this stability, it undoubtedly has an important role in the distribution of forces across the articular surfaces of the joint.[17] Additionally, a normally positioned labrum is critical to normal acetabular development, as animal studies have shown that aberrant positioning of the labrum leads to dysplasia and osteoarthritis.[19]

Seldes et al. reported in detail the anatomy, histologic features, and vascularity of the adult acetabular labrum.[20] They described that the capsule attaches directly to the bony rim of the acetabulum with a distinct separation from the labrum (Figure 2.5). Thus, integrity of the labrum does not appear to be as critical to stability of the hip as compared with the capsulolabral complex in the shoulder. It is likely that the labrum still has a role as a fluid seal, creating a vacuum effect to enhance stability, but labral lesions do not appear to be as synonymous with instability of the hip as compared with the shoulder. These authors also observed that labral degeneration occurs as part of the aging process and identified microvascular proliferation in conjunction with tears, suggesting some capacity for healing.

McCarthy et al. correlated their clinical observations on labral tears with an anatomic study and made the following observations.[21] Tears begin at the articular labral junction, an area that they term the *watershed region*. They observed that the labrum receives its blood supply from the obturator, superior gluteal, and inferior gluteal arteries. These vessels en-

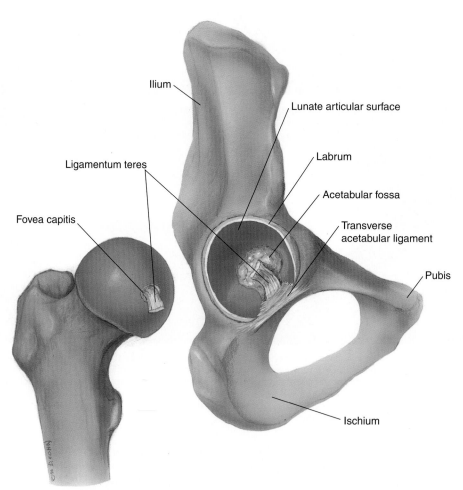

FIGURE 2.4. Acetabulum and the fibrocartilaginous labrum.

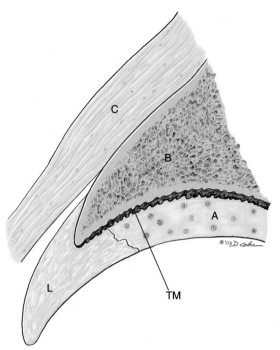

FIGURE 2.5. Relationship of the acetabular labrum and capsule as described by Seldes, including the bone of the acetabulum (B), labrum (L), articular cartilage (A), the tide mark (TM), and capsule (C).

ter through the synovium at the reflection of the capsule onto the peripheral surface of the labrum, penetrating only the outermost layer of the labrum on its capsular side. They also observed that labral lesions are almost uniformly present in elderly cadaver specimens.

Arthroscopy has defined considerable morphologic variation of the labrum. Sometimes it is thin and hypoplastic and other times robust in size. This variation is most evident in the presence of acetabular dysplasia in which the labrum is markedly enlarged, assuming a weight-bearing role and importance in stability of the joint.

The greatest variability of the labrum is found lateral and anterior. The posterior labrum exhibits the most consistent morphology and is the least often damaged. Early arthroscopic literature from Japan reported a propensity for posterior labral tears.[22–24] However, this observation has not been supported by more recent literature in which most tears have been observed laterally and anteriorly.[23–25] This discrepancy may reflect unique aspects of the population or may simply be aberrant because of the small study groups reported.

Villar et al. have developed a classification system for labral tears categorized according to etiology (traumatic, degenerative, idiopathic, congenital, or dysplastic), morphology (radial flap, radial fibrillated, longitudinal, peripheral, or unstable), and location (anterior, posterior, or superior).[25] However, regardless of the tear pattern, these lesions uniformly occur at the articular labral junction. Accompanying articular damage has variously been reported to be present in 50% of the cases by Glick, 48% of the cases by Villar, 55% of cases by Byrd, and 73% of cases by McCarthy.[12,21,26,27] McCarthy also found that only 6% of articular lesions did not have accompanying labral pathology.

The labrum is also susceptible to abnormal variations such as inverted position entrapped within the joint. Inversion can occur with or without accompanying acetabular dysplasia. The exact mechanism by which the labrum becomes inverted is unclear, whether it is congenital or acquired in early life. By the time symptoms occur as a result of tearing of the inverted portion, it is noted to be a long-standing process. However, we have also observed this as an acute phenomenon in which an intact labrum became trapped and was treated by simple arthroscopic reduction.

Dorrell and Catterall[28] have documented an increased incidence of inverted acetabular labra associated with severe hip dysplasia. We have found that lesser degrees of labral inversion and subsequent tearing may be associated with lesser degrees of dysplasia. This concept has been furthered by Klaue et al.,[29] who also reported labral tearing associated with milder degrees of hip dysplasia. However, they described treatment by periacetabular osteotomy. We suspect that arthroscopic debridement could be equally effective in alleviating symptoms with considerably less morbidity. Arthroscopic debridement in the presence of dysplasia should be performed in a conservative fashion. Excessive debridement could potentiate instability and accelerate secondary degenerative wear. However, debridement of the damaged portion can result in significant symptomatic improvement with results comparable with those seen in nondysplastic hips.

Harris et al. reported the presence of an inverted acetabular labrum as a source for subsequent development of osteoarthritis.[30] More recently, we have defined clinical and radiographic features characteristic of osteoarthritis due to an inverted labrum.[31] This condition may occur with or without accompanying radiographic evidence of acetabular dysplasia. Once osteoarthritis has developed, the results of arthroscopy are no better in the presence of an inverted labrum than for other forms of degenerative arthritis. It is an intriguing concept that perhaps early arthroscopic intervention for the inverted labrum could delay the subsequent development of osteoarthritis; however, currently no data support that earlier intervention appreciably alters the natural course of this degenerative process. Debridement may improve the symptoms, but will not necessarily change the long-term outlook.

Detachment of the acetabular labrum has been reported in the literature. Nishina et al. described this by arthrography in a series of patients undergoing

Chiari pelvic osteotomy.[32] Klaue et al. observed this in a series of periacetabular osteotomies performed for acetabular rim syndrome, and Fitzgerald reported on this in his 20-year experience of acetabular lesions treated by both arthrotomy and arthroscopy.[29,33] However, we have observed a labral cleft to occur as a common normal variant (Figure 2.6).[34] The separation of the labrum and acetabulum can be deep without representing a pathologic lesion. It is important not to misinterpret this normal variant as a traumatic detachment.

The pathomechanics of acute labral tears are incompletely understood but are most commonly attributed to a twisting injury. Acute tearing of a healthy labrum seems to represent a minority of cases; thus, underlying degeneration should be suspected with most cases. Degeneration may be present even in relatively young adults. The ability of magnetic resonance imaging (MRI) and gadolinium arthrography with magnetic resonance imaging (MRA) to detect labral pathology is improving, with sensitivities greater than 90%. However, the specificity is more suspect, with false-positive interpretations as high as 20% among MRAs in our series. Additionally, the study by Lecouvet et al. demonstrated MRI evidence of labral pathology in asymptomatic volunteers, and the incidence increased with age.[35] Tanabe has shown by electron microscopy that the labrum is susceptible to senile degenerative changes associated with the aging process, which is consistent with the work of Seldes et al. and McCarthy et al., who, in separate cadaveric studies, each demonstrated 96% prevalence of labral lesions in specimens averaging 78 years of age.[17,20,21] Also of note, although MRIs are improving

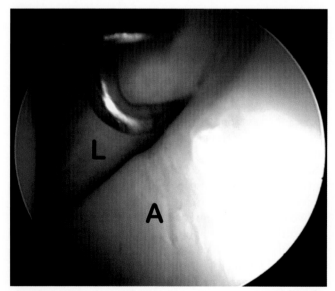

FIGURE 2.6. Example of a normal labral cleft. Viewing the right hip from the anterior portal, the probe has been placed in the separation between the labrum (L) and lateral aspect of the bony acetabulum (A).

at showing labral tears, they remain poor at detecting any accompanying articular damage. Subtle radiographic findings, such as slight joint space narrowing, are often a harbinger of advanced articular wear.

The results of labral debridement (partial labrectomy) are often gratifying but are not uniformly successful even among experienced surgeons. Glick reported only 46% good results at an average 34-month follow-up, but the presence of radiographic evidence of arthritis was a significant influencing variable.[26] In the absence of arthritis, there were 71% good results, and only 21% when arthritis was present. Villar reported 67% patient satisfaction at an average 3.5 years follow-up with this procedure.[27] Moderate chondral damage was present in 48% of cases, but in his series this did not influence the results. We reported an average 20-point improvement (modified Harris hip score) among patients with 5-year follow-up.[12] Fifty-five percent had associated chondral lesions. No statistical difference was identified between those with and without chondral damage, but the power of the study may have been insufficient to detect a difference.

Case 4

A 29-year-old woman presented with a 2-year history of persistent mechanical left hip pain. She attributed the onset of her symptoms to childbirth. Otherwise, no specific episode of trauma occurred. Examination findings were consistent with hip joint pathology. Radiographs were unremarkable for any underlying disease, and an MRA revealed evidence of tearing of the anterior labrum (Figure 2.7A). She also experienced temporary pain relief from the anesthetic effect of the marcaine used to dilute the intraarticular contrast. Arthroscopy substantiated the labral tearing (Figure 2.7B), which was debrided. No significant associated articular pathology was seen, and the patient experienced prompt symptomatic improvement.

Case 5

A 21-year-old male collegiate baseball player developed acute onset of right hip pain doing squats while working out with weights. His symptoms persisted for 3 months despite restricting his activities and participation in a trial of physical therapy and nonsteroidal antiinflammatory medications. Radiographs were unremarkable, but an MRI revealed evidence of labral pathology (Figure 2.8A). With the history of injury, persistent mechanical symptoms refractory to conservative measures, and imaging findings, arthroscopy was recommended. Labral damage was identified as well as an associated area of articular fragmentation at the articular labral junction not evident on MRI (Figure 2.8B). Labral debridement and chondroplasty

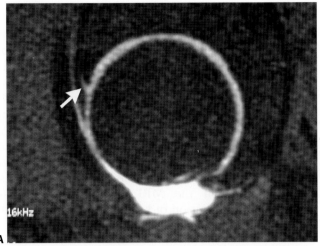

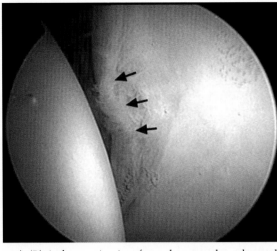

FIGURE 2.7. A 29-year-old woman with pain and catching of the left hip. (A) A sagittal gadolinium arthrography with magnetic resonance imaging (MRA) image reveals a tear of the anterior labrum (arrow). (B) Arthroscopic view from the anterolateral portal demonstrates isolated tearing of the anterior labrum (arrows). (JWT Byrd. Sports Med Arthrosc Rev 10:153, 2002, with permission.)

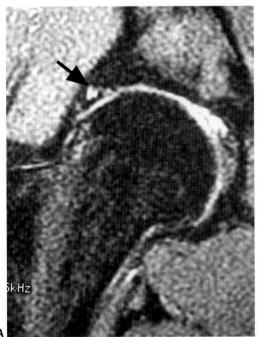

FIGURE 2.8. A 21-year-old collegiate baseball player with acute onset of right hip pain doing squats. (A) Coronal MRI image demonstrates evidence of labral pathology (arrow). (B) Arthroscopic view demonstrates labral pathology (arrows). (C) As the labrum is debrided, associated articular damage at the articular labral junction is uncovered (arrows).

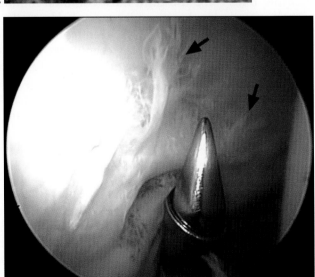

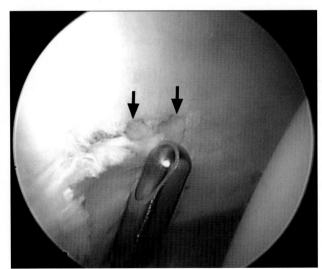

were performed (Figure 2.8C) with prompt symptomatic resolution.

CHONDRAL INJURIES

Chondral lesions exist on a spectrum from acute isolated fragments to diffuse degenerative disease. Acute articular fragmentation is increasingly recognized as a cause of hip pain following trauma.[36] Propagation of a displaced fragment superimposed on underlying degenerative disease may also occur and sometimes explains the acute exacerbation of symptoms in the presence of degenerative arthritis. Preexisting degeneration should always be suspected when the history of trauma is minimal.

A common mechanism for acute articular fragmentation is a direct blow to the greater trochanter, such as that sustained from a fall landing on the lateral aspect of the hip.[36] This trauma is especially seen in athletic young adult men. These individuals are apt to be participating in contact and collision activities in which this type of mechanism is common. Physically fit men have less adipose tissue directly over the trochanter; thus, there is less soft tissue to cushion the blow and, with solid bone structure, the force is delivered unchecked to the joint surface. This trauma results in either a full-thickness articular fragment from the medial aspect of the femoral head, due to the shear forces, or chondrocyte cell death and focal chondromalacia in the superomedial acetabulum as a result of the impact. Elderly patients or patients with osteopenia would more likely sustain a hip fracture.

As noted previously, 48% to 73% of acetabular labral tears have associated articular damage.[12,21,26,27] These lesions occur at the articular labral junction. The extent of articular damage may be the limiting factor in the response to arthroscopy and should be suspected in almost any patient undergoing arthroscopy with an identifiable labral tear. Also, remember that investigative studies are best at showing labral pathology and poorest at showing articular damage. Noguchi et al. have shown that, in the presence of dysplasia, articular wear uniformly begins at the anterolateral margin of the acetabulum.[37] We have observed this to be a common site of origin of articular deterioration both with and without associated acetabular dysplasia. Grade IV articular lesions in this area with surrounding healthy articular surface are sometimes amenable to microfracture. With critical patient selection, as much as 35 points improvement (100-point modified Harris Hip Score) has been reported.[31] For these lesions, microfracture may actually influence the natural history of the process, slowing the degeneration that eventually occurs.

Case 6

A 20-year-old male basketball player presented with an 8-month history of mechanical pain and popping in the left hip following a fall in which he landed directly on the lateral aspect of the hip. Radiographs revealed no acute bony changes (Figure 2.9A). MRI on three previous occasions each showed signal changes in the medial aspect of the femoral head (Figure 2.9B).

Arthroscopy revealed a large full-thickness unstable flap of articular cartilage, displacing from the medial side of the joint, corresponding to the area of signal changes on the MRI (Figure 2.9C). Excision resulted in alleviation of his symptoms (Figure 2.9D).

DISRUPTION OF THE LIGAMENTUM TERES

The exact function of the ligamentum teres remains an enigma. Although its accompanying artery contributes to the vascularity of the epiphysis in childhood, its importance in the adult is less clear. The vessel remains patent in a variable percentage of adults and likely does little to contribute to the vascularity of the femoral head.[38,39] The ligament contributes little to the stability of the joint, but it has been proposed that it has a windshield wiper effect that may facilitate lubrication and nutrition of the joint surfaces.[40] It may well have proprioceptive and nocioceptive importance as well.

Lesions of the ligamentum teres have been rare enough to be published only as isolated case reports.[41–44] These are normally associated with major trauma such as dislocation of the joint. These lesions went unmentioned in the arthroscopic literature before Villar's classification system (partial, complete, and degenerative ruptures) published in 1997.[40] In our series of athletes, we found disruption of the ligamentum teres to be the third most common finding, and these individuals responded remarkably well to arthroscopic debridement with results comparable with loose body removal.[45] More recently, we reported our overall experience in traumatic ruptures of the ligamentum teres.[46] Only 8% of these ligament tears were diagnosed on preoperative studies. However, our ability to recognize these lesions will undoubtedly improve as we have become more aware of their existence.

Disruption is expected in association with a dislocation of the hip but, more commonly, we have found the ligament to tear from a twisting injury. Among 24 cases, 40% were isolated lesions, whereas 60% had other associated pathology. Regardless of associated pathology, the results were remarkably good, with an average 43-point improvement and 96% demonstrating more than 20 points of improvement. Degenerative rupture of the ligament may coexist with de-

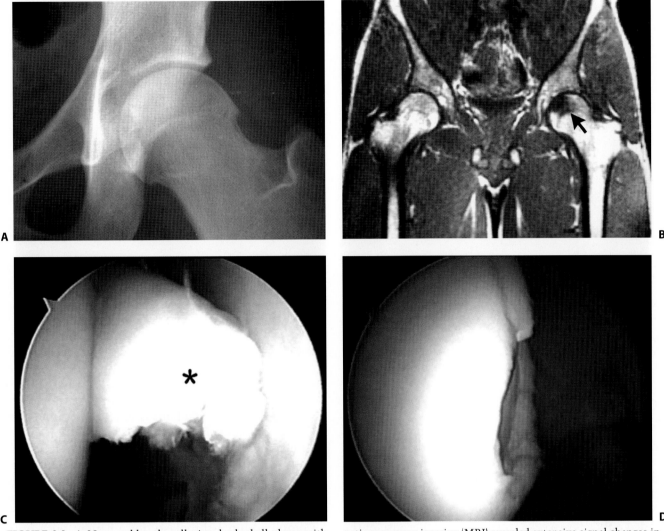

FIGURE 2.9. A 20-year-old male collegiate basketball player with painful catching of the left hip following a fall with lateral impaction of the joint. (A) AP radiograph reveals no acute findings, but there is subtle evidence of underlying congenital changes, characterized by slight lateral uncovering of the femoral head. (B) Mag- netic resonance imaging (MRI) revealed extensive signal changes in the medial aspect of the femoral head (arrow) characterizing the subchondral injury associated with his fall. (C) A full-thickness chondral flap lesion (*) associated with the injury is identified. (D) The unstable portion has been excised.

generative disease. Although debridement may be beneficial, for this circumstance the results are more likely to be determined by the extent of global degeneration.

In the presence of dysplasia, the ligamentum teres is known to hypertrophy.[47,48] This hypertrophic tissue may be more susceptible to disruption and be a source of pain. Among a population of patients with dysplasia, lesions of the ligamentum teres were present in 27%, which is a higher incidence than has been reported in other arthroscopy patient cohorts.[49] The results of debridement were still quite good, with an average improvement of 36 points.

The results of arthroscopic debridement have been encouraging, but the long-term significance of these lesions is still uncertain. Debridement should be limited to only the disrupted fibers. Indiscriminate debridement of the ligamentum teres should be avoided, especially when its exact function and importance remain to be elucidated.

Case 7

A 25-year-old professional softball player sustained an injury to her right hip when she collided with the catcher while trying to steal home plate. Subsequently, she experienced persistent pain and catching, unresponsive to 7 months of conservative treatment including activity modification and supervised physical therapy. Radiographs and MRI were unremarkable. Because of her history of trauma, mechanical symptoms, examination findings, and failure to respond to conservative treatment, arthroscopy was performed, which revealed a traumatic rupture of the ligamentum teres (Figure 2.10) that was debrided. Postoperatively, she experienced pronounced improvement

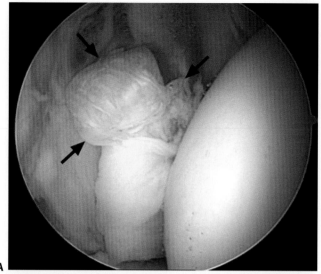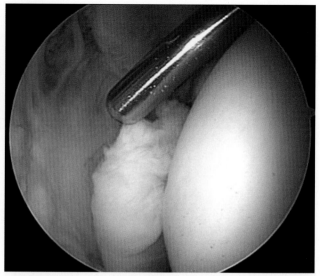

A   B

FIGURE 2.10. A 25-year-old female softball player with pain and catching in her right hip following an acute injury. (A) Arthroscopic view from the anterolateral portal demonstrates disrupted fibers of the ligamentum teres (arrows). (B) The disrupted portion is debrided with a shaver introduced from the anterior portal. (JWT Byrd. Arthroscopy, December 2003, with permission.)

with resolution of her symptoms and was able to return to competitive sports without limitations.

Case 8

A 61-year-old man presented with a 6-month history of progressively worsening mechanical right hip pain, now symptomatic with simple daily activities. Radiographs revealed evidence of degenerative disease (Figure 2.11A), which was further substantiated by an MRI. An intraarticular injection of corticosteroid provided only a few weeks worth of relief. Because of the magnitude and duration of symptoms, arthroscopy was offered as an option. Degenerative labral and articular damage was identified in addition to a degenerate rupture of the ligamentum teres (Figure 2.11B). Debridement included removal of the deteriorated ligament fibers (Figure 2.11C) as well as damaged articular and labral tissue.

DEGENERATIVE ARTHRITIS

Many patients suffer from degenerative disease of the hip, yet few are candidates for arthroscopic intervention. The results are often unpredictable in terms of patient satisfaction. However, some patients may respond moderately well. The following are general parameters that may be useful in patient selection.

1. Age. The younger the patient, the more likely arthroscopy is to be considered as a palliative and temporizing procedure to delay the eventual need for a total hip arthroplasty. The concerning ramifications of hip replacement in the young population are well known.[50]

2. Radiographic findings. The less advanced the radiographic evidence of disease, the more likely the patient is to be considered for arthroscopic debridement. Advanced radiographic disease, especially when bone-on-bone contact is present, often precludes consideration of this procedure.

3. Relatively recent onset of symptoms. Occasionally, a patient may have moderately advanced radiographic evidence of disease or be elderly but only recently has developed the onset of symptoms. In this setting, one may be hesitant to recommend hip arthroplasty for a patient with only relatively recent onset of symptoms.

4. Mechanical symptoms. As with other disorders, symptoms such as locking, catching, or sharp stabbing pain are more indicative of a process that may be improved with arthroscopic debridement. Simply pain with activity in absence of mechanical symptoms is a poor indicator of the benefits of arthroscopy.

5. Failure of response to conservative treatment. This is perhaps the most important parameter, including the roles of activity modification, physical therapy, and antiinflammatory medications.

6. Reasonable expectations. It is important that the patient have a clear understanding regarding the limitations of what can be accomplished with arthroscopic debridement. The goal is simply to reduce discomfort with low-impact activities. Because the success of the procedure is determined by the level of patient satisfaction, unreasonable expectations ensure an unsuccessful result.

Typically, arthroscopic debridement is considered only if the patient's symptoms have progressed to the point that otherwise the surgeon would be consider-

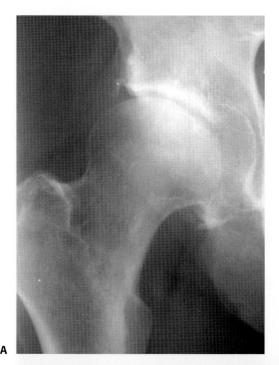

A

FIGURE 2.11. A 61-year-old man with a 6-month history of progressively worsening right hip pain. (A) AP radiograph reveals evidence of degenerative changes with underlying dysplasia but partial joint space preservation. (B) Arthroscopy reveals a hypertrophic degenerate ligamentum teres (*). (C) The deteriorated fibers are debrided.

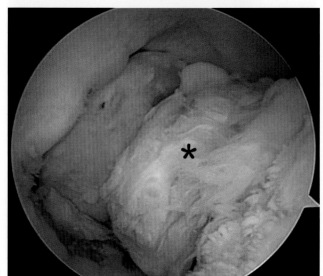

B

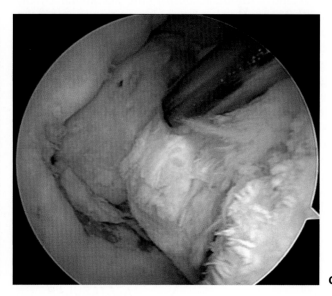

C

ing total hip arthroplasty. Arthroscopy is only an alternative to hip replacement, not a procedure to be considered for milder symptoms associated with the disease. This is important for two reasons. First, if an adequate response is not achieved, the patient must be prepared for whether he or she is subsequently ready to consider hip replacement. Second, some patients are able to live in a delicate equilibrium with the underlying degenerative changes for years. There is always the risk that attempted arthroscopic debridement may aggravate the process and inadvertently accelerate the need for arthroplasty.

A moderately successful result of arthroscopic debridement can only be gauged as some improvement for some length of time. The subjective gauge is whether improvement is adequate enough to be satisfactory to the patient and of sufficient duration to have been deemed worthwhile. Jackson reports that arthroscopic debridement for degenerative disease of the knee results in approximately an 80% likelihood of some improvement.[51] With proper patient selection, it is hoped that this percentage could be approached for the hip. Thus far, published results of arthroscopy for arthritis of the hip remain inferior to those of the knee. Sampson (personal communication) attributes this inability to achieve comparable results between the knee and hip to the differences in the joint architecture. The knee is a tricompartmental joint, whereas the hip is a unicompartmental joint. Patients can selectively unload the medial or lateral compartments of the knee simply by altering the way they walk and can avoid loading the patellofemoral joint in flexion. The hip, as a unicompartmental joint, cannot be as selectively unloaded.

Villar, in a preliminary report, described 60% improvement among patients undergoing arthroscopy for osteoarthritis.[52] Glick et al. reported only 34% patient satisfaction among patients with degenerative disease followed for a minimum of 2 years.[53] In a subsequent study of labral lesions, good results were reported in only 21% of patients when there was coexistent arthritis.[26] In our prospective study of patients with 5-year follow-up, 50% of those with arthritis demonstrated significant improvement at 2 years, and this diminished to 35% at 5-year follow-up.[12] Although the statistical success rate is not encouraging, some patients have continued to do remarkably well.

Harris et al. were the first to report inversion of the acetabular labrum as a cause of osteoarthritis (Figure 2.12).[30] More recently, we have reported on osteoarthritis due to an inverted labrum that can occur with and without accompanying acetabular dysplasia.[31] The cardinal radiographic feature is superolateral joint space narrowing (Figure 2.13). This condition has been implicated in cases that experience acute exacerbation of symptoms despite chronic radiographic findings and has also been identified in cases which demonstrate rapid radiographic evidence of joint space loss (Figure 2.14). The results of arthroscopic debridement in this condition are no better than the results reported for other causes of arthritis, but recognizing the radiographic features may help avoid a more extensive, and unnecessary, workup when the symptoms seem poorly explained by the radiographic findings. In this condition, the articular de-

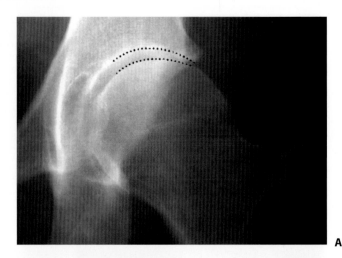

A

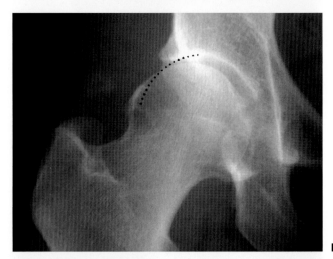

B

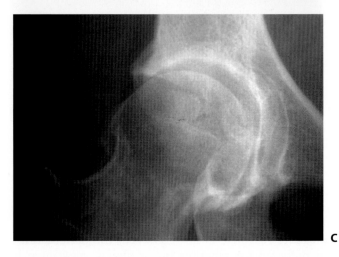

C

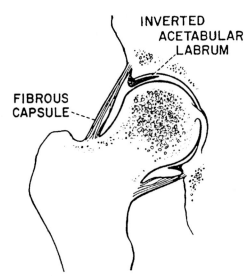

FIGURE 2.12. Etiology of osteoarthritis secondary to an inverted acetabular labrum as depicted by Harris. (WH Harris. Clin Orthop 213:31, 1986, with permission.)

FIGURE 2.13. The cardinal radiographic feature of osteoarthritis due to an inverted labrum is superolateral joint space narrowing. (A) Narrowing of the superolateral joint space creates a convergence laterally of the normally parallel lines created by the radius of curvature of the subchondral bone of the acetabulum and the convex surface of the femoral head. (B) Another method of visually interpreting narrowing of the joint space is that the arc created by the radius of curvature of the acetabulum intersects the femoral head. (C) Secondary features of osteoarthritis including osteophyte formation are present, but the cardinal radiographic feature of asymmetric superolateral joint space narrowing is also evident. (From Byrd and Jones,[31] with permission of Arthroscopy.)

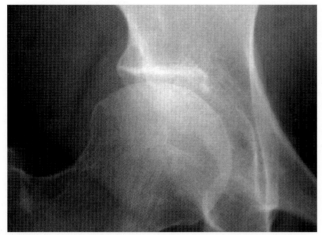
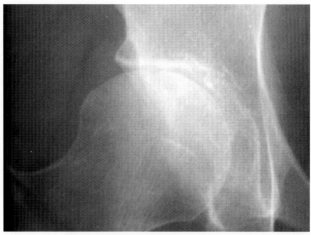

A

B

FIGURE 2.14. A 63-year-old woman developed relatively sponta- neous onset of right hip pain. (A) Initial radiographs are fairly un- remarkable. (B) Follow-up radiographs 3 months later show a pro- nounced change with loss of the superolateral joint space. (From Byrd and Jones,[31] with permission of Arthroscopy.)

terioration uniformly begins laterally on the acetabu- lar side and then secondarily involves the femoral head. Occasionally, grade IV acetabular lesions with healthy surrounding articular cartilage may be candi- dates for microfracture and represent a small subpop- ulation of patients who may respond remarkably well. The postoperative rehabilitation protocol for this pro- cedure includes 10 weeks of strict protective weight bearing, with emphasis on range of motion during the early fibrocartilaginous healing phase.

Another pattern of primary osteoarthritis begins with articular wear on the medial aspect of the femoral head. Radiographs demonstrate medial joint space nar- rowing and often remarkably good preservation of the superior weight-bearing surface (Figure 2.15A). The ar- throscopic findings are consistent with the radio- graphic findings. The most lateral articular surface of the femoral head is remarkably well preserved, but the entire medial half is void of articular surface with eburnated bone and similar findings on the medial as- pect of the acetabulum (Figure 2.15B,C). The princi- pal feature is not to be encouraged by the apparent su- perior joint space preservation because the results of arthroscopy, again, do not appear to be superior to other causes of arthritis.

Case 9

A 59-year-old man presented with progressive me- chanical left hip pain, obligating him to a sedentary lifestyle. Radiographs revealed evidence of osteoarthri- tis and features suggesting an underlying inverted labrum (Figure 2.16A). Arthroscopy demonstrated the chronically inverted position of the acetabular labrum as well as associated degenerative changes (Figure 2.16B). Debridement resulted in significant improve- ment for more than 2 years, after which the patient opted for total hip arthroplasty.

SYNOVIAL DISEASE

As with other joints, arthroscopic synovectomy has a recognized role in the hip. A variety of synovial dis- orders may be addressed, including various inflam- matory arthritides and miscellaneous synovial con- ditions such as synovial osteochondromatosis, pig- mented villonodular synovitis, and possibly hemo- philiac arthropathy.[54]

Synovial lesions of the hip may demonstrate either a focal or a diffuse pattern. Focal lesions emanate from the pulvinar of the acetabular fossa. The pulvinar nor- mally consists of adipose tissue covered by synovium that resides above the ligamentum teres within the fossa. Lesions in this area are sometimes quite painful and respond remarkably well to arthroscopic debride- ment. In this author's estimation, the pulvinar is the neural equivalent of the fat pad in the knee. The tis- sue seems to be quite sensitive, and lesions of this area are painful. The diffuse pattern involves the sy- novial lining of the capsule. An adequate synovectomy of this area necessitates arthroscopy of the peripheral compartment.[55] The synovectomy is still subtotal, but is at least as complete as can be achieved by any tech- nique other than dislocating the hip in association with an open approach. Gondolph-Zink et al. have de- scribed a technique of semiarthroscopic synovectomy, but this procedure offers no advantage over arthros- copy that addresses both the intraarticular and pe- ripheral compartments.[56]

Rheumatoid arthritis represents the most com- monly encountered inflammatory arthritis. Synovec- tomy is indicated in the presence of disabling pain unresponsive to conservative measures including ac- tivity modification, physical therapy, and intraarticu- lar injections. Significant symptomatic improvement has been noted even in the presence of advanced ra- diographic changes. However, in general, the extent of

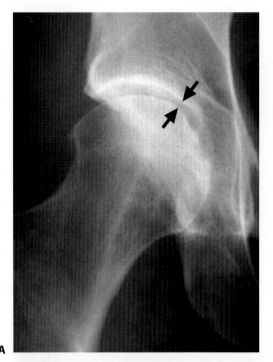

FIGURE 2.15. A 56-year-old woman with a 6-month history of progressively worsening right hip pain. (A) AP radiograph demonstrates minimal features of osteoarthritis. The superior joint space is relatively well preserved, while subtle evidence of medial space narrowing (arrows) is identified. (B) Arthroscopic view of the medial portion of the joint reveals diffuse erosive articular loss of the medial femoral head (arrows). (C) Viewing from the anterior portal, the lateral articular surface of both the femoral head and acetabulum are intact (left side), while a line of demarcation (arrows) is evident with the adjoining articular erosion (asterisk) of the medial acetabulum.

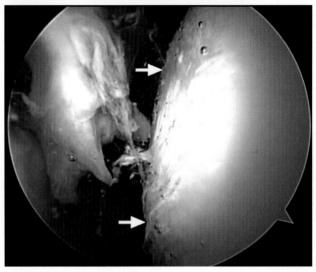

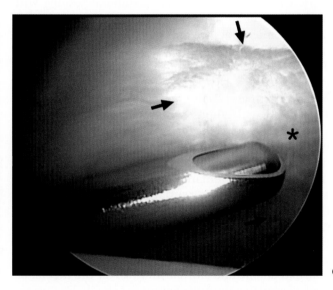

accompanying articular surface damage is usually an indicator of the likely success of arthroscopy.

It is important to be aware that radiographic evidence of joint space preservation may belie the presence of advanced articular surface damage. Arthroscopic inspection has discerned the presence of this advanced damage in cases of disabling hip pain unexplained by seemingly healthy radiographs. This potential discrepancy between radiographic findings and the extent of joint deterioration is important to consider. In these circumstances, the results of arthroscopy may be poor, but information is gained to explain the disproportionate symptoms. Definitive treatment such as with a total hip arthroplasty is then recognized as an option.

Hajdu[57] developed a classification system for soft tissue tumors based on the tissue of origin. Tumors of tendosynovial tissue seem to have the greatest predilection for the hip and include synovial chondromatosis and pigmented villonodular synovitis.[58]

Milgram has described three phases of synovial chondromatosis based on a temporal sequence.[59] During phase I, the synovial disease is active but no loose bodies are yet present. The second phase is transitional, in which there is active synovial proliferation and loose bodies are present. During the third phase, the synovium becomes quiescent with no demonstrable disease, but the loose bodies remain. Because of the insidious nature of the disease, by the time symptoms become significant enough to incite diagnosis

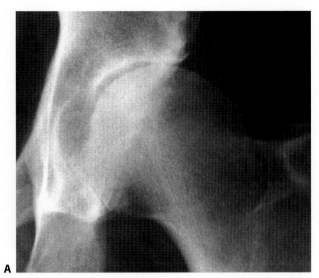

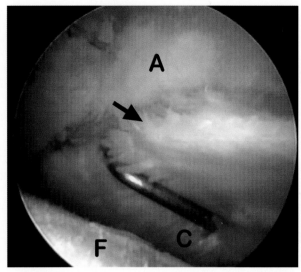

FIGURE 2.16. A 59-year-old man with a painful left hip. (A) AP radiograph shows moderate osteoarthritis. (B) Arthroscopic view illustrates a probe entered through the capsule (C) defining an inverted labrum (arrow) with associated diffuse articular wear of the acetabulum (A) and femoral head (F). (B, from Byrd,[34] with permission of Arthroscopy.)

and surgical intervention, the synovial process has usually long since receded, leaving behind only the loose bodies to create symptoms. Thus, the histologic diagnosis is often in limbo unless synovium can be identified actively producing loose bodies. Recurrence of disease is possible, but recurrence of symptoms following arthroscopy is usually more accurately the result of residual disease because it can be difficult to ensure that an absolutely thorough debridement has been performed.

The hip is surpassed only by the knee and the elbow as the site of involvement of synovial chondromatosis.[60,61] However, in the hip, the diagnosis is often much more elusive. The loose bodies may be small and entirely radiolucent. In the study by McCarthy et al., at least half these cases were unrecognized before arthroscopy.[4]

Pigmented villonodular synovitis has been reported in both a nodular and diffuse pattern.[62] The hip is the second most frequent site of involvement of this disease, with both patterns having been encountered.[61,63] Synovectomy has been proposed as the treatment of choice for patients with preserved articular cartilage.[64] The nodular pattern presents as more discrete lesions and can be completely resected with greater reliability. The diffuse pattern requires a much more extensive synovectomy. A generous synovectomy can still be accomplished arthroscopically with less surgical morbidity than an open procedure.

Hemophiliac arthropathy rarely involves the hip. In other joints, synovectomy has been used for the treatment of recurrent bleeds and early degenerative changes, but this has not been recommended for the hip.[65] The reluctance regarding surgical intervention in the hip may be due to the presence of fibrosis or the potential morbidity of an open synovectomy in this population. Arthroscopy may offer a less invasive approach, but this role has not yet been explored for this disease.

Case 10

A 17-year-old girl presented with a 2-year history of progressively worsening right hip pain without any specific precipitating event. Workup revealed a well-circumscribed intracapsular lesion in the posterior aspect of the joint (Figure 2.17A). Arthroscopy defines the lesion (Figure 2.17B), which was excised, revealing a nodular pattern of pigmented villonodular synovitis.

Case 11

A 19-year-old woman was referred with a 7-year history of gradually worsening right hip pain. She described pain with activity, but also a sharp stabbing sensation with twisting maneuvers. Radiographs revealed evidence of synovial chondromatosis (Figure 2.18A), which was further substantiated by a CT scan (Figure 2.18B,C). Lesions were noted to be present within the intraarticular and peripheral portions of the joint. Arthroscopy substantiated the intraarticular loose bodies, which were debrided (Figure 2.18D,E). Numerous loose bodies resided in the peripheral compartment (Figure 2.18F,G), which were excised in addition to performing a synovectomy.

Case 12

A 52-year-old woman was referred for bilateral hip pain of 2 years duration following a high-concentra-

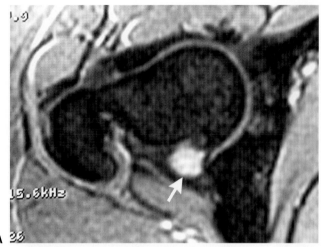

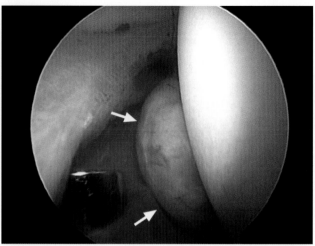

FIGURE 2.17. A 17-year-old girl presents with a 2-year history of ill-defined right hip pain. (A) MRI suggested a posterior intraarticular cyst (arrow). (B) Arthroscopy reveals a nodular form of pigmented villonodular synovitis (arrows). Excision resulted in resolution of symptoms. (Byrd JWT: Arthroscopy of the hip: overview. In: McGinty JB (ed). Operative Arthroscopy, 3rd ed. Phildelphia: Lippincott Williams & Wilkins, 2003:821–842, with permission.)

tion external exposure to organophosphate insecticides. She developed a persistently elevated sedimentation rate and multiple organ disease involving the liver and kidneys as well as hip pain that had been responsive only to repeated intraarticular injections of corticosteroids. Radiographs were normal (Figure 2.19A). Arthroscopy revealed a proliferative reactive synovitic process emanating from the pulvinar of the acetabular fossa (Figure 2.19B). Significant symptomatic improvement following debridement of the right hip subsequently led to debridement of the left, which did equally well.

Case 13

A 30-year-old woman was referred for consideration of arthroscopy. She had a long-standing history of rheumatoid arthritis managed with chronic oral prednisone suppressions. She has experienced right hip symptoms for 3 years, but the hip has become increasingly painful over the past 6 months. An intraarticular injection of corticosteroid failed to provide protracted relief.

Radiographs revealed modes underlying osteopenia, consistent with her disease, but the joint space has been well maintained (Figure 2.20A). With the chronicity and magnitude of her symptoms and failure of response to conservative treatment including an intraarticular injection, she was thought to be an appropriate candidate for arthroscopy.

At arthroscopy, the articular surfaces were remarkably well maintained, but a proliferative villous synovial process emanated from the capsular lining (Figure 2.20B). This process was debrided with a full-radius synovial resector approaching the synovium

from all three portals. Postoperatively, the patient experienced marked improvement of her symptoms.

IMPINGING OSTEOPHYTES

Osteophytes, or bone fragments, can impinge on the joint, causing pain. These can often be excised arthroscopically. Excision of osteophytes or fragments caused by previous trauma are the most likely to result in successful patient satisfaction.[66] This procedure may necessitate an extracapsular as well as extraarticular dissection. Principles for effectively and safely performing this procedure are as follows.

1. Thorough knowledge of the normal anatomy is necessary to accurately assess anatomy altered by trauma.
2. Constant orientation to the extraarticular anatomy is important, especially the neurovascular structures, relative to the area of dissection.
3. When dissecting outside the capsule, keep the soft tissue debridement directly on bone and avoid straying into the surrounding soft tissues. Remember that "bone is home."
4. Optimal visualization is best achieved with a high-flow fluid management system. Blood and debris hinder visualization in the absence of adequate flow. A high-flow system is necessary to achieve adequate flow without having to use excessive pressure. Increased pressure results in inordinate fluid extravasation; this cannot be modulated well with a gravity-flow system alone.
5. Maintain hemostasis: hypotensive anesthesia (systolic BP < 100 mm Hg); add epinephrine to the fluid; and employ an electrocautery device.

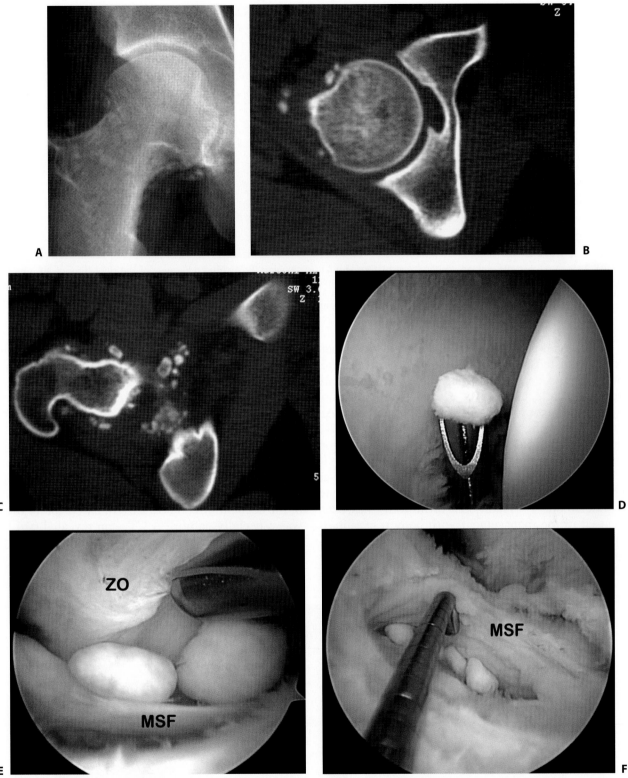

FIGURE 2.18. A 19-year-old woman with a 7-year history of worsening right hip pain. (A) AP radiograph reveals findings of synovial chondromatosis characterized by numerous loose bodies. (B, C) CT scan further substantiates the presence of loose bodies within the joint and within the peripheral compartment. (D) Intraarticular loose bodies are debrided. (E) Viewing the peripheral compartment, large loose bodies are identified between the medial synovial fold (MSF) and zona orbicularis (ZO). (F) Lifting the medial synovial fold (MSF), numerous small loose bodies are identified along the medial neck.

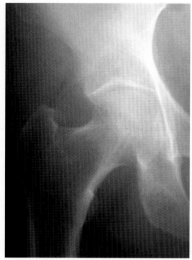

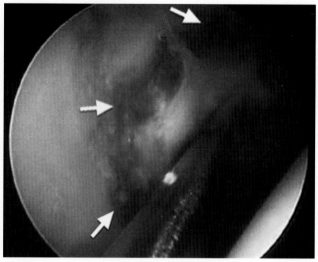

FIGURE 2.19. A 52-year-old woman with a 2-year history of bilateral hip pain following high-dose cutaneous exposure to organophosphate insecticides. (A) AP radiograph of the right hip is unremarkable with well-maintained joint space and no evidence of bony changes. (B) Arthroscopic view of the right hip reveals a proliferative reactive synovitic process obliterating the acetabular fossa (arrows), which is being debrided.

Osteophytes are commonly encountered in association with osteoarthritis but rarely benefit from excision. The osteophytes evident radiographically are rarely the sole cause of pain but are simply a radiographic indicator of the degenerative process. Although debridement in the presence of degenerative disease is sometimes appropriate, osteophyte excision alone is rarely a productive undertaking.

The concept of femoroacetabular impingement as a consequence of hip joint morphology is beginning to be understood.[67,68] Traditional arthrotomy has been proposed in the management with bony resection. It is likely that most of these can be addressed arthroscopically with equal success. However, an apprecia-tion for the pathomechanics of these specific lesions is just beginning to unfold. Many overlap with associated osteoarthritis, in which case excision of the impinging lesion may be of limited benefit.

Case 14

A 46-year-old man was referred for persistent left hip pain 18 months following closed treatment of a posterior fracture-dislocation involving the posterior lip of the acetabulum (Figure 2.21A). Extension of the hip was especially painful. A CT scan revealed two large fragments residing posterior to the joint, impinging on the femoral head (Figure 2.21B).

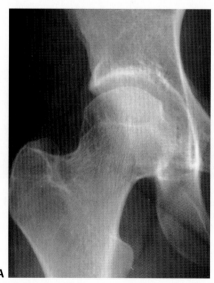

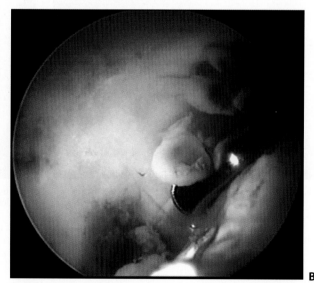

FIGURE 2.20. A 30-year-old woman with rheumatoid arthritis and protracted right hip pain. (A) AP radiograph reveals mild osteopenia with excellent joint space preservation. (B) Proliferative villous synovial disease is present, which responded well to arthroscopic synovectomy.

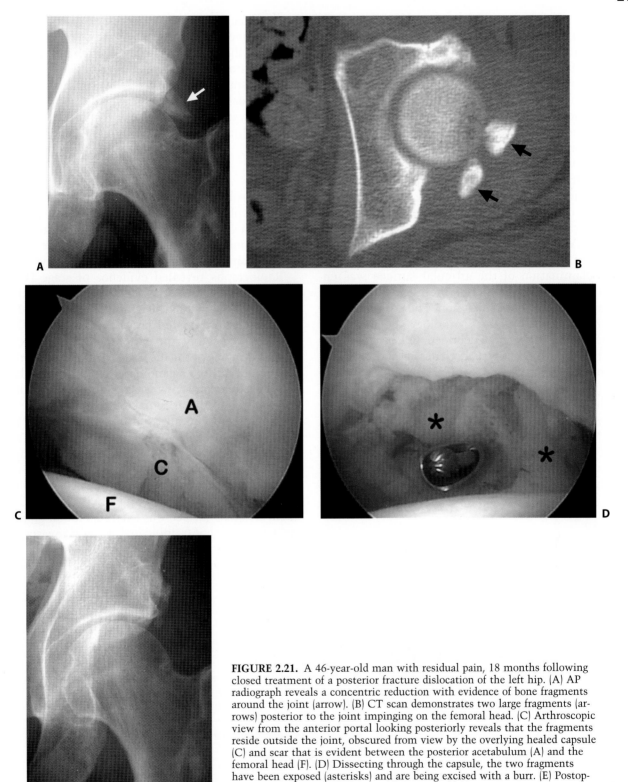

FIGURE 2.21. A 46-year-old man with residual pain, 18 months following closed treatment of a posterior fracture dislocation of the left hip. (A) AP radiograph reveals a concentric reduction with evidence of bone fragments around the joint (arrow). (B) CT scan demonstrates two large fragments (arrows) posterior to the joint impinging on the femoral head. (C) Arthroscopic view from the anterior portal looking posteriorly reveals that the fragments reside outside the joint, obscured from view by the overlying healed capsule (C) and scar that is evident between the posterior acetabulum (A) and the femoral head (F). (D) Dissecting through the capsule, the two fragments have been exposed (asterisks) and are being excised with a burr. (E) Postoperative radiograph demonstrates the extent of bony excision.

Arthroscopy revealed the fragments to be extra-capsular (Figure 2.21C). Dissecting through the capsule, around the bony fragments, allowed them to be excised with significant symptomatic improvement postoperatively (Figure 2.21D).

AVASCULAR NECROSIS OF THE FEMORAL HEAD

The role of arthroscopic debridement in the management of avascular necrosis (AVN) of the femoral head is limited. Arthroscopic debridement has been used for end-stage disease in young patients as an effort to delay the eventual need for total hip replacement. For this circumstance, the results are uniformly poor.[69,70] Symptomatic improvement, at best, is brief and rarely justifies the procedure. Ruch et al. explored the role of arthroscopy in staging of AVN of the femoral head.[71] They found arthroscopy to be of no benefit in the evaluation of stage II (precollapse) disease or in young patients (<30 years of age) with stage III (subchondral fracture) disease. These are thought to be the best candidates for free-vascularized fibular grafting, and none of these cases had delamination of the articular surface. They advocate diagnostic arthroscopy for stage IV (postcollapse) patients who are otherwise candidates for osteotomy or vascularized graft. If complete delamination of the articular surface was encountered, they would debride the fragment and perform a simple core decompression. These patients also often have coexistent labral pathology and acetabular fragmentation that can be debrided. O'Leary et al. reported their retrospective experience in patients with osteonecrosis.[72] In general, osteonecrosis was found to be a poor prognostic indicator but was not a contraindication to arthroscopy. Accompanying mechanical symptoms were a better prognostic indicator of potentially treatable pathology, delaying the eventual need for arthroplasty. However, they would not recommend arthroscopy in the presence of osteonecrosis and absence of mechanical symptoms.

Case 15

This case highlights the radiographic and corresponding arthroscopic appearance of stage IV AVN of the femoral head (Figure 2.22). The arthroscopic findings may be diverse. There are varying degrees of delamination of the articular surface of the femoral head or chondral fragmentation of the femoral head and acetabular surfaces. Despite the variable arthroscopic findings, debridement for stage IV disease results in only modest improvement for a brief period of time and is of limited benefit.

Case 16

A 28-year-old man is referred for consideration of arthroscopy of his right hip. He presented with acute exacerbation of right hip pain. He recounted mild symptoms off and on for years, but despite this he was fully active, including running 2 to 3 miles 3 days a week.

Radiographs revealed evidence of stage IV AVN (Figure 2.23A). An MRI scan further defined the extent of involvement of the femoral head (Figure 2.23B). A contradiction existed between the modest symptoms experienced by the patient and the advanced radiographic stage of the disease. To determine if the patient might still be a candidate for a free-vascularized fibular graft, arthroscopy was recommended to discern the integrity of the articular surfaces.

Arthroscopy revealed that the entire articular surface overlying the area of the lesion was unstable, having delaminated off the underlying necrotic bone (Figure 2.23C). This included the medial portion of the femoral head, extending superiorly and laterally to the area marked with the probe (Figure 2.23D,E). The unstable articular surface was excised. Fibular grafting of the defect was contraindicated. Even if revascularization of the bone could be achieved, there was no remaining overlying articular surface.

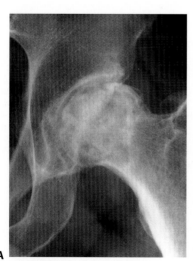
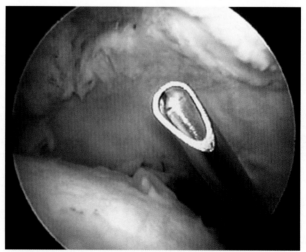

FIGURE 2.22. (A) AP radiograph of the left hip of a 44-year-old man with stage IV avascular necrosis (AVN). (B) Arthroscopic view demonstrates areas of grade IV chondral fragmentation from both the femoral head and acetabulum.

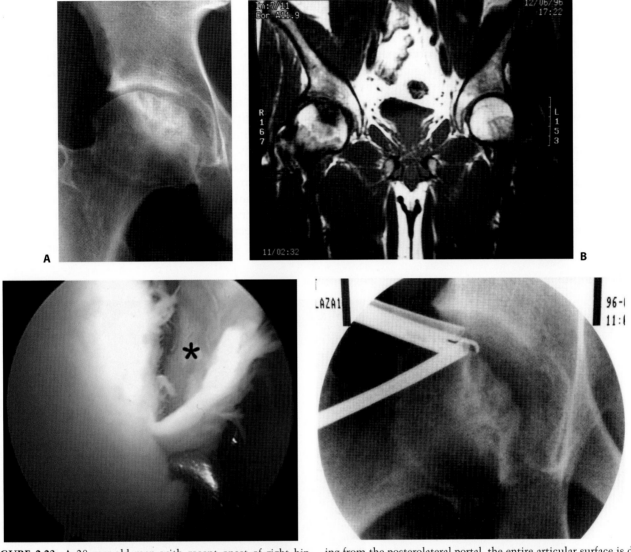

FIGURE 2.23. A 28-year-old man with recent onset of right hip symptoms, but no restriction in activities. (A) An AP radiograph reveals evidence of stage IV AVN characterized by joint space preservation and no apparent acetabular involvement. (B) An MRI scan further defines the extent of femoral head involvement. (C) View-ing from the posterolateral portal, the entire articular surface is delaminated off the medial aspect of the femoral head (asterisk). The lateral extent is marked with the probe. (D) The position of the probe is evident on the fluoroscopic image and corresponds with the lateral margin of the lesion evident on the radiograph.

INSTABILITY

Instability of the hip has variously been reported as isolated case reports, mostly in association with trauma, but occasionally in absence of a precipitating injury.[66,73] Open capsulorrhaphy has been proposed for recurrent episodes. More recently, Philippon has postulated that instability may accompany labral pathology and has advocated thermal capsulorrhaphy in conjunction with debridement of the damaged labrum.[74] The reasoning is hypothetical and, although there may be some logic for this in select cases, currently no data exist to suggest that the results of partial labrectomy are improved by adjunct thermal capsular shrinkage. Also, as documented by Seldes et al., the relationship of the capsule and labrum in the hip is different than the capsulolabral complex encountered in the shoulder.[20] The capsule attaches directly to the bony acetabulum separate from the labrum and thus the labrum is not an integral part of the capsular structure.

Although the role for thermal capsulorrhaphy is limited, we have observed remarkable success in properly selected cases. Arthroscopy of the peripheral compartment with the traction released allows excellent access to the capsule for performing this procedure. More energy is necessary than that used in the shoulder due to the thicker hip capsule. Principally, we reserve this technique for cases of recalcitrant instability caused by an incompetent capsule with normal joint geometry. In cases with severe acetabular dysplasia, it seems unlikely that a soft tissue procedure alone will accomplish a successful long-term result. Caution must also be taken when assessing potential candidates because many patients may describe a sensation of subluxation in the absence of true joint instability. The diagnosis can be elusive, but is most easily suspected in hyperlax individuals who have demonstrated previous instability of other joints, especially the shoulder. This is most commonly encountered in collagen disorders such as Ehlers–Danlos syndrome. Patient compliance with the postoperative rehabilitation protocol is imperative to a successful result. We advocate hip spica bracing with a limited arc of motion for 8 weeks postoperatively. With this protocol, all patients have still been able to regain range of motion while none have demonstrated recurrence of instability.

Case 17

A 16-year-old girl was referred for symptomatic instability of her left hip. Her medical history is remarkable for Ehlers–Danlos syndrome, and she had undergone previous successful capsulorrhaphy of both shoulders. She had experienced intermittent episodes of instability for 3 years. Six months previously, she had sustained a more serious injury when she fell down steps. She experienced incapacitating hip pain that resolved when her hip was reduced in the emergency room. Since then, she was plagued by persistent mechanical symptoms. Radiographs demonstrated a concentric reduction with good coverage of the femoral head (Figure 2.24A). An MRA suggested labral pathology, and she experienced pain relief from the

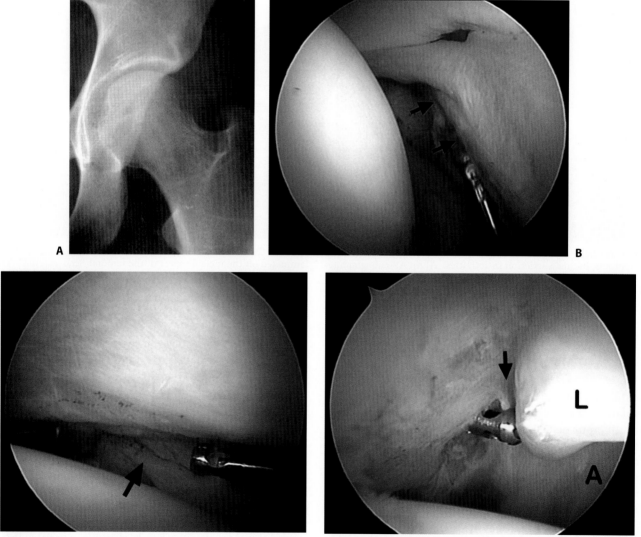

FIGURE 2.24. A 16-year-old girl with symptomatic instability of her left hip. (A) AP radiograph demonstrates a concentric reduction with good coverage of the femoral head. (B) Viewing posteriorly from the anterolateral portal, thermal capsulorrhaphy is begun with the laser introduced from the posterolateral portal. A band of tissue (arrows) illustrates the capsular response. (C) Viewing laterally from the anterior portal, treatment of the lateral capsule is identified (arrow). (D) Now viewing anteriorly from the anterolateral portal, tightening of the capsule at the capsulolabral reflection (arrow) is being performed. The capsular surface of the labrum (L) is seen; the acetabulum (A) is far to the right.

anesthetic effect of the intraarticular injection. Arthroscopy was recommended to address her intraarticular damage as well as to perform thermal capsulorrhaphy for her laxity. At arthroscopy, the labrum was found to be intact, but her capsular laxity was addressed (Figure 2.24B–D). Postoperatively, she was maintained in a hip spica brace with the extension–flexion arc blocked from 15 to 70 degrees for 8 weeks. She then progressed with a supervised rehabilitation program focusing on stabilization exercises and experienced complete resolution of her symptoms.

ADHESIVE CAPSULITIS

Adhesive capsulitis of the hip has previously been described in the literature as case reports.[75–79] The following profile of this condition is presented based on our experience and previously published information. Adhesive capsulitis of the hip presents and behaves similar to adhesive capsulitis in the shoulder. There may or may not be associated intraarticular pathology. Some respond to conservative treatment including oral antiinflammatory medication and physical therapy emphasizing range of motion. It is likely that there are numerous cases that resolve spontaneously without getting treatment. Also, adhesive capsulitis of the hip may not present to the physician as frequently as adhesive capsulitis of the shoulder because the accompanying dysfunction may not be as severe. Patients are able to compensate for restricted range of motion in the hip much better than they can for restriction in the shoulder.

The cardinal presenting feature is painful, restricted range of motion. Radiographs rule out limited motion caused by advanced degenerative disease, but the examiner must differentiate whether restricted motion is truly due to capsular adhesions or self-limited by the patient because of painful guarding. Often there may be a history of trauma such as a twisting injury or fall, but this is not very helpful in determining whether there is coexistent intraarticular damage.

As with other hip disorders, MRI is variable in its ability to detect accompanying intraarticular pathology. Murphy et al. reported arthrography to be diagnostic due to reduced intracapsular volume, but we have not found this to be uniformly reliable.[75] Accompanying pathology may include labral or articular injury. There are also several reports of synovial chondromatosis presenting with adhesive capsulitis, and we have observed this relationship as well.[75,76]

For recalcitrant cases, manipulation under anesthesia with concomitant arthroscopy has been quite successful. It is likely that some cases might respond to simple manipulation alone but, with the uncertainty of investigative studies to identify intraarticular damage, we have routinely employed arthroscopy for this condition.

In fact, manipulation is essential to being able to carry out successful arthroscopy in the presence of adhesive capsulitis. There is one report of failed attempted arthroscopy for adhesive capsulitis that subsequently underwent an open capsulectomy.[78] It is likely that with manipulation and attention to the details of the technique, arthroscopy could have been successfully employed, avoiding an open procedure.

Examination under anesthesia confirms the presence of adhesive capsulitis characterized by restricted rotational motion in both directions. Manipulation is then performed by placing the leg in the figure of 4 position. Stabilizing the pelvis, gentle pressure is applied to the medial aspect of the ipsilateral knee, pressing the knee down toward the table. The crepitus associated with the adhesions breaking loose can be felt and heard just as when performing manipulation of a shoulder. After performing this maneuver, it is then easier to gently stretch the hip in internal and external rotation to regain full motion. As with the shoulder, this manipulation must be performed in a judicious fashion to minimize the risk of fracture, which could be a disastrous complication.

After completing the manipulation, arthroscopy is performed in a standard fashion. Hemorrhagic fibrinous debris is identified within the joint similar to that encountered in the shoulder after manipulation.

Postoperative rehabilitation emphasizes range of motion more so than other hip procedures. As motion is regained, patients typically experience marked gratification in terms of reduced pain and improved function.

Case 18

A 42-year-old woman presented with a 10-month history of left hip pain that developed during an exercise program. Her symptoms have steadily worsened despite modifying her activities. On examination, she has painful limited motion in all planes. Her radiographs are unremarkable. An MRA shows evidence of a small anterior labral tear, and she obtained pronounced temporary pain relief from the anesthetic effect of the intraarticular injection. Arthroscopy was recommended. On examination under anesthesia, she had markedly reduced rotational motion of the left hip compared with the right. However, by placing the hip in a figure of 4 position and applying gentle pressure to the medial aspect of the knee, adhesions could be felt releasing. This procedure resulted in regaining full rotational motion of the joint. Arthroscopy revealed a small anterior labral tear (Figure 2.25A), which was conservatively debrided. Also present was hemorrhagic fibrinous debris consistent with adhesive capsulitis (Figure 2.25B–D). Postoperatively, she had immediate and complete alleviation of her symptoms. This relief was believed to be mostly attributable to

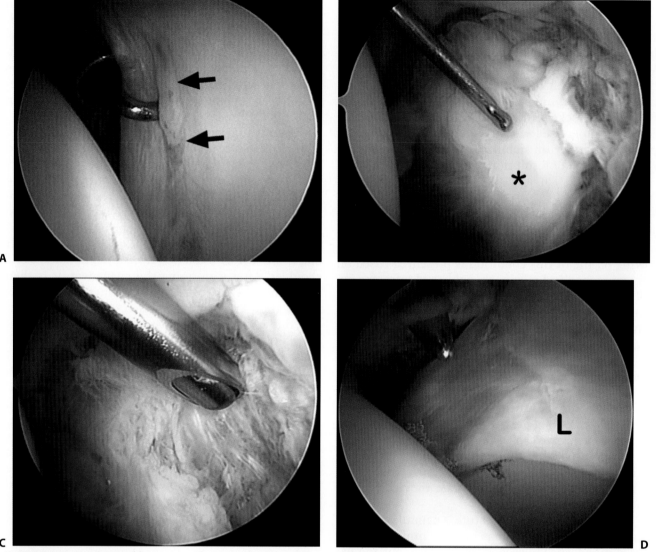

FIGURE 2.25. A 42-year-old woman with pain and restricted motion of the left hip. (A) Arthroscopy reveals a small peripheral longitudinal tear of the anterior labrum (arrows). (B) Dense fibrous adhesions are evident in the acetabular fossa (asterisk). (C) De-bridement of the fibrotic tissue is performed. (D) Viewing peripheral to the labrum (L) illustrates the hemorrhagic fibrotic tissue characteristic of adhesive capsulitis.

the adhesive capsulitis and, only to a lesser extent, the labral tear.

SEPSIS

Arthroscopic lavage for acute bacterial sepsis of the hip has been described in the pediatric literature by Chung et al.[80] Blitzer described similar indications for lavage and debridement in an adult population, and Bould et al. have published a case report as well.[81,82] Arthroscopic visualization of the joint is better than can be accomplished with an open approach unless the hip is dislocated intraoperatively. More important, the morbidity of arthroscopy is significantly less and may be especially important when joint infection occurs in a medically compromised patient. A seriously ill patient may be capable of withstanding an arthro-

scopic procedure better than an open operation. Appropriate patient selection may be a factor in choosing this procedure as a successful outcome is more likely when early intervention is performed for an acute infectious process caused by a bacterial organism that demonstrates sensitivity to antibiotics. These parameters especially apply for infection in the presence of a total hip arthroplasty, as reported by Hyman et al.[83]

Case 19

A 57-year-old man presented with a 1-week history of spontaneous onset disabling left hip pain. There was no attributable injury. His recent medical history was remarkable for an episode of acute gastroenteritis 1 week prior. Radiographs were unremarkable (Figure 2.26A). The same day, an MRI showed evidence of a

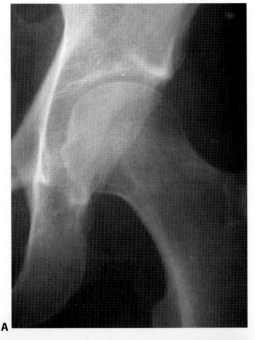

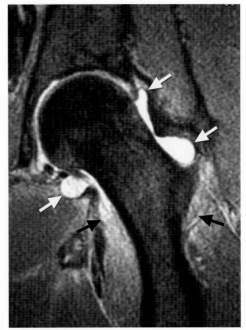

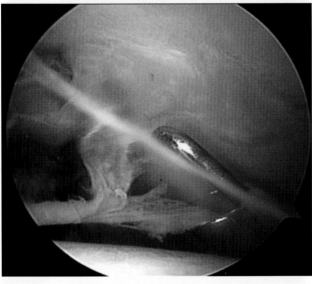

FIGURE 2.26. A 59-year-old man with evidence of a septic hip. (A) AP radiograph is unremarkable. (B) Coronal MRI demonstrates a pronounced effusion (white arrows) and surrounding soft tissue edema (black arrows). (C) Arthroscopy revealed diffuse exudated material throughout the joint.

significant effusion with surrounding soft tissue edema (Figure 2.26B), and aspiration demonstrated turbid fluid with gram-positive cocci. His Westergren sedimentation rate was markedly elevated at 62. He underwent emergent arthroscopy with debridement and lavage (Figure 2.26C). Cultures grew *Escherichia coli*. He was maintained on intravenous antibiotics for 2 weeks, followed by 4 weeks of oral medication. There was no recurrence of infection.

STATUS POST TOTAL HIP ARTHROPLASTY

Case reports of arthroscopy for removal of entrapped foreign material following total hip arthroplasty have been described with successful results.[84–86] Arthros-

copy has a role in other problems associated with hip arthroplasty but should always be viewed cautiously as there are few sources of a painful hip prosthesis that are amenable to arthroscopic intervention.[87] Hyman et al. have reported successful arthroscopic management of eight consecutive patients with late, acutely infected total hips.[83] The important parameters included early diagnosis, prompt intervention, a sensitive microorganism, and appropriate antibiotic therapy. Another area in which arthroscopy may gain an increasing role is with the growing awareness of the problems associated with polyethylene wear debris.[88]

Case 20

A 59-year-old man was referred for arthroscopic assessment of a painful left total hip arthroplasty. A press-fit prosthesis had been placed 3 years earlier. Five months previously, he had fallen, landing in the seated position, and had experienced pain ever since. An extensive workup had failed to reveal any evidence of fracture, loosening, or infection. Arthroscopy was requested to see if there was any undetected failure of the acetabular liner or other occult findings. Arthroscopy was carried out with a standard distraction technique (Figure 2.27A). There was noted to be turbid, but sterile fluid, in addition to fibrinous material, which was biopsied and debrided (Figure 2.27B). This material revealed granulomatous infiltrates. Otherwise, the prosthesis was intact (Figure 2.27C,D).

UNRESOLVED HIP PAIN

Diagnostic arthroscopy is not a substitute for clinical diagnostic skills and appropriately coordinated investigative studies. As stated by Dr. Jack Hughston, "looking is not a substitute for thinking." Considered casually, unresolved hip pain would certainly be an easily abused indication.

Arthroscopy has defined many elusive and often treatable causes of hip pain. This success has done much to stimulate advancements among noninvasive investigative studies. As various imaging methods continue to improve, the role of diagnostic arthroscopy should diminish. Numerous situations still ex-

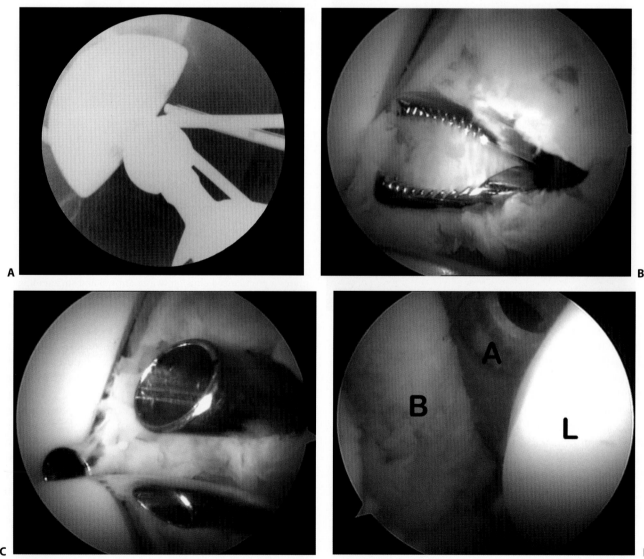

FIGURE 2.27. A 59-year-old man with a painful left total hip arthroplasty. (A) AP fluoroscopic view demonstrates distraction of the joint allowing placement of the three standard arthroscopic portals. (B) Fibrinous tissue is present and being biopsied. (C) Viewing from the anterior portal, the relationship of the lateral two portals is demonstrated within the joint, also illustrating the intact articulating surfaces of the prosthesis. (D) The interface of the bone (B) and acetabular shell (A) is visualized behind the acetabular liner (L).

ist in which arthroscopy is contemplated without a clear diagnosis, but at least with a high degree of suspicion that the problem is intraarticular and potentially amenable to arthroscopic intervention or, as stated by Burman in 1931, " . . . a good differential of various lesions that may be amenable to arthroscopic intervention."[89] Under appropriate circumstances, the literature still supports the role of diagnostic arthroscopy. In the study by Baber et al., arthroscopy altered the diagnosis in more than half of 328 patients undergoing the procedure.[90]

ASSOCIATED WITH OPEN PROCEDURES

In varied examples, arthroscopy has been described either in conjunction with open procedures or as a prelude to a subsequent open procedure. Futami et al.[91] described the role of arthroscopy in coordination with pinning for slipped capital femoral epiphysis, and Ruch has described arthroscopic guidance in positioning for core decompression in the presence of AVN.[91,92] Hawkins described arthroscopically assisted debridement of the hip via a miniarthrotomy, and Sekiya et al. have reported a similar method of arthroscopy via a limited anterior approach.[93,94] Osteotomy is occasionally performed for a variety of hip disorders.[95] Arthroscopy may be a useful adjunct in the planning process for selecting candidates for osteotomy.[5] Its role in staging of AVN and addressing coexistent intraarticular pathology has also been described.[71]

CONTRAINDICATIONS

Many contraindications exist for hip arthroscopy for reasons other than the hip itself. Medical illness or disease may preclude the patient from being an adequate risk for surgery. An active focus of infection contraindicates this relatively elective procedure. However, these contraindications are not unique to hip arthroscopy.

The clearest contraindication to hip arthroscopy is ankylosis of the joint characterized by a fixed position on attempted range of motion. Lesser degrees of arthrofibrosis or capsular constriction may, similarly, preclude arthroscopy when the joint cannot be adequately distracted or distended for introduction of the instruments. Marked limitation of rotational motion is often a harbinger of this type of process. Acetabular protrusio may also be a radiographic indicator of limited distractability of the joint, which can make it difficult to safely place the instruments.

Open wounds, ulcerative lesions, and superficial infections contraindicate the passage of arthroscopic instruments into the joint due to risk of secondarily creating a pyarthrosis. Similarly, other sources of soft tissue compromise may contraindicate instrumentation of the joint when there may be a concern regarding potential wound healing. Heterotopic ossification within the surrounding soft tissues may also create difficulties for access.

Appreciation of the bony architecture and neurovascular anatomy about the hip is critical to safe arthroscopy and, thus, any significant alteration in the normal anatomy of the bones or soft tissues, whether from previous trauma or surgery, may contraindicate arthroscopy.

One must also keep in mind potential stress risers in the bone, whether from disease, trauma, or previous surgery. A significant stress riser that could propagate a fracture may contraindicate the use of distraction forces often necessary for arthroscopy.

Severe obesity may be a relative contraindication to hip arthroscopy, more than arthroscopy for any other joint. Extra-length instruments are routinely needed, even for moderate-sized patients, and extremely dense soft tissues may overcome the effective operating length of currently available instruments.

Advanced disease states with destruction of the hip joint are also a contraindication to arthroscopy. This reflects poor patient selection and emphasizes the importance of proper indications.

SUMMARY

There are many indications for hip arthroscopy. However, the patients who adequately fit these indications are few. Be critical in your patient selection process. When you are clear on the indications, even then, expect surprises. Use each case as a learning tool to interpret normal variations and the significance of suspected pathological lesions.

References

1. Byrd JWT: Hip arthroscopy for post-traumatic loose fragments in the young active adult: three case reports. Clin Sport Med 1996;6:129–134.
2. Okada Y, Awaya G, Ikeda T, Tada H, Kamisato S, Futami T: Arthroscopic surgery for synovial chondromatosis of the hip. J Bone Joint Surg 1989;71B:198–199.
3. Witwity T, Uhlmann RD, Fischer J: Arthroscopic management of chondromatosis of the hip joint. Arthroscopy 1988;4:55–56.
4. McCarthy JC, Bono JV, Wardell S: Is there a treatment for synovial chondromatosis of the hip joint. Arthroscopy 1997;13:409–410.
5. Bowen JR, Kumar VP, Joyce JJ, Bowen JC: Osteochondritis dissecans following Perthes' disease: arthroscopic-operative treatment. Clin Orthop 1986;209:49–56.
6. Medlock V, Rathjen KE, Montgomery JB: Hip arthroscopy for the late sequelae of Perthes disease. Arthroscopy 1999;15:552–553.

7. Glick JM: Hip arthroscopy. In: McGinty JB (ed) Operative Arthroscopy. New York: Raven Press, 1991:663–676.

8. Cory JW, Ruch DS: Arthroscopic removal of a .44 caliber bullet from the hip. Arthroscopy 1998;14:624–626.

9. Teloken MA, Schmietd I, Tomlinson DP: Hip arthroscopy: a unique inferomedial approach to bullet removal. Arthroscopy 2002;18:E21.

10. Epstein H: Posterior fracture-dislocations of the hip: comparison of open and closed methods of treatment in certain types. J Bone Joint Surg 1961;43A:1079–1098.

11. Epstein H: Posterior fracture-dislocations of the hip: long-term follow-up. J Bone Joint Surg 1974;56A:1103–1127.

12. Byrd JWT, Jones KS: Prospective analysis of hip arthroscopy with five year follow up. Presented at AAOS 69th Annual Meeting, Dallas, Texas, February 14, 2002.

13. Paterson I: The torn acetabular labrum: a block to reduction of a dislocated hip. J Bone Joint Surg 1957;39B:306–309.

14. Dameron TB: Bucket-handle tear of acetabular labrum accompanying posterior dislocation of the hip. J Bone Joint Surg. 1959;41A:131–134.

15. Rashleigh-Belcher HJC, Cannon SR: Recurrent dislocation of the hip with a "Bankart-Type" lesion. J Bone Joint Surg 1986;68B:398–399.

16. Altenberg AR: Acetabular labrum tears: a cause of hip pain and degenerative arthritis. South Med J 1977;70:174–175.

17. Tanabe H: Aging process of the acetabular labrum—an electron-microscopic study. J Jpn Orthop Assoc 1991;65:18–25.

18. Chevrot A, Adamsbaum C, Gailly G, et al: The labrum acetabulare based on 121 arthrographies of the hip in adults. J Radiol 1988;69:711–720.

19. Kim YH: Acetabular dysplasia and osteoarthritis developed by an eversion of the acetabular labrum. Clin Orthop 1987;215:289–295.

20. Seldes RM, Tan V, Hunt J, Katz M, Winiarsky R, Fitzgerald RH Jr: Anatomy, histologic features, and vascularity of the adult acetabular labrum. Clin Orthop 2001;382:232–240.

21. McCarthy JC, Noble PC, Schuck MR, Wright J, Lee J: The watershed labral lesion: its relationship to early arthritis of the hip. J Arthroplasty 2001;16(8 Suppl 1):81–87.

22. Ueo T, Suzuki S, Iwasaki R, Yosikawa J: Rupture of the labra acetabularis as a cause of hip pain detected arthroscopically, and partial limbectomy for successful pain relief. Arthroscopy 1990;6:48–51.

23. Ikeda T, Awaya G, Suzuki S, Okada Y, Tada H: Torn acetabular labrum in young patients. J Bone Joint Surg 1988;70B:13–16.

24. Suzuki S, Awaya G, Okada Y, Maekawa M, Ikeda T, Tada H: Arthroscopic diagnosis of ruptured acetabular labrum. Acta Orthop Scand 1986;57:513–515.

25. Lage LA, Patel JV, Villar RN: The acetabular labral tear: an arthroscopic classification. Arthroscopy 1996;12:269–272.

26. Farjo LA, Glick JM, Sampson TG: Hip arthroscopy for acetabular labrum tears. Arthroscopy 2001:15:132–137.

27. Santori N, Villar RN: Acetabular labral tears: result of arthroscopic partial limbectomy. Arthroscopy 2000;16:11–15.

28. Dorrell JH, Catterall A: The torn acetabular labrum. J Bone Joint Surg 1986;68B:400–403.

29. Klaue K, Durnin CW, Ganz R: The acetabular rim syndrome. J Bone Joint Surg 1991;73B:423–429.

30. Harris WH, Bourne RB, Oh I: Intraarticular acetabular labrum: a possible etiological factor in certain cases of osteoarthritis of the hip. J Bone Joint Surg 1979;61A:510–513.

31. Byrd JWT, Jones KS: Osteoarthritis caused by an inverted acetabular labrum: radiographic diagnosis and arthroscopic treatment. Arthroscopy 2002;18:741–747.

32. Nishina T, Saito S, Ohzono K, Shimizu N, Hosoya T, Ono K: Chiari pelvic osteotomy for osteoarthritis: the influence of the torn and detached acetabular labrum. J Bone Joint Surg 1990;72B:765–769.

33. Fitzgerald RH: Acetabular labrum tears. Clin Orthop 1995;311:60–68.

34. Byrd JWT: Labral lesions: an elusive source of hip pain: case reports and review of the literature. Arthroscopy 1996;12:603–612.

35. Lecouvet FE, VandeBerg BC, Malghen J, Lebon CJ, Moysan P, Jamart J, Maldague BE: MR imaging of the acetabular labrum: variations in 200 asymptomatic hips. Am J Roentgenol 1996;167:1025–1028.

36. Byrd JWT: Lateral impact injury: a source of occult hip pathology. Clin Sports Med 200;20:801–816.

37. Noguchi Y, Miura H, Takasugi S, Iwamoto Y: Cartilage and labrum degeneration in the dysplastic hip generally originates in the anterosuperior weight-bearing area: an arthroscopic observation. Arthroscopy 1999;15:496–506.

38. Howe WW Jr, Lacey T II, Schwartz RP: A study of the gross anatomy of the arteries supplying the proximal portion of the femur and the acetabulum. J Bone Joint Surg 1950;32A:856–866.

39. Wertheimer LG, Lopes SDLF: Arterial supply of the femoral head, a combined angiographic and histological study. J Bone Joint Surg 1953;35B:442–461.

40. Gray AJR, Villar RN: The ligamentum teres of the hip: an arthroscopic classification of its pathology. Arthroscopy 1997;13:575–578.

41. Delcamp DD, Klarren HE, VanMeerdervoort HFP: Traumatic avulsion of the ligamentum teres without dislocation of the hip. J Bone Joint Surg 1988;70A:933–935.

42. Barrett IR, Goldberg JA: Avulsion fracture of the ligamentum teres in a child. A case report. J Bone Joint Surg 1989;71A:438–439.

43. Glynn TP Jr, Kreipke DL, DeRossa GP: Computed tomography arthrography in traumatic hip dislocation. Skeletal Radiol 1989;18:29–31.

44. Ebraheim NA, Savolaine ER, Fenton PJ, Jackson WT: A calcified ligamentum teres mimicking entrapped intraarticular bony fragments in a patient with acetabular fracture. J Orthop Trauma 1991;5:376–378.

45. Byrd JWT, Jones KS: Hip arthroscopy in athletes. Clin Sports Med 2001;20:749–762.

46. Byrd JWT, Jones KS: Traumatic rupture of the ligamentum teres as a source of hip pain. Arthroscopy 2002;18:SS–26.

47. Michaels G, Matles AL: The role of the ligamentum teres in congenital dislocation of the hip. Clin Orthop 1970;71:199–201.

48. Ippolito E, Ishii Y, Ponseti IV: Histologic, histochemical, and ultrastructural studies of the hip joint capsule and ligamentum teres in congenital dislocation of the hip. Clin Orthop 1980;146:246–258.

49. Byrd JWT, Jones KS: Hip arthroscopy in the presence of dysplasia. Arthroscopy 2001;17:S1.

50. Callaghan JJ: Results of primary total hip arthroplasty in young patients. Instr Course Lect 1994;43:315–321.

51. Jackson RW: Arthroscopic treatment of degenerative arthritis. In: McGinty J (ed). Operative Arthroscopy. New York: Raven Press, 1991:319–323.

52. Villar RN: Arthroscopic debridement of the hip: a minimally invasive approach to osteoarthritis. J Bone Joint Surg 1991;73B:170–171.

53. Farjo LA, Glick JM, Sampson TG: Hip arthroscopy for degenerative joint disease. Arthroscopy 1998;14(4):435.

54. Sim FH: Synovial proliferative disorders: role of synovectomy. Arthroscopy 1985;1:198–204.

55. Dienst M, Godde S, Seil R, Hammer D, Kohn D: Hip arthroscopy without traction: in vivo anatomy of the peripheral hip joint cavity. Arthroscopy 2001;17:924–931.

56. Gondolph-Zink B, Puhl W, Noack W: Semiarthroscopic synovectomy of the hip. Int Orthop 1988;12:31–35.

57. Hajdu SI: Tumors of tendosynovial tissue. In: Hajdu SI (ed). Pathology of Soft Tissue Tumors. Philadelphia: Lea & Febiger, 1979:165–226.

58. Lange TZ: Tumors and tumorous conditions. In: Steinberg MD (ed). The Hip and Its Disorders. Philadelphia: Saunders 1991: 571.

59. Milgram JW: Synovial osteochondromatosis. J Bone Joint Surg 1977;59B:792–801.

60. Villacin AB, Brigham LN, Bullough PG: Primary and secondary synovial chondrometaplasia. Hum Pathol 1979;10:439–451.

61. Spjut JH, Dorfmann HD, Fechner RD, Ackerman LV, Firminger HI (eds): Tumors of bone and cartilage. In: Atlas of Tumor Pathology, Second Series. Washington DC: Armed Forces Institute of Pathology, 1983:391–410.

62. Enneking WF: Musculoskeletal Tumor Surgery. New York: Churchill Livingstone, 1983:1167–1174.

63. Danzig LA, Gershuni DH, Resnick D: Diagnosis and treatment of diffuse pigmented villonodular synovitis of the hip. Clin Orthop 1982;168:42–77.

64. DellaValle AG, Piccaluga F, Potter HG, Salvati EA, Pusso R: Pigmented villonodular synovitis of the hip. Clin Orthop 2001;388:187–199.

65. Goodman SB, Schurman DJ: Miscellaneous disorders. In: Steinberg ME (ed) The Hip and Its Disorders. Philadelphia: Saunders, 1991:683–704.

66. Byrd JWT: Hip arthroscopy: patient assessment and indications. Instr Course Lect 2003;52:711–719.

67. Millis MB, Kim YJ: Rationale of osteotomy and related procedures for hip preservation: a review. Clin Orthop 2002;405:108–121.

68. Siebenrock KA, Schoeniger R, Ganz R: Anterior femoroacetabular impingement due to acetabular retroversion: treatment with periacetabular osteotomy. J Bone Joint Surg Am 2003;85-A(2):278–286.

69. Sampson TG, Glick JM: Indications and surgical treatment of hip pathology. In: McGinty J, Caspari R, Jackson R, Poehling G (eds). Operative Arthroscopy, 2nd ed. New York: Raven Press, 1996:1067–1078.

70. Byrd JWT, Jones KS: Prospective analysis of hip arthroscopy with 2-year follow-up. Arthroscopy 2000;16:578–587.

71. Ruch DS, Sekiya J, Dickson SW, Loman LA, Pope TL, Poehling GG: The role of hip arthroscopy in the evaluation of avascular necrosis. Orthopedics 2001;24:339–343.

72. O'leary JA, Berend K, Vail TP: The relationship between diagnosis and outcome in arthroscopy of the hip. Arthroscopy 2001;17:181–188.

73. Bellabarba C, Sheinkop MB, Kuo KN: Idiopathic hip instability. An unrecognized cause of coxa saltans in the adult. Clin Orthop 1998;355:261–271.

74. Philippon MJ: The role of arthroscopic thermal capsulorrhaphy in the hip. Clin Sports Med 2001;20:817–830.

75. Murphy WA, Siegel MJ, Gilula LA: Arthrography in the diagnosis of unexplained chronic hip pain with regional osteopenia. Am J Roentgenol 1977;129:283–287.

76. Griffiths HJ, Utz R, Burke J, Bonfiglio T: Adhesive capsulitis of the hip and knee. Am J Roentgenol 1985;144:101–105.

77. Modesto C, Crespo E, Villas C, Aquerreat D: Adhesive capsulitis. Is it possible in childhood? Scand J Rheumatol 1995;24:255–256.

78. Mont MA, Lindsey JM, Hungerford DS: Adhesive capsulitis of the hip. Orthopaedics 1999;22:343–345.

79. McGrory BJ, Endrizzi DP: Adhesive capsulitis of the hip after bilateral adhesive capsulitis of the shoulder. Am J Orthop 2000;29:457–460.

80. Chung WK, Slater GL, Bates EH: Treatment of septic arthritis of the hip by arthroscopic lavage. J Pediatr Orthop 1993;13: 444–446.

81. Blitzer CM: Arthroscopic management of septic arthritis of the hip. Arthroscopy 1993;9:414–416.

82. Bould M, Edwards D, Villar RN: Arthroscopic diagnosis and treatment of septic arthritis of the hip joint. Arthroscopy 1993; 9:707–708.

83. Hyman JL, Salvati EA, Laurencin CT, et al: The arthroscopic drainage, irrigation, and debridement of late, acute total hip arthroplasty infections: average 6-year follow-up. J Arthroplasty 1999;14:903–910.

84. Nordt W, Giangarra CE, Levy IM, Habermann ET: Arthroscopic removal of entrapped debris following dislocation of a total hip arthroplasty. Arthroscopy 1987;3:196–198.

85. Vakili F, Salvati EA, Warren RF: Entrapped foreign body within the acetabular cup in total hip replacement. Clin Orthop 1980;150:159–162.

86. Shifrin LZ, Reis ND: Arthroscopy of a dislocated hip replacement: a case report. Clin Orthop 1980;146:213–214.

87. Turner RH, Schiller AD: Revision Total Hip Arthroplasty. New York: Grune & Stratton, 1982.

88. Bankston AB, Cates H, Ritter MA, Keating EM, Faris PM: Polyethylene wear in total hip arthroplasty. Clin Orthop 1995;317: 7–13.

89. Burman M: Arthroscopy or the direct visualization of joints. J Bone Joint Surg 1931;13:669–694.

90. Baber YF, Robinson AH, Villar RN: Is diagnostic arthroscopy of the hip worthwhile? A prospective review of 328 adults investigated for hip pain. J Bone Joint Surg [Br] 1999;81:600–603.

91. Futami T, Kasahara Y, Suzuki S, Sata Y, Ushikubo S: Arthroscopy for slipped capital femoral epiphysis. J Pediatr Orthop 1992;12:592–597.

92. Ruch DS, Satterfield W: The use of arthroscopy to document position of core decompression of the hip. Arthroscopy 1998;14:617–619.

93. Hawkins RB: Arthroscopy of the hip. Clin Orthop 1989;249: 44–47.

94. Sekiya JK, Wojtys EM, Loder RT, Hensinger RN: Hip arthroscopy using a limited anterior exposure: an alternative approach for arthroscopic access. Arthroscopy 2000;16:16–20.

95. Millis MB, Poss R, Murphy SB: Osteotomies of the hip in the prevention and treatment of osteoarthritis. Instr Course Lect 1992;51:145–154.

3

Physical Examination

J.W. Thomas Byrd

Examination of a painful hip is fairly succinct. Much of the examination focuses on assessing for extraarticular sources of hip pain. In fact, in the author's center, only approximately 20% of all patients who present with a chief complaint of hip problems actually have an intraarticular source of their symptoms, with the most common being degenerative arthritis. Also, for those who do genuinely have an intraarticular source of their symptoms, only a small percentage are candidates for any type of arthroscopic intervention.

Common extraarticular sources of hip-related symptoms begin remote from the joint itself. These complaints include symptoms referred from the lumbar spine, sacroiliac joint, and sciatic nerve. Hamstring and ischial symptoms are usually readily differentiated. However, hip flexor or adductor muscle strains may closely mimic hip joint symptoms. Lateral symptoms such as trochanteric bursitis or hip abductor muscle injury are usually characteristic. Deep tendinous involvement such as the piriformis or iliopsoas tendon may be difficult to differentiate from mechanical hip symptoms and may also occur in conjunction with intraarticular pathology.

An occult femoral hernia produces groin symptoms. Pain localization suggests hip pathology, but symptoms are not generated by examination of the hip. Nor do symptoms correlate with weight bearing or walking as much as with Valsalva-type maneuvers.

Consequently, it is often a challenge to differentiate musculoskeletal problems from visceral or nervous system disorders. After determining that the problem is musculoskeletal, the next step is to differentiate intraarticular (or intracapsular) sources from extraarticular disorders. Even then, many intraarticular sources of hip pain are not amenable to arthroscopic intervention. Examples include femoral neck stress fracture seen in active individuals, early-stage avascular necrosis frequently plaguing the younger population, and advanced arthritic disorders that are usually apparent radiographically. Thus, various imaging studies are often important in ruling out some of these disease states as much as in confirming a diagnosis (see Chapter 4).

HISTORY

Because there are various disorders that can result in a painful hip, the history may be equally varied as far as onset, duration, and severity of symptoms. For example, acute labral tears associated with an injury have gone undiagnosed for decades, presenting as a chronic disorder. Conversely, patients with a degenerative labral tear may describe the acute onset of symptoms associated with a relatively innocuous episode and gradual progression of symptoms.

In general, a history of a significant traumatic event is a better prognostic indicator of a problem potentially correctable with arthroscopy.[1] Insidious onset of symptoms is a poorer prognostic indicator. This situation suggests either underlying degenerative disease or some predisposition to injury, which is not likely to be completely correctable with arthroscopy. Patients may recount a minor precipitating episode such as a twisting injury; however, even under these circumstances, be wary that there may be underlying susceptibility of the joint to damage and, again, a less certain prognosis.

Mechanical symptoms such as locking, catching, popping, or sharp stabbing in nature are better prognostic indicators of a problem correctable by arthroscopy.[2] Simply pain in absence of mechanical symptoms is a poorer predictor. However, the presence of a *pop* or *click* is an often overrated feature of the hip examination. This sensation may indicate an unstable lesion inside the joint, but many painful intraarticular problems never demonstrate this finding, and popping and clicking can occur due to many extraarticular causes, most of which are normal.

There are characteristic features of the history that often indicate a mechanical hip problem (Table 3.1). These signs are helpful in localizing the hip as the source of trouble but are not specific for the type of pathology. As expected, the pain is worse with activities, although the degree is variable. Straight plane activities such as straight-ahead walking are often well tolerated while twisting maneuvers such as simply turning to change direction may produce sharp pain, especially when turning toward the symptomatic side,

TABLE 3.1. Characteristic Hip Symptoms.

Symptoms worse with activities
Twisting, such as turning, changing directions
Seated position may be uncomfortable, especially with hip flexion
Rising from seated position often painful (catching)
Difficulty ascending and descending stairs
Symptoms with entering and exiting an automobile
Dyspareunia
Difficulty with shoes, socks, hose, and so forth

which places the hip in internal rotation. Sitting may be uncomfortable, especially if the hip is placed in excessive flexion. Rising from the seated position is especially painful, and the patient may experience an accompanying catch or sharp stabbing sensation. Symptoms are worse with ascending or descending stairs or other inclines. Entering and exiting an automobile is often difficult with accompanying pain as this loads the hip in a flexed position along with twisting maneuvers. Dyspareunia is often an issue due to hip joint pain; this is commonly a problem among female patients, but may be a difficulty for male patients as well. Difficulty with shoes, socks, or hose may simply result from pain or may reflect restricted rotational motion and more advanced hip joint involvement.

Based on the information obtained in the history, a preliminary differential diagnosis should be formulated. The history assists the examiner in performing an appropriately directed physical examination.

PHYSICAL EXAMINATION

The information obtained in the history is just a screening tool. It helps direct the examination, but it should not unduly prejudice the approach. The examiner must be systematic and thorough to avoid potential pitfalls and missed diagnoses (Figure 3.1). In reference to examination of the hip, Otto Aufranc[3] noted that "more is missed by not looking than by not knowing."

INSPECTION

The most important aspect of inspection is stance and gait. The patient's posture is observed in both the standing and seated positions. Any splinting or protective maneuvers used to alleviate stresses on the hip joint are noted. While standing, a slightly flexed position of the involved hip and concomitantly the ipsilateral knee is common (Figure 3.2). In the seated position, slouching or listing to the uninvolved side avoids extremes of flexion (Figure 3.3).

An antalgic gait is often present, but dependent on the severity of symptoms. Typically, the stance phase is shortened and hip flexion appears accentuated as extension is avoided during this phase (Figure 3.4). Varying degrees of abductor lurch may be present as the patient attempts to place the center of gravity over the hip, reducing the forces on the joint (Figure 3.5A,B).

Observation is made for any asymmetry, gross atrophy, spinal malalignment, or pelvic obliquity that may be fixed or associated with a gross leg length discrepancy.

MEASUREMENTS

Certain measurements should be recorded as a routine part of the assessment. Leg lengths should be measured from the anterior superior iliac spine to the me-

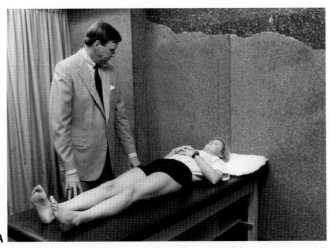

A

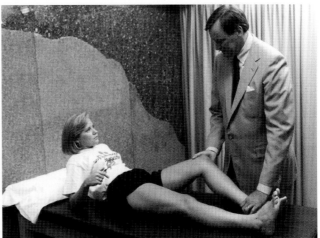

B

FIGURE 3.1. (A) It is important that both hips be examined. This necessitates that the examination table be positioned so that the examiner can approach the patient from both sides. (B) Always begin the examination with the uninvolved extremity.

This approach can gain the patient's confidence and provide potentially useful information for comparison when examining the involved hip. Failure to do so can result in missing useful information.

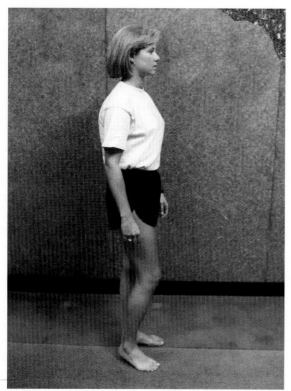

FIGURE 3.2. During stance, the patient with an irritated hip tends to stand with the joint slightly flexed. Consequently, the knee will be slightly flexed as well. This combined position of slight flexion creates an effective leg length discrepancy. To avoid dropping the pelvis on the affected side, the patient tends to rise slightly on his or her toes.

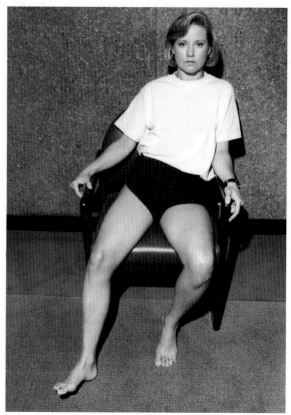

FIGURE 3.3. In the seated position, slouching and listing to the uninvolved side allows the hip to seek a slightly less flexed position. This is usually combined with slight abduction and external rotation, which relaxes the capsule.

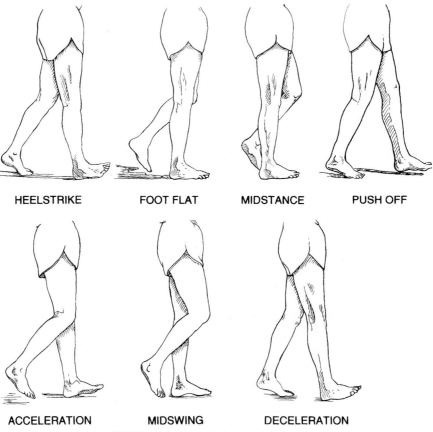

HEELSTRIKE   FOOT FLAT   MIDSTANCE   PUSH OFF

ACCELERATION   MIDSWING   DECELERATION

FIGURE 3.4. Normal phases of gait.

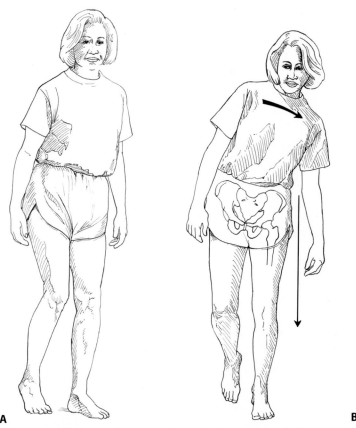

A **B**

FIGURE 3.5. (A) During ambulation, the stance phase of gait is shortened. Hip extension is avoided by keeping the joint in a slightly flexed position. This slight flexion creates a functional leg length discrepancy with shortening on the involved side and partially creates a lurch. (B) Further abductor lurch may occur as a compensatory mechanism to reduce the forces across the joint. Shifting the torso over the involved hip moves the center of gravity closer to the axis of the hip, shortens the lever arm moment, and reduces compressive joint force.

dial malleolus (Figure 3.6). Significant leg length discrepancies (greater than 1.5 cm) may be associated with a variety of chronic conditions. Typically, if this appears to be a contributing factor, we try to correct for half of the recorded discrepancy in the course of conservative treatment, preferably with an insert that is cosmetically more acceptable than a built-up shoe.

Thigh circumference, although a crude measurement, may reflect chronic conditions and muscle atrophy (Figure 3.7). It is important to measure the involved compared with the uninvolved side. Sequential measurement on subsequent examination may be helpful as an indicator of response to therapy. Again, this is a crude measure that only indirectly reflects hip function, but hip disease conversely usually affects the entire lower extremity.

It is important to accurately record range of motion of the hip in a consistent and reproducible fashion. Although reduced range of motion itself is rarely an indication for arthroscopic intervention, it is often a good indicator of the extent of disease and response to treatment.

The degree of flexion and the presence of a flexion contracture are determined by using the Thomas test (Figure 3.8). Extension is recorded with the patient in the prone position, raising the leg (Figure 3.9).

There are several effective mechanisms for recording rotational motion of the hip. It is important to select one and be consistent. Flexing the hip 90 degrees and then internally and externally rotating the joint is an easy and reproducible method for recording rotational motion (Figure 3.10). Abduction and adduction are recorded as well (Figure 3.11).

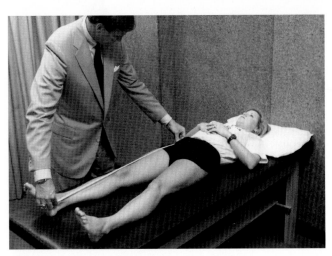

FIGURE 3.6. Leg lengths are measured from the anterior superior iliac spine to the medial malleolus.

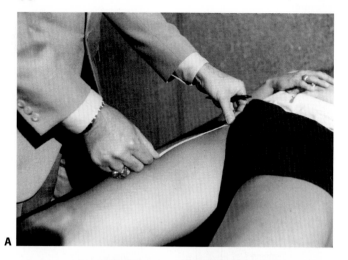

A

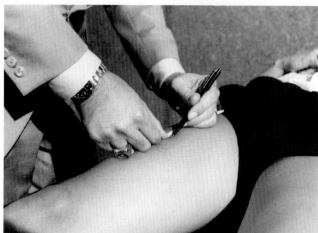

B

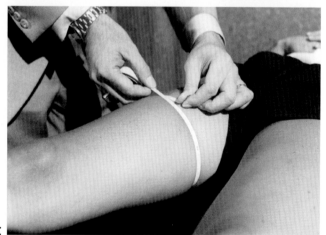

C

FIGURE 3.7. Thigh circumference should be measured at a fixed position, both for consistency of measurement of the affected and unaffected limbs and for consistency of measurement on subsequent examinations. (A) A tape measure is placed from the anterior superior iliac spine (ASIS) toward the center of the patella. (B) A selected distance below the anterior superior iliac spine is marked (typically 18 cm). (C) Thigh circumference is then recorded at this fixed position.

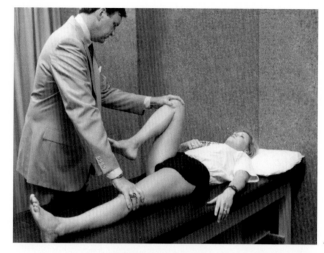

A

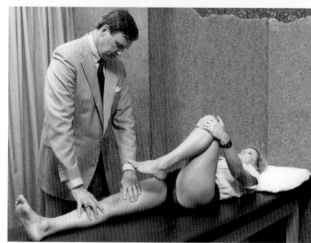

B

FIGURE 3.8. (A) In the supine position, the uninvolved hip is kept in maximal extension. This stabilizes the pelvis and avoids contribution of pelvic tilt to hip flexion. The affected hip is then maximally flexed and motion recorded. (B) To check extension or presence of a flexion contracture, the unaffected hip is brought into maximal flexion and held by the patient, locking the pelvis. The affected hip is then brought out toward extension and motion recorded.

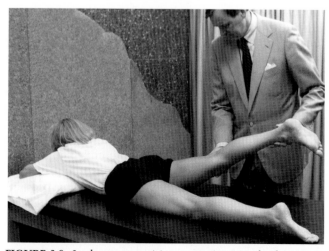

FIGURE 3.9. In the prone position, extension can also be quantitated in an assisted fashion.

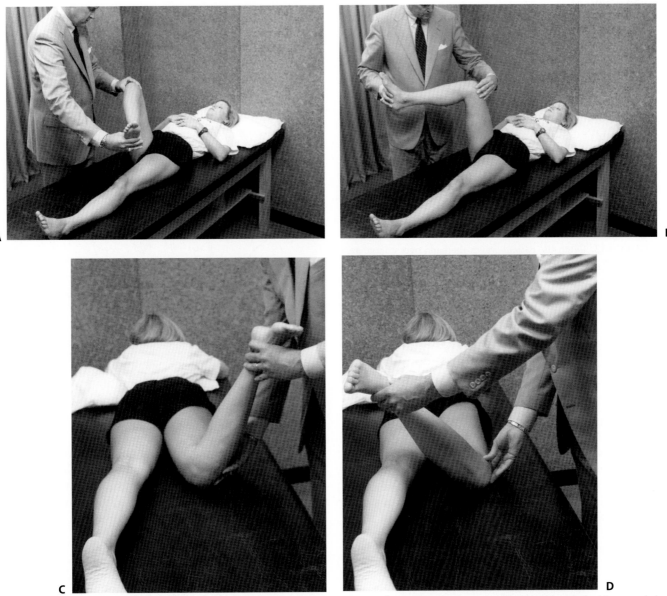

FIGURE 3.10. (A, B) Supine, with the hip flexed 90 degrees, the hip is maximally rotated internally and externally with motions recorded. This method is simple, quick, and reproducible. (C, D) Al-ternatively, rotational motion can be recorded with the hip extended in the prone position. Whatever method is chosen, it is important to be consistent on sequential examinations.

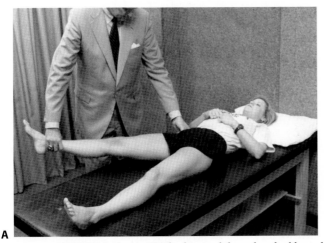

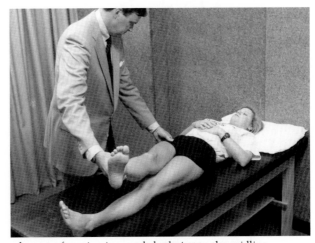

FIGURE 3.11. (A, B) The hip is abducted and adducted, and range of motion is recorded relative to the midline.

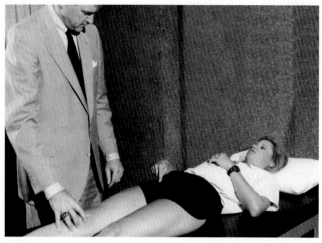

FIGURE 3.12. Often the patient waves the hand over a large area of involvement. However, the patient is asked, with encouragement and instruction, to point with one finger to the area of maximal involvement.

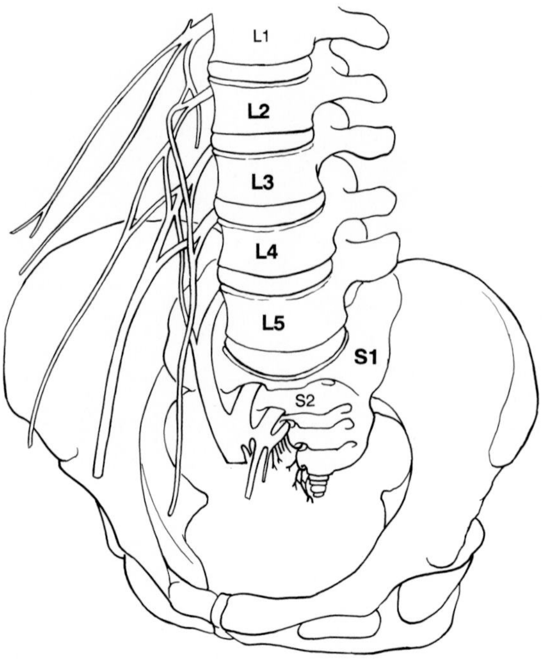

SYMPTOM LOCALIZATION

The One-Finger Rule

Although this is less well applied to the hip than to other joints, such as the knee, it is still important to ask the patient to use one finger and point to the spot that hurts the worst (Figure 3.12). This test provides much useful information before beginning palpation. It allows the examiner to discern the point of maximal tenderness. Consequently, this area is reserved until last when performing the examination. This forces the examiner to be more systematic, exploring uninvolved areas first, and enhances the patient's trust

FIGURE 3.14. The hip joint receives innervation from branches of L2 to S1 of the lumbosacral plexus, but predominantly from the L3 nerve root.

by not stimulating pain at the beginning of the examination (Figure 3.13).

Hilton's law states that "the same trunks of nerves whose branches supply the groups of muscles moving a joint furnish also a distribution of nerves to the skin over the insertion of the same muscles, and the interior of the joint receives its nerves from the same

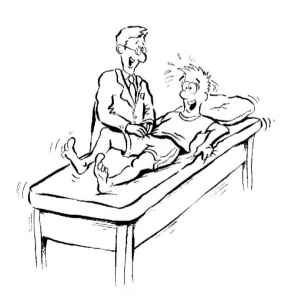

FIGURE 3.13.

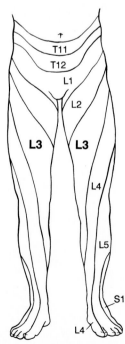

FIGURE 3.15. The L3 dermatome crosses the anterior thigh and extends distally along the medial thigh to the level of the knee.

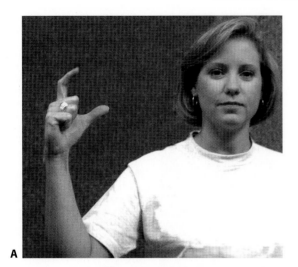

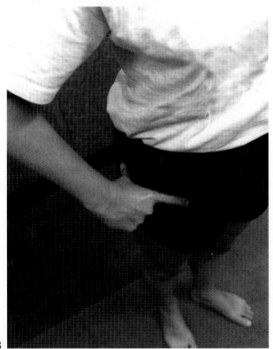

FIGURE 3.16. (A, B) The C sign. This term reflects the shape of the hand when a patient describes deep interior hip pain. The hand is cupped above the greater trochanter with the thumb posterior and the fingers gripping deep into the anterior groin.

sensation of deep, lateral discomfort or posterior pain, but usually only in conjunction with a predominant anterior component.

The C Sign

The classic complaint of patients with hip pathology is "groin pain." However, the author has identified a common characteristic sign of patients presenting with hip disorders. The patient cups his or her hand above the greater trochanter when describing deep interior hip pain. The hand forms a C and thus this has been termed the *C sign* (Figure 3.16). Because of the position of the hand, this can be misinterpreted as indicating lateral pathology such as the iliotibial band or trochanteric bursitis, but quite characteristically, the patient is describing deep interior hip pain.

Palpation

Palpation is usually unrevealing as far as any specific areas of discomfort related to an intraarticular source of hip symptoms (Figure 3.17). Obviously, one must

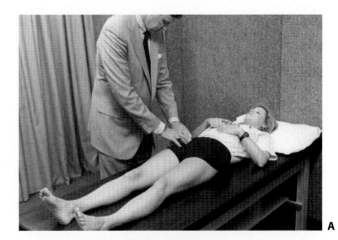

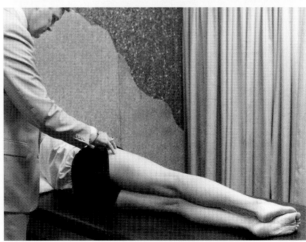

FIGURE 3.17. Palpation requires a systematic approach. It also requires a knowledge and orientation of the topographic anatomy about the hip and surrounding structures. Palpation is performed with the patient (A) supine and (B) in the lateral decubitus position.

source."[4] Although this may ensure physiologic harmony among the various structures, it also explains why muscle spasms and cutaneous sensations may accompany joint irritation.

Classic mechanical hip pain is described as being anterior, typically emanating from the groin area. The hip joint receives innervation from branches of L2 to S1 of the lumbosacral plexus, predominantly L3 (Figure 3.14). Consequently, hip symptoms may be referred to the L3 dermatome, explaining the presence of symptoms referred to the anterior and medial thigh, distally to the level of the knee (Figure 3.15).

Intracapsular hip pathology almost always has a component of anterior hip pain. There may also be a

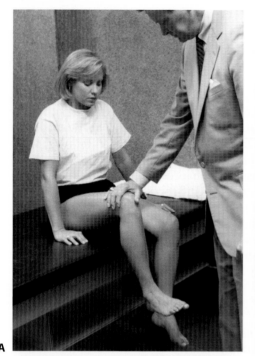

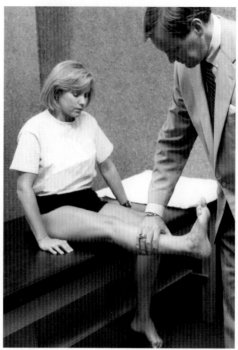

FIGURE 3.18. (A) Resisted hip flexion with the knee flexed isolates the iliopsoas tendon. Contribution from the sartorius is minimal as this is a very weak muscle. (B) Resisted hip flexion combined with knee extension recruits the rectus femoris, which crosses both joints as a hip flexor and knee extensor. (C) Resisted hip extension can be tested with the patient prone. (D) Another useful test for extensor weakness is to simply have the patient rise from the seated position with the arms crossed; this is difficult when significant extensor muscle weakness is present. (E) Manual testing of abductor strength is most easily performed in the lateral position. (F) Manual testing of adductor strength can similarly be tested, but with the patient supine.

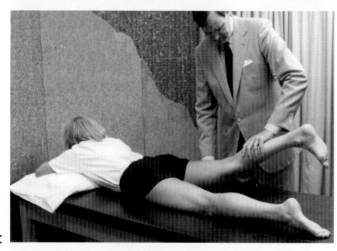

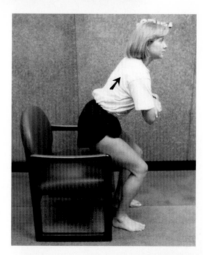

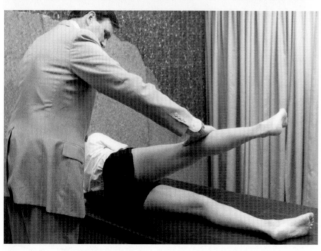

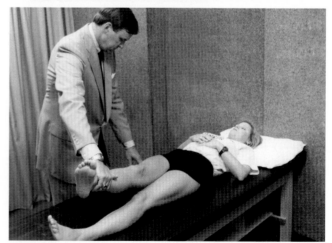

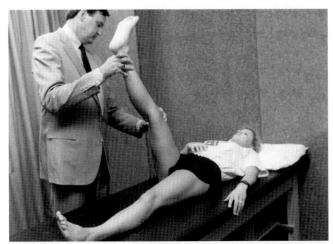

FIGURE 3.19. The classic straight leg raise (SLR) test is performed to assess tension signs of lumbar nerve root irritation. A positive interpretation is characterized by reproduction of radiating pain along a dermatomal distribution of the lower extremity. It may also recreate local joint symptoms or discomfort in stretching of the hamstring tendons.

be familiar with the topographic and deep anatomy to correlate the structures being palpated. Aufranc[3] noted that "a continuing study of anatomy marks the difference between good and expert ability."

Palpation is used more to assess potential sources of hip-type pain, other than the joint itself. It is important to be systematic, palpating the lumbar spine, sacroiliac (SI) joints, ischium, iliac crest, lateral aspect of the greater trochanter and trochanteric bursa, muscle bellies, and even the pubic symphysis, each of which may elicit information regarding a potential source of hip symptoms.

MUSCLE STRENGTH

Manual muscle testing is a crude measure of hip function, but it may elicit useful information (Figure 3.18). If injury to a specific muscle group is suspected, resisted contraction should reproduce localized symptoms.

Active range of motion and resisted active range of motion may also reproduce joint symptoms. However, when carefully interpreted, a distinction can be made between symptoms of a muscle strain and hip pain. This differentiation may be least clear with a strain of the hip flexors. In this setting, active hip flexion reproduces pain while passive flexion should not.

SPECIAL TESTS

Special tests include those maneuvers used to define other sources of symptoms as well as those used to define symptoms localized to the hip. There also needs to be an appreciation of how tests for other sources may also affect a painful hip.

The straight leg raise is important for assessing signs related to lumbar nerve root irritation (Figure 3.19). It may also provoke local joint symptoms. The Patrick or Faber test (flexion, abduction, external rotation) has been described both for stressing the SI joint looking for symptoms localized to this area and for isolating symptoms to the hip (Figure 3.20). Differentiation between pain localized to the SI joint and the hip is usually easy.

The single most specific test for hip pain is log rolling of the hip back and forth (Figure 3.21). This test moves only the femoral head in relation to the acetabulum and the surrounding capsule. There is no significant excursion or stress on myotendinous structures or nerves. Absence of a positive log roll test does not preclude the hip as a source of symptoms, but its presence greatly raises the suspicion.

Forced flexion combined with internal rotation is a more sensitive maneuver that may elicit symptoms associated with even subtle hip pathology (Figure 3.22). Sometimes there may be an accompanying pop or click, but more important is whether the maneuver reproduces the type of hip pain that the patient experiences with activities. This maneuver may normally be uncomfortable, so it is important to compare the response on the symptomatic and asymptomatic sides. Alternatively, forced abduction with external rotation sometimes produces symptoms (Figure 3.23).

An active straight leg raise or straight leg raise against resistance also often elicits hip symptoms (Figure 3.24). This maneuver generates a force of several times body weight across the articular surfaces and actually can generate more force than walking.

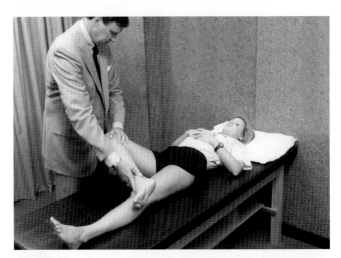

FIGURE 3.20. With the patient supine, the Patrick or Faber test is performed by crossing the ankle over the front of the contralateral knee and then forcing the knee of the involved extremity down on the table. This combination of flexion, abduction, and external rotation stresses the sacroiliac (SI) joint, and when injury or inflammation is present, this movement markedly enhances symptoms localized to the SI area. This same maneuver can irritate the hip joint as well, but with distinctly different localization of symptoms.

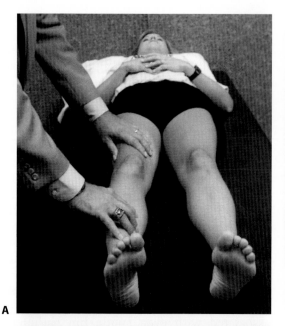

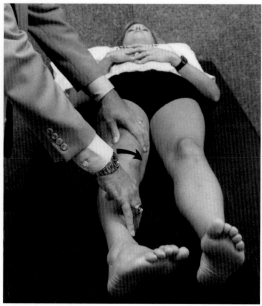

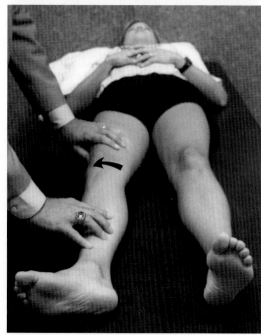

FIGURE 3.21. The log roll test is the single most specific test for hip pathology. With the patient supine (A), gently rolling the thigh internally (B) and externally (C) moves the articular surface of the femoral head in relation to the acetabulum but does not stress any of the surrounding extraarticular structures.

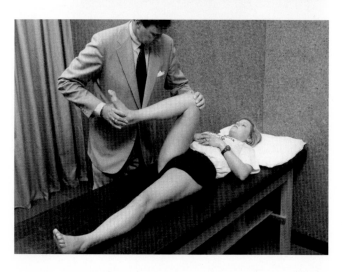

FIGURE 3.22. Forced flexion combined with internal rotation is often very uncomfortable and usually elicits symptoms associated with even subtle degrees of hip pathology.

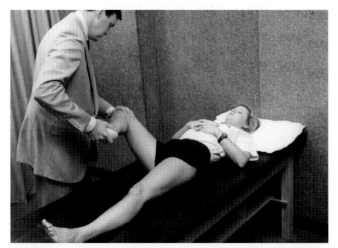

FIGURE 3.23. Flexion combined with abduction and external rotation similarly is often uncomfortable and may reproduce catching-type sensations associated with labral or chondral lesions.

Various maneuvers may create a click or popping sensation, which may reflect an unstable labral tear or chondral fragment. However, the origin of these clicks or pops is often unclear, and they do not uniformly reflect an intraarticular lesion.

Snapping of the iliopsoas tendon is a common condition that occasionally can be difficult to distinguish from an intraarticular problem. The characteristic maneuver for creating this type of snap is bringing the hip from a flexed, abducted, externally rotated position into extension with internal rotation.[5,6] The snapping occurs as the iliopsoas tendon transiently lodges on the anterior aspect of the hip capsule or pectineal eminence. Although it is important not to misinterpret snapping of the iliopsoas tendon as an intraarticular problem, it is likely that numerous intraarticular disorders get misdiagnosed as a *snapping hip syndrome.* For recalcitrant cases, snapping due to the iliopsoas tendon can often be substantiated by reproducing the snap

under fluoroscopy with iliopsoas bursography. Ultrasound is another method for inspecting the iliopsoas tendon that may be advantageous because producing the snap is less encumbered by the overlying fluoroscopy unit, it is noninvasive, and the contralateral side can be examined for comparison.

Snapping due to the iliotibial band is more easily distinguished from hip joint disorders because of its lateral location.[6–8] These patients frequently present with a sensation that their hip is subluxing and can dynamically produce a maneuver that grossly suggests hip joint instability. However, this visual appearance is uniformly created by the tensor fascia lata flipping back and forth across the greater trochanter. If necessary, stability of the hip can be substantiated by obtaining plain films with the hip in the position that grossly looks subluxed, confirming a concentric reduction.

RADIOGRAPHY

Plain radiographs are an integral part of the routine assessment of any hip problem. Typically, an anteroposterior (AP) radiograph of the pelvis and frog lateral view of the affected hip represent the minimum radiographic assessment (Figure 3.25). The AP pelvis film is centered low over the hips, and this is used rather than just an AP of the affected hip for two reasons. First, it allows radiographic examination of closely related areas, including the sacrum, sacroiliac joints, ilium, ischium, and pubis (Figure 3.26). Second, it allows a comparison view of the contralateral hip to help assess subtle variations in the bony architecture. The frog lateral, while not a true lateral of the hip, does provide a good lateral view of the femoral head, often the area of most concern. Although a crosstable lateral represents a more true lateral radiograph

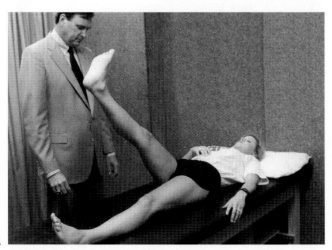

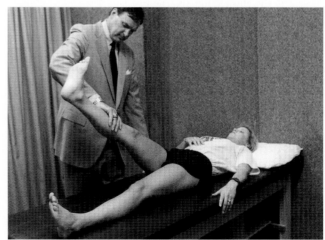

A   **B**

FIGURE 3.24. (A, B) An active straight leg raise, or especially a leg raise against resistance, generates compressive forces of multiple times body weight across the hip joint. Consequently, this is often painful, especially when there is even an mild degree of underlying degenerative disease.

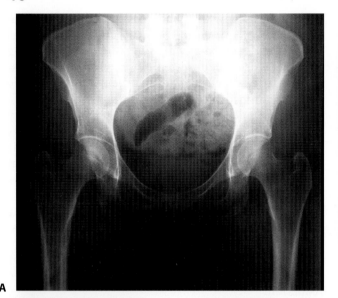

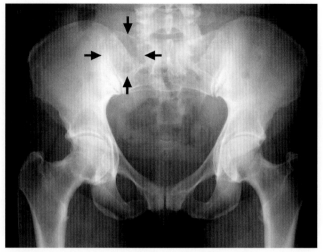

FIGURE 3.26. AP pelvis radiograph of a 50-year-old woman with a chief complaint of "right hip pain." Chronic bony changes are apparent around both hips, but an aggressive lytic lesion is identified in the right sacrum (arrows).

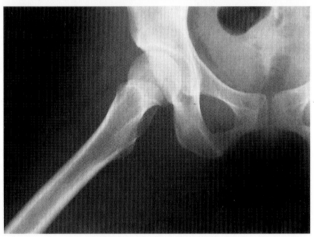

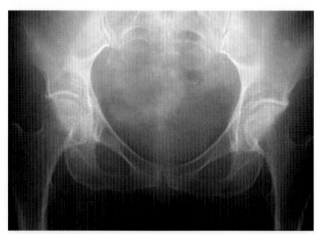

FIGURE 3.25. (A) An anteroposterior (AP) radiograph of the pelvis is centered low to include the hips. Performed properly, this provides good radiographic assessment of the hip in the AP plane. Additionally, it allows radiographic visualization of the surrounding structures, including the lumbosacral junction, sacrum, coccyx, sacroiliac joint, ilium, ischium, and pubis. Of equal importance, it provides a comparison view of the contralateral hip, which is often helpful when trying to interpret subtle irregularities or variations present in the affected hip. (B) The frog lateral provides an excellent radiographic view of the proximal femur in a perpendicular plane to the AP film.

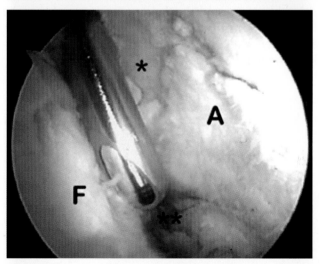

of the joint, it provides less useful information about the proximal femur and adds little to interpretation of the acetabulum as a routine screening tool.

Varying degrees of degeneration may be apparent radiographically with either inflammatory or oteoarthritic disorders and are readily recognized. However, subtle findings may be associated with various forms of intraarticular pathology. Just as is commonly seen in the knee, significant articular surface damage apparent at arthroscopy may be related to only subtle radiographic evidence of joint space narrowing on radiographs that could be superficially interpreted as normal (Figure 3.27).

FIGURE 3.27. (A) AP pelvis radiograph of a 74-year-old woman with chronic rheumatoid arthritis who presented with recent onset of intractable mechanical left hip pain. Radiographs were reported as superficially normal with only modest evidence of inflammatory degenerative changes, insufficient to solely explain the magnitude of her symptoms. (B) Arthroscopic view of the left hip from the anterolateral portal revealing extensive articular surface erosion of both the femoral head (F) and acetabulum (A) with area of exposed bone (*) and extensive synovial disease.

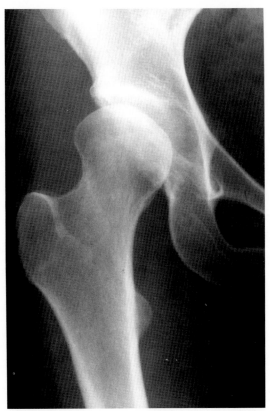

FIGURE 3.28. AP radiograph of the right hip of a 50-year-old woman, demonstrating classic characteristics of acetabular dysplasia.

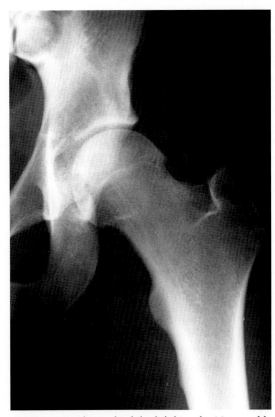

FIGURE 3.30. AP radiograph of the left hip of a 20-year-old collegiate basketball player with mild long-standing activity-related hip pain. There is subtle joint space narrowing in the superior weight-bearing portion of the hips and malformation of the femoral head that is distinct, but not classic, for the common developmental disorders of the hips.

The relationship of congenital hip dysplasia and labral pathology has been well defined.[9,10] Severe dysplasia carries a significant incidence of an inverted acetabular labrum (Figure 3.28). Milder degrees of dysplasia, characterized by slight lateral uncovering of the femoral head, or slight valgus position of the femoral neck may be associated with milder degrees of labral disease (Figure 3.29). Additionally, subtle congenital or developmental changes such as those associated with mild Legg–Calvé–Perthes disease or mild untreated slipped capital femoral epiphysis may be associated with symptomatic labral or chondral lesions in adulthood (Figure 3.30).

Traditionally, the single most definitive test for differentiating an intraarticular (or intracapsular) source of hip pain from an extraarticular source has been a fluoroscopically guided injection of anesthetic into the joint. Contrast is used to confirm the intracapsular position, followed by instillation of 8 to 10 ml bupivicaine. Temporary alleviation of symptoms for several hours is usually indicative of intraarticular pathology. The potential for extravasation or communication with surrounding bursas precludes this test from being 100% reliable. However, lack of response to the injection should lead one to look elsewhere for the source of pathology. Also, for older patients with a

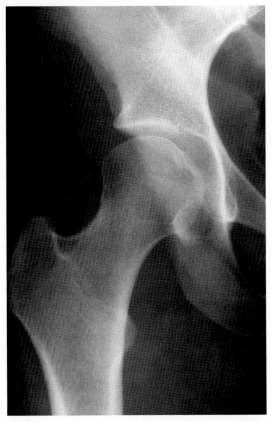

FIGURE 3.29. AP radiograph of the right hip of a 24-year-old woman with mechanical catching, suggestive of labral pathology. Signs of mild dysplasia include a slight valgus position of the femoral neck and slight lateral uncovering of the femoral head.

principal diagnosis of degenerative disease, concomitant use of a solution containing corticosteroid occasionally provides protracted pain relief analogous to injection of an arthritic knee. Currently, with the development of gadolinium arthrographic techniques with magnetic resonance imaging (MRI) (MRA), this anesthetic injection test can now be combined with the contrast medium used for imaging. It is imperative for the treating surgeon to specify to the radiologist when performing MRA to be certain to include bupivicaine. Response to the anesthetic may provide more reliable information than the images.

References

1. Byrd JWT, Jones KS: Prospective analysis of hip arthroscopy with two year follow up. Arthroscopy 2000;16:578–587.

2. O'Leary JA, Berend K, Vail TP: The relationship between diagnosis and outcome in arthroscopy of the hip. Arthroscopy 2001;17:181–188.

3. Aufranc OE: The patient with a hip problem. In: Aufranc OE (ed). Constructive Surgery of the Hip. St. Louis: Mosby, 1962:15–49.

4. Hilton J: Rest and Pain. London: Bell, 1863.

5. Jacobsen T, Allen WC: Surgical correction of the snapping iliopsoas tendon. Am J Sport Med 1990;18:1470–1474.

6. Allen WC, Cope R: Coxa saltans: the snapping hip revisited. J Am Acad Orthop Surg 1995;3:303–308.

7. Zoltan DJ, Clancy WG Jr, Keene JS: A new operative approach the snapping hip and refractory trochanteric bursitis in athletes. Am J Sports Med 1986;14:201–204.

8. Brignall CG, Stainsby GD: The snapping hip: treatment by Z-plasty. J Bone Joint Surg 1991;73B:253–254.

9. Dorrell J, Catterall A: The torn acetabular labrum. J Bone Joint Surg 1986;68B:400–403.

10. Klaue K, Durnin DW, Ganz R: The acetabular rim syndrome. J Bone Joint Surg 1991;73B:423–429.

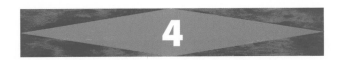

Adult Hip Imaging

Roy E. Erb

The role of diagnostic imaging in the evaluation of unexplained hip pain has been expanded recently by advances in computed tomography (CT) and magnetic resonance imaging (MRI)[1–3] and the efforts of several investigators toward improving detection of labral pathology.[4–17] Of particular interest to the arthroscopist, MR arthrography has proven accurate in the detection of injuries of the acetabular labrum[4–16] and can also demonstrate chondral damage, loose bodies, and abnormalities of the ligamentum teres.[17] This chapter is tailored to the arthroscopist and includes a brief review of imaging modalities used in the evaluation of adult hip pain followed by a discussion and illustration of the imaging features of hip disorders.

DIAGNOSTIC IMAGING MODALITIES AND PROCEDURES

Plain Radiography

Plain radiography remains the mainstay in initial imaging of suspected hip disease. Standard hip radiographic series include an anteroposterior (AP) view of the pelvis and coned-down AP and *frog lateral* views of the affected hip. The AP view of the pelvis is obtained to allow evaluation of symmetry of the hips, to detect concomitant contralateral hip disease, and to exclude abnormalities of the pelvis that could present clinically as hip pain. The AP views of the pelvis and hip are obtained with the X-ray beam aligned in the AP plane with the feet internally rotated.[18] The frog lateral view of a hip is obtained with the hip abducted and the X-ray beam oriented in the AP direction.[18] A groin lateral view (surgical lateral view) of the hip, instead of the frog lateral view, may be used in cases of an acute proximal femur fracture as the affected hip remains in neutral position. In this examination, the unaffected leg is abducted and elevated, and the X-ray beam is aligned parallel to the table with 20 degrees cephalad angulation.[19] Oblique or Judet[20] views are used to better demonstrate acetabular fractures and are obtained with the X-ray beam oriented in the AP plane with the patient in the supine position with rotation of the pelvis. The anterior Judet view depicts the anterior column and posterior acetabular rim and is obtained with the affected hip rotated 45 degrees anteriorly. The posterior Judet view demonstrates the posterior column and anterior acetabular rim and is taken with the affected hip rotated 45 degrees.

Historically, plain tomography of the hip was most commonly used in the evaluation of healing or nonunion of a proximal femur fracture treated with open reduction and internal fixation,[21] collapse of the femoral head in osteonecrosis, or the depiction of a suspected osteoid osteoma. The basis for the use of plain tomography in the setting of an open reduction and internal fixation was decreased metallic artifact relative to CT. With the advent of multislice, multidetector, helical CT, thin collimation CT with two-dimensional (2D) reformatting has essentially replaced the use of plain tomograms, providing similar resolution and information with a much shorter examination time and less metallic artifact than conventional CT.

Computed Tomography

CT is used to further characterize bony abnormalities of the hip detected on plain radiographs by providing cross-sectional information not present on plain radiographs. CT of the hip is employed primarily in the setting of trauma or in characterizing neoplasm of the proximal femur or acetabulum. Occasionally, it is used in the evaluation of congenital hip dysplasia and preoperative prosthesis planning. The emergence of helical and multislice helical CT has revolutionized our ability to acquire rapid high-resolution images of the hip and has several advantages over conventional CT, including improved resolution, shorter examination time, and lower radiation dose.[1] CT of the hip in trauma is used primarily to better characterize a fracture or fracture/dislocation detected on plain radiography. CT can reveal the spatial relationship of fractures, articular surface fractures of the femoral head and acetabulum (Figure 4.1), and the presence of intraarticular loose fragments (Figure 4.2) and can yield information used in predicting hip instability in injuries involving posterior wall fractures.[22] In the evaluation of neoplasm of the proximal femur or acetabulum, CT is typically used to help characterize the nature of the tumor matrix and demonstrate cortical thinning or destruction.

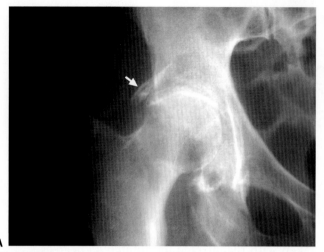

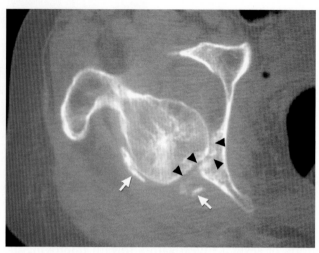

A   B

FIGURE 4.1. Impaction fractures of the femoral head and acetabulum associated with posterior dislocation of the right hip. (A) Plain radiograph demonstrates overlap of the cortex of the superior femoral head and acetabulum, internal rotation of the femur, and fracture fragments adjacent to the lateral acetabulum (arrow). (B) Computed tomography (CT) scan reveals impaction fractures of the femoral head and posterior wall of the acetabulum (arrowheads) as well as fracture fragments from the posterior wall (arrows).

CT examination of the hip at our institution is performed using a multislice helical scanner (General Electric, Milwaukee, WI). Imaging is performed in the axial plane and extends from just cephalad to the anterior inferior iliac spine to just caudal to the lesser trochanter. A bone algorithm is used with 2.5-mm collimation at 1.25-mm intervals at a table speed of 0.75 seconds. Two-dimensional (2D) coronal and sagittal reformations are often generated from the data set to aid in spatial orientation. Three dimensional (3D) images are less often generated but may be helpful for surgical planning.

Magnetic Resonance Imaging

MRI has become the secondary imaging examination of choice in the evaluation of unexplained hip pain. MRI has the unique ability to demonstrate soft tissue and marrow-based abnormalities that cannot be seen on plain radiographs or CT. The spectrum of pathology of the hip demonstrated with MRI has expanded well beyond detecting osteonecrosis, for which hip MRI gained its initial success. MRI is effective in demonstrating intraarticular and extraarticular pathology. Extraarticular disorders that are well demonstrated with MRI include muscle injuries,[23,24] iliopsoas and trochanteric bursitis,[25,26] sacroiliitis, and pelvic neoplasms. Intraarticular hip disorders depicted on MRI include joint effusions,[27] osteonecrosis,[28,29] stress fractures,[30,31] occult fractures,[32–35] osteoarthritis, and inflammatory arthropathies.[36] Unfortunately, conventional MRI has had poor success with demonstrating articular surface cartilage[37] and acetabular labral[5] abnormalities. Future development and improvements in MRI technology may lead to successful noninvasive evaluation of these structures.

Protocols for MRI of the hip vary among institutions and with the type of scanner used. Likewise, the information gained from MRI of the hip greatly depends on the field strength of the scanner, selection of sequences, and the experience and knowledge of the radiologist interpreting the examination. Currently, low-field-strength scanners do not provide the image quality of high-field-strength scanners. Examinations that do not include high-resolution small field of view images of the affected hip do not allow accurate evaluation of articular surface and labral abnormalities. Although there is no correct set of sequences, some important principles exist when developing protocols. MRI of the hip should include at least one coronal T1-weighted sequence and preferably at least one T2-weighted sequence that includes the pelvis and both hips. This protocol is based on the need to evaluate for occult pelvic pathology (insufficiency fractures,

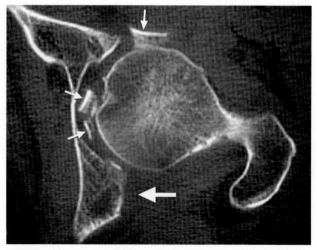

FIGURE 4.2. Intraarticular fracture fragments after reduction of a posterior hip dislocation. CT scan reveals multiple intraarticular fragments (arrows) and large defect (large arrow) in the posterior wall of the acetabulum.

sacroiliitis, and tumors) that may manifest clinically as hip pain and to evaluate the contralateral femoral head, because osteonecrosis is often bilateral. A T2-weighted sequence is also helpful in comparing the amount of joint fluid present in the hips. At least one small field of view high-resolution sequence of the affected hip should be obtained to allow better visualization of chondral, subchondral, and labral abnormalities.[17]

At our institution, MRI of the hip is performed using a General Electric (Milwaukee) 1.5-T superconducting magnet. A torso coil (General Electric, Milwaukee) is used for the images of both hips and an extremity coil (General Electric, Milwaukee) is used for high-resolution images of the affected hip. Coronal T1-weighted images (TR = 550, TE = minimum, 4.0 mm, 1.0-mm gap, 256X192, 2 NEX, FOV = 34 cm) of both hips depict anatomy and marrow-based abnormalities (osteonecrosis, occult fractures, and so forth). Fat-suppressed T2-weighted fast spin echo (FSE) images of both hips in the coronal (TR = 3300, TE = 102, 4.0 mm, 1.0-mm gap, ET = 8, 256X192, 3NEX, FOV = 34 cm) and axial (TR = 5000, TE = 102, 4.0 mm, 1.0-mm gap, ET = 14, 256X224, 3 NEX, FOV = 34 cm) planes are helpful in demonstrating intraarticular and extraarticular fluid collections, osteonecrosis, marrow edema, stress fractures, sacroiliitis, and paraarticular muscle injuries. High-resolution proton density fat-suppressed FSE images (TR = 3500, TE = 34, 3.0 mm, 1.0-mm gap, ET = 8, 256X192, 3 NEX, FOV = 16 cm) are helpful in assessing the acetabular labrum, articular cartilage, and articular surface of the femoral head.

Magnetic Resonance Arthrography

Several reports have documented the success of MR arthrography of the hip in detecting labral pathology.[4,5,,8,9,12,14] In addition to labral pathology, this examination has the potential to demonstrate loose bodies and abnormalities of the articular cartilage[10] and ligamentum teres.[17] MR arthrography allows better visualization of normal intraarticular anatomy (Figure 4.3) and pathology than conventional MRI by distending the capsule from the underlying bone and surrounding normal structures. MR arthrography of the hip is thus helpful when conventional MRI is noncontributory and there is clinical suspicion for labral injury or other intraarticular abnormality.

MR arthrography of the hip involves intraarticular injection of either a dilute solution of gadolinium (1–2 mmol) or saline under fluoroscopic guidance followed by multiplanar MRI of the hip. Concomitant injection of anesthetic[15,17] as a diluent adds the advantage of providing clinical information helpful in distinguishing intraarticular from extraarticular pathology. At our institution, if the patient has not undergone conventional MRI before MR arthrography, precontrast

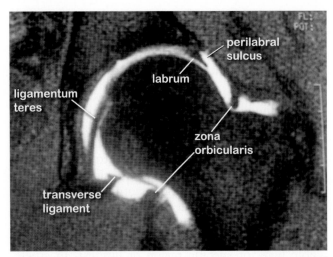

FIGURE 4.3. Normal anatomy seen on magnetic resonance (MR) arthrography. Coronal T1-weighted fat-suppressed image of the left hip demonstrates the lateral labrum, perilabral sulcus, transverse ligament, ligamentum teres, and zona orbicularis.

imaging of the hip is performed similar to the protocol outlined previously. This step can yield useful information regarding the presence or absence of a joint effusion and may demonstrate obvious intraarticular or extraarticular pathology that obviates the need for MR arthrography. Written informed consent is obtained on all patients undergoing MR arthrography of the hip. The technique for gaining access to the hip is identical to that described later in this chapter using a 22-gauge spinal needle. Approximately 1 mL iodinated contrast (Conray 60; Mallinkcrodt, St. Louis, MO) is injected to verify an intraarticular position of the needle. After verification of an intraarticular position of the needle, a mixture of 0.05 mL gadolinium (Omniscan, Nycomed, Princeton, NJ) and 3 mL iodinated contrast is administered into the joint, followed by the injection of 5 to 6 mL 0.5% bupivacaine HCl. This combination results in an intraarticular dilution of gadolinium of approximately 1:200. MRI is performed within 45 minutes of the injection. Postinjection imaging using the extremity coil includes fat-suppressed T1-weighted images (TR = 750, TE = minimum, 4.0 mm, 0 gap, 256X256, 2 NEX, FOV = 16 cm) in the axial, coronal, sagittal, and oblique axial[10] (image plane oriented parallel to the femoral neck) planes. Although radial reconstructions can be obtained and have been reported to improve detection of labral pathology,[38] we have not employed this technique on a routine basis.

In cases in which MRI is contraindicated, CT arthrography can be used. Single-contrast technique should be adequate to evaluate the labrum and to identify loose bodies. At our institution, a combination of 5 mL 0.5% bupivicaine HCL and 5 mL Conray 60 (Mallinkcrodt, St Louis, MO) is used for single-contrast hip CT arthrography. CT is performed similar to the method outlined previously with coronal and sagittal reformations.

Nuclear Scintigraphy

With the advent of MRI, nuclear scintigraphy has had a diminished role in the evaluation of hip pain. The bone scan is the most common scintigraphic examination used in the evaluation of skeletal disorders. Radionuclide bone scanning is sensitive to bone turnover and may reveal information regarding local blood flow and can help distinguish monostotic from polyostotic disease.[39] This examination employs the use of radiopharmaceutically labeled bone-avid agents and gamma camera technology to produce images of the whole body or specific region of interest. In single-phase examinations, a radiopharmaceutically labeled diphosphonate agent (typically technetium-99 methylene diphosphonate, MDP) is injected intravenously, and planar images are obtained 2 to 4 hours after injection. Although seldom used to evaluate the hip, the triple-phase bone scan is a variant of this method typically used to distinguish cellulitis from osteomyelitis. The triple-phase examination includes immediate sequential images of a specified region to evaluate blood flow, immediate static imaging to assess blood pool activity, and delayed images to evaluate bone turnover. Osteomyelitis is distinguished from cellulitis by demonstrating focal increased osseous activity on the delayed images. Other variations in radionuclide bone scanning that may improve lesion detection include the use of pinhole collimation and single photon emission computed tomography (SPECT).[39] SPECT yields multiplanar tomographic images that also may also aid in lesion localization. The use of tumor- and inflammation-avid agents in imaging hip disease is beyond the scope of this text.

Hip Arthrography, Injection, and Aspiration

Historically, conventional arthrography of the hip in adults was used in cases of suspected hip infection, intraarticular loose bodies, and synovial proliferative disorders and to evaluate potential loosening or infection of a hip prosthesis.[40] Today, a limited form of conventional arthrography (Figure 4.4) is still used in conjunction with hip injections and aspirations and CT and MR arthrography. At our institution, an anterior approach is used (Figure 4.5) to gain intraarticular access using sterile technique, buffered 1% lidocaine HCl as a local anesthetic, and small-gauge spinal needles (3.5 inch). Diagnostic aspirations are typically performed in cases of suspected septic arthritis or infected hip prosthesis. In the case of a native hip, an entry site mark is placed on the skin lateral to the vascular bundle directly anterior to the lateral portion of the femoral neck. Using sterile technique and local anesthetic, a 20-gauge needle is advanced to the lateral aspect of the junction of the femoral head and neck. Aspiration with a 10- to 12-mL syringe is then performed. A small amount (1–2 mL) of iodinated contrast is injected to verify an intraarticular position of the needle. When an aspiration of a total hip arthroplasty is performed, an entry site is chosen just lateral to the base of the neck of the femoral component so that the needle can be visualized. If a *dry tap* occurs, 10 to 20 mL sterile water (nonbacteriostatic) is injected into the joint and reaspirated.

Intraarticular injection of a long-acting anesthetic and corticosteroid can be used to distinguish intraar-

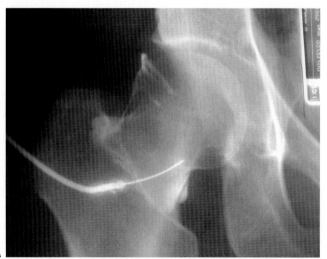
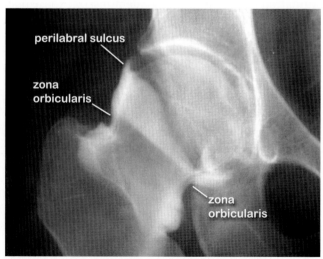

FIGURE 4.4. Intraarticular contrast injection and arthrogram. (A) Spinal needle positioned over medial femoral neck and early filling of the joint capsule. (B) Normal distribution of contrast demonstrating the paralabral sulcus and linear indentation of the zona orbicularis.

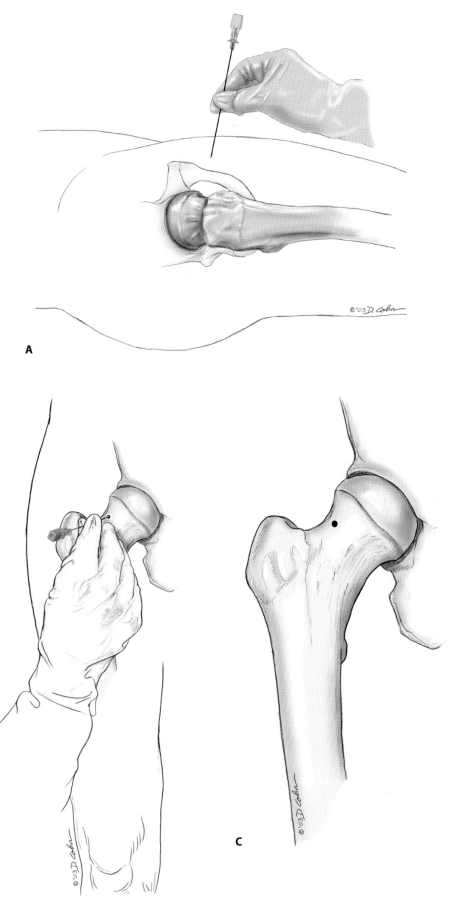

FIGURE 4.5. (A–C) Technique for fluoroscopic hip injection. Note the needle entry is directly anterior to the femoral neck.

ticular from extraarticular symptoms and to reduce pain and inflammation accompanied with arthritis. The choice of steroid and anesthetic used is largely dependent on personal experience and preference of either the radiologist or referring physician.[41] At our institution, we typically use 40 mg methylprednisolone acetate (Depomedrol) and 7 mL 0.5% bupivacaine HCl. The technique used is similar to that outlined previously for diagnostic aspirations, with the exception that a 22-gauge spinal needle is used. Aspiration is performed before contrast administration to exclude overt evidence for infection and to evacuate a joint effusion. Again, a small amount (1–2 mL) of iodinated contrast is injected to verify an intraarticular position of the needle. The steroid and anesthetic are then injected as a mixture into the joint. The patient is then assessed for evidence of symptom improvement and to report any clinical improvement to the referring physician.

Iliopsoas Bursography

Iliopsoas bursography has been successfully used to diagnose iliopsoas tendon snapping syndrome.[42] The examination is considered diagnostic of iliopsoas snapping syndrome if a jerking motion of the iliopsoas tendon is observed fluoroscopically as the patient reproduces the snapping or popping sensation. In our institution, this procedure has been replaced with ultrasound. Ultrasound has proven successful in a relatively recent report of a small group of patients examined for iliopsoas snapping syndrome[43] and has been useful in our clinical practice. Ultrasound has the advantages of being noninvasive, lacks ionizing radiation, and allows concomitant evaluation of the contralateral side.

The technique for iliopsoas bursography (Figure 4.6) is similar to that of a fluoroscopically guided hip injection. With the patient on the fluoroscopic table in the supine position, a skin mark is placed directly anterior to the middle of the femoral neck. Using sterile technique and 1% buffered lidocaine HCl as a local anesthetic, a 22-gauge spinal needle is advanced toward the upper portion of the femoral head. After making contact with the anterior acetabular rim, the needle is withdrawn 2 to 3 mL. Approximately 5 mL iodinated contrast is then injected and should course in a longitudinal direction and outline the iliopsoas tendon. Additionally, 5 mL 0.5% bupivicaine is administered into the bursa. The tendon is then observed under fluoroscopy as the patient reproduces the snapping sensation, typically with straightening the leg from the flexed, externally rotated, and abducted position.[44] The tendon should glide normally over the anterior capsule and iliopectineal eminence. A jerking movement of the tendon at the time the patient experiences symptoms is considered diagnostic of iliop-

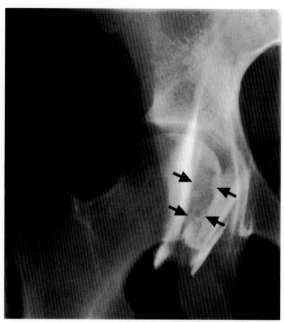

FIGURE 4.6. Iliopsoas bursogram. Contrast outlines the tendon (arrows) and myotendinous junction of the right iliopsoas muscle. (Courtesy of E. Paul Nance, MD.)

soas tendon snapping syndrome. Video recording of this portion of the examination is preferred for documentation purposes and enables the referring physician to review the tendon motion.

IMAGING FEATURES OF HIP PATHOLOGY

Osteonecrosis

Osteonecrosis of the femoral head is an important cause of hip pain that may be idiopathic or seen in association with a number of underlying risk factors such as trauma, sickle cell disease, steroid use, alcohol abuse, radiation, and pancreatitis. MRI has assumed the leading role among other imaging modalities in the evaluation of osteonecrosis.[1,3] With its ability to demonstrate fatty marrow and tissue water, MRI readily depicts changes in marrow content and marrow-based pathology (Figure 4.7). MRI is preferable to nuclear scintigraphy in the workup of osteonecrosis as it is generally considered more sensitive and specific in detecting the disorder,[28] and findings seen on MRI can have prognostic and therapeutic implications.[45–47]

Clinical staging of osteonecrosis is typically based on a modification[48, 49] of the work by Ficat. The most common MRI classification used in the evaluation of osteonecrosis was proposed by Mitchell et al.[28] This system correlates the MRI appearance of the osteonecrotic focus with histopathology and is believed to correspond to the temporal evolution of osteonecrosis and degree of clinical symptoms. Common to all of the appearances of osteonecrosis in this classification is a rim of low signal on T1-weighted

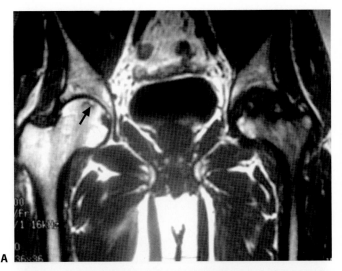

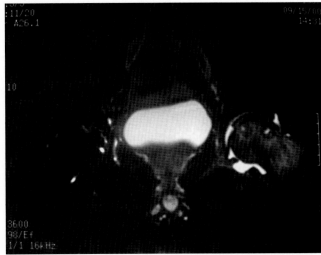

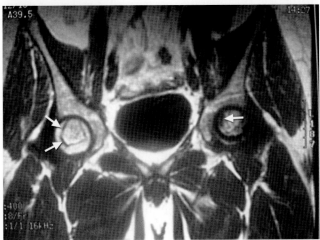

FIGURE 4.7. Bilateral osteonecrosis of the femoral head. (A) Coronal T1-weighted image of both hips demonstrates a linear focus of decreased signal (arrow) parallel to the articular surface in the right femur defining the margin of the osteonecrotic segment. Also, a large heterogeneous area of decreased signal is seen in the left femoral head extending into the left femoral neck. (B) Coronal T2-weighted fat-suppressed images of both hips reveals a large left hip effusion, increased signal in the left femoral head and neck (class C), and small focal areas of increased signal in both femoral heads. (C) Coronal T1-weighted image of both hips anteriorly demonstrates a linear ring (arrows) of low signal defining the margin of the osteonecrotic focus that is isointense with fat (class A).

images along the margin of the osteonecrotic focus. The osteonecrotic focus demonstrates signal intensities on MRI as follows: class A, signal intensity isointense to fat on T1-weighted and T2-weighted images (Figure 4.7A–C); class B, signal intensity isointense to blood, high signal intensity on T1- and T2-weighted images; class C, signal intensity isointense to fluid, low signal on T1-weighted images and high signal on T2-weighted images; class D, signal intensity isointense to fibrous tissue, low signal on T1- and T2-weighted images. On T2-weighted images, the transition between normal and necrotic bone may appear as a *double line* composed of an inner band of high signal corresponding to granulation tissue adjacent to an outer band of low signal thought to represent sclerosis from bone repair.[28] In advanced osteonecrosis, subchondral fracture of the femoral head may be seen on MRI as a curvilinear area of low signal on T1- or T2-weighted images immediately beneath and parallel to the articular surface.

A diffuse bone marrow edema pattern on MRI involving the femoral head and extending to the intertrochanteric region has been described.[50] Distinction of this pattern of osteonecrosis from transient

osteoporosis of the hip is important if core decompression is contemplated. Several authors recommend a careful search for a subchondral focal lesion indicating osteonecrosis.[29,46,47] Correlation with plain radiography may be helpful as well as transient osteoporosis typically demonstrates osteopenia on radiographs 4 to 8 weeks after the initial onset of symptoms.[51] Ultimately, clinical and imaging follow-up may be necessary to distinguish these two entities.

Evidence exists that MRI can be helpful in predicting future collapse of the articular surface[45–47] in osteonecrosis. Beltran et al. reported a correlation in future collapse of the femoral head after core decompression with the preoperative size of the osteonecrotic focus.[45] In this series, femoral head collapse occurred in 87% of cases involving greater than 50% of the weight-bearing articular surface (WBAS), 43% of cases involving 25% to 50% WBAS, and in no cases involving less than 25% WBAS. Shimizu et al.[47] reported similar observations in which collapse did not occur in patients with an osteonecrotic focus compromising less than 25% of the diameter of the femoral head. In their series, collapse occurred in 74% of patients with lesions greater than 25% of the femoral head diameter and involving greater than 67% WBAS.[47] In a prospective study of patients with steroid-induced osteonecrosis, Iida et al.[46] found that marrow edema seen on MRI correlated well with pain and subsequent collapse of the femoral head.

Osteoarthritis

Osteoarthritis is the most common arthropathy encountered in adults and can be primary or secondary. Secondary osteoarthritis occurs from a number of underlying conditions including trauma, infection, crystal deposition disease, osteonecrosis, and acetabular dysplasia. The initial plain radiographic finding of osteoarthritis is nonuniform superolateral joint space narrowing that results from cartilage loss (Figure 4.8). This pattern is easily distinguished from the uniform joint space narrowing seen in inflammatory arthropathies that typically occurs in an axial direction. As joint space loss progresses in osteoarthritis, reactive bone formation (subchondral sclerosis and osteophytosis) occurs in response to altered mechanical stresses. Osteophytes may develop along the medial femoral head and lateral acetabulum, and new bone formation may occur along the medial femoral neck. Subchondral cyst formation develops primarily in the subchondral bone of the lateral acetabulum and femoral head.[52] More advanced osteoarthritis leads to remodeling of the femoral head and acetabulum.

Although not often used in the evaluation of osteoarthritis, CT may be helpful in the localization of paraarticular calcification or ossification and in the detection of loose bodies. Lack of contrast in the joint, however, can limit its ability to distinguish intraarticular and extraarticular calcifications. In cases of end-stage osteoarthritis, CT can be used for preoper-

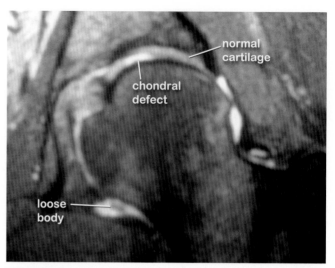

FIGURE 4.9. Osteoarthritis. Noncontrasted coronal proton density fat-suppressed image of the left hip demonstrates a full-thickness defect in the articular surface cartilage of the superior femoral head with a loose cartilaginous fragment in the inferior joint recess. Note the cartilage demonstrates intermediate signal (brighter than subjacent cortical bone and less intense than joint fluid).

ative planning and prosthesis fitting for total hip arthroplasty.

Conventional MRI of the hip has had modest to poor success with evaluating cartilage thickness[37] and demonstrating cartilage abnormalities of the femoral head and acetabulum. The detection of cartilage abnormalities of the hip with MRI is hindered by the configuration of the articular surfaces and the close apposition of the femoral and acetabular cartilage. In an early investigation of cadaver hips, Hodler et al. reported that conventional MRI with fat-suppressed T1-weighted images was not accurate in determining cartilage thickness.[37] A relatively recent study using a 3D spoiled gradient echo (SPGR) pulse sequence and hip traction reported success in detecting discontinuity of cartilage at the junction of normal and necrotic foci of the femoral head in osteonecrosis.[53] Based on our clinical success with depicting cartilaginous abnormalities of the knee and ankle with fat-suppressed proton density FSE imaging, we employ this sequence in our investigation of the hip to assess cartilage and labral pathology. Normal cartilage on this sequence appears as an intermediate signal structure that has higher signal intensity than subjacent bone and less signal intensity than joint fluid (Figure 4.9). In addition, this sequence demonstrates a distinct junction of the acetabular cartilage and labrum where the labrum is lower in signal than the adjacent cartilage.

In the absence of a joint effusion, conventional MRI is limited in its ability to demonstrate loose bodies. The presence of a joint effusion or introduction of intraarticular fluid with MR arthrography improves the sensitivity of detecting intraarticular cartilage and os-

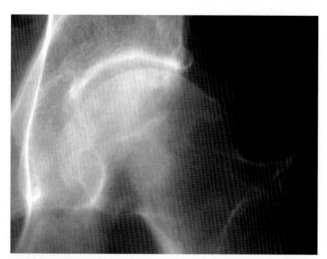

FIGURE 4.8. Osteoarthritis of the left hip. Plain radiograph shows superolateral joint space narrowing, subchondral sclerosis, and subchondral cyst formation. Early osteophytes are noted on the lateral acetabulum and medial femoral head.

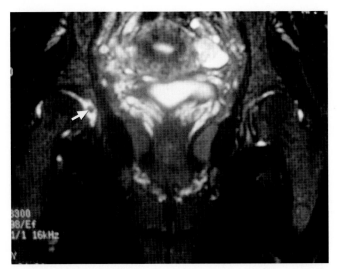

FIGURE 4.10. Loose body in osteoarthritis. Coronal T2-weighted fat-suppressed image of both hips demonstrates a small loose body (arrow) in the medial right hip joint outlined by joint fluid.

seous fragments by outlining these structures with fluid (see Figures 4.9, 4.10). Subchondral cysts in the femoral head and acetabulum demonstrate low signal on T1-weighted images and high signal on T2-weighted images and can fill in with contrast on MR arthrography.

Labral Pathology

Injury of the acetabular labrum is now recognized as an important cause of mechanical hip pain that can be surgically treated with resultant symptomatic relief. Recent interest and efforts directed toward improving our ability to diagnose labral tears has resulted in a growing knowledge of the MRI and MR arthrographic appearance of the normal and abnormal labrum.[4,5,7–10,12–15,54] Knowledge of the anatomy of the hip capsule, acetabular labrum, and articular cartilage and an understanding of the location and appearance of labral tears are essential to proper diagnosis of labral pathology. The acetabular labrum is a horseshoe-shaped fibrocartilaginous structure attached to the periphery of the acetabulum that adds depth to the hip joint.[55] Inferiorly the labrum continues as the transverse ligament from the anterior margin to the posterior margin of the acetabulum. In cross section on MRI, the labrum typically has a triangular configuration. Variation in the shape and intrasubstance signal of the labrum and even absence of the labrum on conventional MRI in asymptomatic individuals have been reported.[54–56] In a group of patients with asymptomatic hips, Lecouvet et al. noted that the presence of increased intrasubstance signal in the labrum and absence of the labrum on T1-weighted images increased in incidence with age.[55] Cotton et al., in a study of asymptomatic volunteers, also reported

that increased intrasubstance signal in the acetabular labrum on T1- and T2-weighted images and absence of the labrum was frequently observed.[9] It must be noted, however, that these observations[54,55] regarding absent labra are based on conventional MRI sequences and often lack distension of the perilabral sulcus achieved with MR arthrography, which aids in defining the presence, morphology, and articular surface contour of the labrum. Although debated in the radiologic community, the possibility of a normal sublabral sulcus occurring at the junction of the acetabular cartilage and labrum has been reported[57] and can be problematic when evaluating for labral tears. Although variation exists in the location of labral pathology in documented series,[58,59] it is generally considered that most labral injuries occur in the anterior or anterosuperior portion of the labrum. Lage et al.[59] have classified labral tears with respect to etiology (traumatic, degenerative, idiopathic, and congenital) and morphology (radial flap, radial fibrillated, longitudinal peripheral, and unstable).

Although conventional MRI has not proven successful in detecting labral injuries,[5] MR arthrography has recently been shown to be sensitive (ranging from 57% to 91%) for demonstrating tears and detachment of the labrum.[4,5,9,12,14] Czerny et al. have proposed an imaging classification of labral pathology of the hip based on the morphology of the labrum and labral-capsular relationship, intrinsic MRI signal, and the presence of fluid tracking into the junction of the acetabular cartilage and labrum.[4,5] This classification is based on the severity of injury and the shape of the labrum and configuration of the labral-capsular junction. One caveat to this classification is the assumption that a sublabral sulcus does not exist. To date no report has correlated the MRI or MR arthrography appearance of the morphologic subtypes of labral tears proposed by Lage et al.[59] The most definitive evidence for a labral tear on MR arthrography is the presence of contrast tracking into the substance of the labrum (Figure 4.11). Most authors consider the presence of contrast extending into the junction of the labrum and acetabular cartilage as evidence for a labral tear or detachment.[4,5,7,9,13–15] This author considers that this finding (Figure 4.12) can represent a longitudinal tear, partial labral detachment, or a sublabral sulcus. Although the distinction between a normal sublabral sulcus and injury to the labrum cannot always be made, subjective assessment of the size of the lesion[10] and correlation with the clinical response to intraarticular anesthetic may be helpful. Additional MR arthrographic findings that suggest the presence of a labral tear include a blunted or absent labrum or irregularity of the labral surface.[13] Enlargement of the labrum with increased intrinsic signal on T2-weighted images without leakage of contrast into the labrum is likely the result of intrasubstance degeneration. Par-

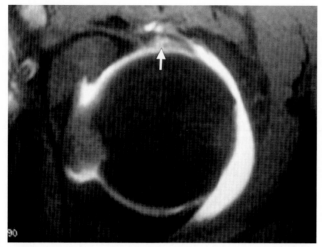

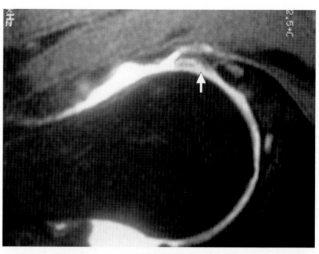

FIGURE 4.11. Longitudinal labral tear. MR arthrogram of the left hip demonstrates direct evidence of a labral tear with contrast extending into the substance of the labrum. (A) Axial T1-weighted fat-suppressed image shows contrast entering the substance of the anterior labrum (arrow). (B) Sagittal T1-weighted fat-suppressed image demonstrates contrast extending into the interface of the anterior labrum and acetabular cartilage (arrow).

alabral cysts are considered to be secondary evidence for underlying labral pathology,[60] theoretically developing as synovial fluid leaks through a labral defect. These cysts are dark on T1-weighted images and bright on T2-weighted images and may fill with contrast on MR arthrography (Figure 4.13).

Ligamentum Teres Pathology

The clinical significance of abnormalities of the ligamentum teres is less well known. The ligament carries a small artery to the fovea of the femoral head but has no known mechanical function. A tear of the ligament with an unstable fragment or enlargement of the ligament theoretically may lead to mechanical hip symptoms. The ligamentum teres is a triangular-shaped structure with a broad-based attachment to the posteroinferior portion of the cotyloid fossa of the acetabulum and courses cephalad to attach to the fovea.[55] Based on arthroscopic findings, injuries of the ligamentum teres result from both major and minor hip trauma.[61] Gray and Villar[61] proposed an arthroscopic classification of abnormalities of the ligamentum teres as follows: complete tears, partial tears, and degenerate ligamentum teres. On MRI and MR arthrography, the normal ligamentum teres appears as a band-like structure that demonstrates low signal intensity on all sequences and courses from the posteroinferior portion of the acetabulum to the fovea (see Figure 4.3). The ligament is best evaluated on the axial and coronal images. A chronic complete tear of the ligament may manifest by absence of this structure on MR arthrography. An acute complete tear may appear as a discontinuity in the ligament fibers or avulsion from the fovea. Partial tears or degenerative ligamentum teres are difficult to discern and typically demonstrate partial thickness tearing, irregularity, or thickening of ligament fibers or increased intrasubstance signal on T2-weighted images (Figure 4.14).[17]

Trauma

Plain radiographs remain the initial imaging examination in the evaluation of trauma to the pelvis and hip. Judet views can be helpful in establishing fracture patterns of the acetabulum. Inlet and outlet views are used to better evaluate fractures of the anterior and posterior pelvic ring. Secondary imaging of the hip with CT may be helpful for surgical planning in complex fractures and fracture/dislocations, and for the evaluation of intraarticular fragments (see Figure 4.2) and associated articular surface fractures in hip dislocations (see Figure 4.1).

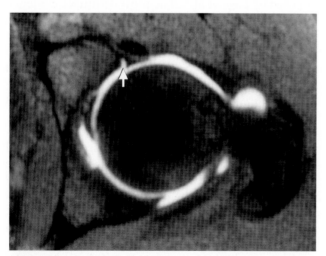

FIGURE 4.12. Detachment of the anterior labrum on MR arthrography. Axial T1-weighted fat-suppressed image demonstrates a large cleft between the anterior labrum and acetabulum (arrow) consistent with labral detachment. Arthroscopy revealed traumatic detachment of the anterior labrum.

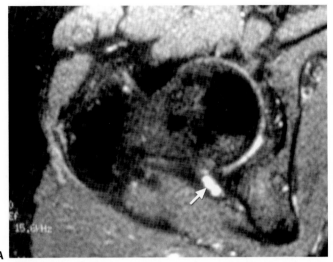

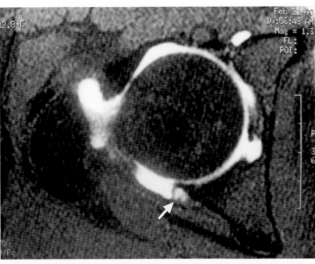

FIGURE 4.13. Posterior paralabral cyst. (A) Axial proton density fat-suppressed image of the right hip reveals a small posterior paralabral cyst (arrow) that is typically indicative of underlying labral pathology. (B) Axial T1-weight fat-suppressed image from an MR arthrogram demonstrates contrast filling the paralabral cyst (arrow).

Although it is not typically used to evaluate hip fractures in patients with normal bone mineralization, Potter et al.[62] reported the ability of MRI to demonstrate occult injuries of the femoral head not seen on CT and injury of the sciatic nerve in patients with acetabular fractures. MRI has had an increasing role in the evaluation of hip trauma in the elderly. Nondisplaced femoral neck or intertrochanteric fractures in elderly patients can be radiographically occult or difficult to diagnose. MRI has proven to be the imaging modality of choice to exclude an occult hip fracture (Figure 4.15) in this patient population.[32–34,63] Radionuclide bone scanning can be normal in the first 48 hours after a fracture in the elderly and is less sensitive than MRI in detecting occult hip fractures.[33] In addition to identifying occult femoral fractures, fractures of the pelvis and soft tissue injuries of the hip can be detected with MRI[23,64] (Figures 4.16, 4.17).

Most protocols used in the evaluation of a potential hip fracture include coronal T1-weighted images and short T1-weighted inversion recovery (STIR) or T2-weighted fat-suppressed images. T1-weighted images demonstrate decreased signal either diffusely or oriented in a linear fashion at the site of a fracture (see Figure 4.15). STIR and T2-weighted images demonstrate increased signal at the fracture site corresponding to bone marrow edema or hemorrhage. A linear focus of decreased signal corresponding to a fracture line may be seen coursing through the area of marrow edema on these latter two sequences. It is now well recognized that a common fracture pattern in the elderly hip is an incomplete intertrochanteric fracture

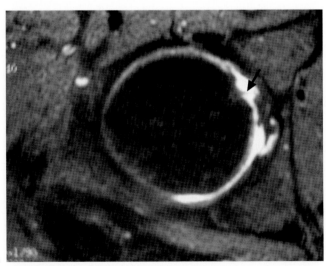

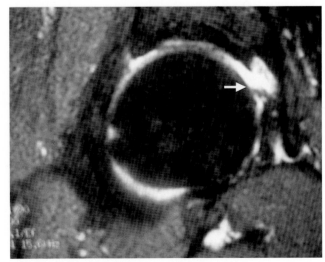

FIGURE 4.14. Partial tear of the ligamentum teres on MR arthrogram. (A) Axial T1-weighted fat-suppressed image reveals irregularity of the anterior fibers of the foveal attachment of the ligamentum teres (arrow). (B) Coronal T1-weighted fat-suppressed image shows a partial tear of the ligamentum teres at the foveal attachment (arrow).

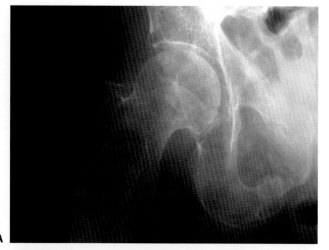

A

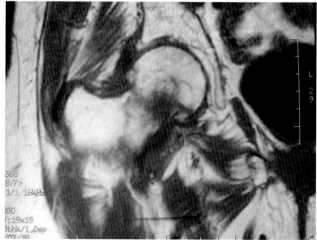

B

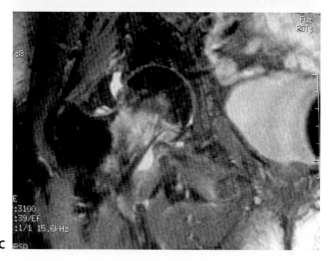

C

FIGURE 4.15. Radiographically occult femoral neck fracture detected by MR. (A) AP radiography of the right hip reveals generalized demineralization and old healed pubic rami fractures but no evidence for a femoral neck fracture. (B) Coronal T1-weighted image demonstrates a broad band of decreased signal traversing the femoral neck consistent with a subcapital femoral neck fracture. (C) Coronal proton density fat-suppressed image reveals a large zone of increased signal throughout the femoral neck consistent with marrow edema and an acute fracture.

that begins in the greater trochanter and extends in a longitudinal fashion into the medullary canal without crossing to the opposite cortex.[63] The results of MRI in such cases can have therapeutic implications by demonstrating the extent to which the fracture crosses the medullary canal.[63]

In addition to osseous injuries of the hip, MRI successfully reveals injuries of the paraarticular soft

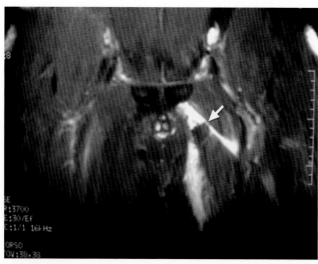

A

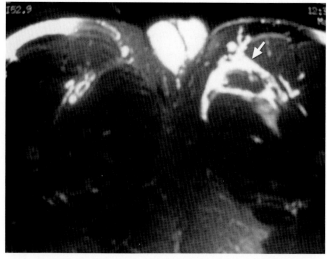

B

FIGURE 4.16. Type III (complete avulsion) injury of the left adductor longus muscle. (A) Coronal proton density fat-suppressed image of both hips shows complete detachment of the proximal adductor longus tendon with approximately 2.5-cm retraction of the tendon (arrow). (B) Axial T2-weighted fat-suppressed image reveals abnormal high signal (indicative of edema or hemorrhage) in and around the left adductor longus muscle belly (arrow).

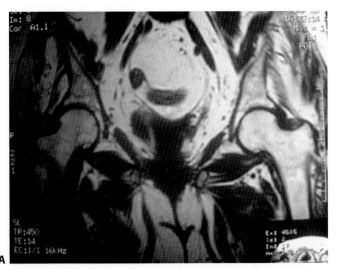

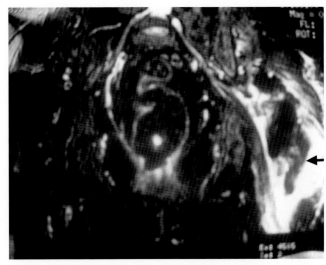

FIGURE 4.17. Soft tissue injury in an elderly patient suspected of having a femoral neck fracture. (A) Coronal T1-weighted image of both hips reveals no femoral neck fracture. (B) Coronal T2- weighted fat-suppressed image demonstrates marked soft tissue edema or hemorrhage (arrow) and rupture of the left gluteus maximus muscle

tissues.[23,24,64] MRI offers an excellent means of identifying, localizing, and determining the severity of muscle and tendon injuries about the hip. Injuries of the myotendinous unit typically occur at the myotendinous junction. On MRI, muscular injuries typically demonstrate increased signal within muscle fibers at the myotendinous junction on T2-weighted or STIR images, indicating intrasubstance hemorrhage or edema. Abnormally increased signal in the tendon on T2-weighted images, myofascial separation, muscle fiber retraction, or wavy-appearing tendon fibers are indicative of a more severe injury. A complete tear involves avulsion of the origin or insertion of the tendon (see Figure 4.16) or complete disruption of muscle fibers.

Stress Fractures

Stress fractures of the femoral neck and pelvis are a common cause of unexplained hip pain and are important to diagnose due to the risk for developing a complete fracture and potentially necessitating surgical intervention. Plain radiographs are typically normal in the early stage of femoral neck stress fractures. The earliest plain radiographic change in a femoral neck stress fracture is an indistinct linear area of sclerosis oriented perpendicular to the major trabeculae or new bone formation along the medial femoral neck. Both nuclear scintigraphy and MRI are more sensitive than plain radiographs in detecting early stress fractures. Bone scanning typically reveals increased activity at the site of the fracture because of increased bone turnover and increased flow. MRI, however, is preferable to nuclear scintigraphy as it typically yields a more specific diagnosis and better spatial resolution and allows simultaneous evaluation of the extraarticular soft tissues.[30] Femoral neck stress fracture appears as a focal poorly defined area of abnormal signal along the medial femoral neck that is dark on T1-

weighted images and bright on T2-weighted or STIR sequences (Figure 4.18). In a study of patients with femoral neck stress fractures, resolution of marrow edema seen on MRI occurred by 6 months in 90% of patients.[31]

Transient Osteoporosis and Transient Bone Marrow Edema

Although originally described in women in their third trimester of pregnancy,[65] transient osteoporosis of the hip is now a well-recognized cause of hip pain that is most commonly seen in middle-aged men. The clinical diagnosis of transient osteoporosis and distinction of this disorder from other causes of bone marrow edema seen on MRI remains a challenge.[29,50,66,67] The plain radiographic hallmark of transient osteoporosis is the presence of osteopenia involving the femoral head and neck. The development of this radiographic finding typically occurs 4 to 8 weeks after the onset of symptoms.[51] Bone scanning is more sensitive than plain radiography and typically demonstrates increased activity in the femoral head and neck extending to the intertrochanteric region. MRI in transient osteoporosis demonstrates a diffuse marrow edema pattern in the femoral head and neck that is dark on T1-weighted images and bright on T2-weighted or STIR images (Figure 4.19). Similar signal changes may be present in the acetabulum, and a joint effusion is usually present.[51]

Another entity described in the radiology literature that parallels the MRI findings of transient osteoporosis is the bone marrow edema syndrome.[51] Although clinically similar to transient osteoporosis, authors distinguish this entity from transient osteoporosis by the lack of osteopenia on plain radiographs.[51] There is probably no reason to distinguish

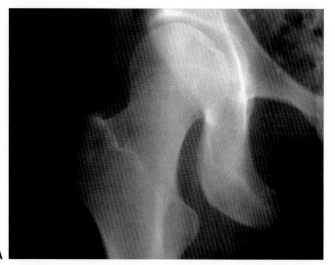
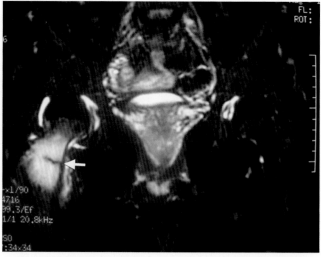

A   B

FIGURE 4.18. Femoral neck stress fracture. (A) Plain radiograph is normal. (B) Coronal T2-weighted fat-suppressed image reveals a linear focus of decreased signal in the medial femoral neck (arrow) surrounded by bright marrow edema indicative of a stress fracture.

these two entities based on imaging as there is no change in outcome or treatment. As alluded to earlier, there can be difficulty in distinguishing transient osteoporosis of the hip from a marrow edema pattern of osteonecrosis seen on MRI.[50] In an effort to identify subtle osteonecrotic foci of the femoral head in cases of diffuse marrow edema, Vande Berg et al.[29] recommend the use of high-resolution T2-weighted images and sagittal imaging. More recently, Iida et al.[46] suggest STIR images may be more helpful than T2-weighted images in identifying subchondral osteonecrotic foci in cases of diffuse marrow edema. Distinction of these two entities may have to rely on clinical follow-up and repeat imaging with MRI.

Snapping Iliopsoas Tendon Syndrome

The snapping iliopsoas tendon syndrome is a reported cause of hip pain associated with a snapping or popping sensation with hip movement.[42,43,68] It is postulated that the iliopsoas tendon jerks over the iliopectineal eminence, anterior joint capsule, or lesser trochanteric bony prominence.[42] At our institution, ultrasound evaluation of the hip (Figure 4.20) has replaced iliopsoas bursography as the initial method of evaluation for iliopsoas snapping syndrome. Ultrasound has appealing advantages of being noninvasive, lacks exposure to ionizing radiation, and allows concomitant assessment of the contralateral hip.[43] The

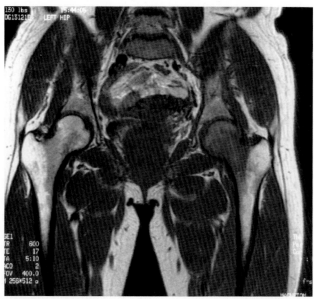
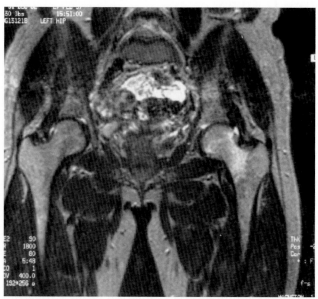

A   B

FIGURE 4.19. Transient osteoporosis of the hip. (A) Coronal T1-weighted image reveals decreased signal in the left femoral head, neck, and extending into the lesser trochanter. (B). Coronal T2-weighted image demonstrates increased signal (marrow edema) in the same distribution. (Courtesy of E. Paul Nance, MD.)

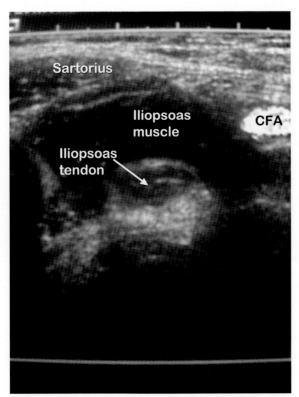

FIGURE 4.20. Normal hip anatomy on ultrasound. Transverse image at the level of the femoral head using a linear array 8-MHz transducer demonstrates the normal appearance of the iliopsoas tendon, right common femoral artery (CFA), iliopsoas muscle, and sartorius muscle.

examination is performed using a high-frequency linear or curved array transducer. The tendon is best evaluated in the transverse plane with the transducer immediately anterior to the hip at the level of the femoral head and anterior acetabular rim. Scanning is performed as the patient reproduces the popping sensation typically with extension of the leg from the

flexed, externally rotated, and abducted position. A cine clip of the tendon motion can be stored and potentially downloaded to CD for future review by the referring physician.

Bursitis

Inflammation of bursa around the hip can be an important extraarticular source of hip pain. MRI and CT have the ability to demonstrate abnormal accumulation of bursal fluid around the hip, but MRI is better suited to demonstrate these collections due to better soft tissue contrast.[25,26,69] An abnormal amount of fluid in the iliopsoas bursa or greater trochanteric bursa may imply bursitis, although a small amount of fluid in bursa can be seen in asymptomatic patients.[69] Fluid accumulating in a bursa is dark on T1-weighted images and bright on T2-weighted images. In the iliopsoas bursa, this fluid collection courses in a longitudinal fashion posterior to the iliopsoas muscle (Figure 4.21).[25,26,69]

Septic Arthritis

Acute septic arthritis is an uncommon cause of hip pain in the adult, but one that needs to be diagnosed expediently to avoid the consequences of delayed therapy. Plain radiographs are typically normal in early septic arthritis or at best may show widening of the joint space. Radionuclide bone scanning may demonstrate increased activity in the hip but is nonspecific. Much of the experience with MRI and septic arthritis of the hip has been in children focused on efforts to distinguish transient synovitis from septic arthritis.[70] In septic arthritis MRI may demonstrate a pathologic effusion and may show edema in the paraarticular soft tissues (Figure 4.22). MRI cannot distinguish a sterile

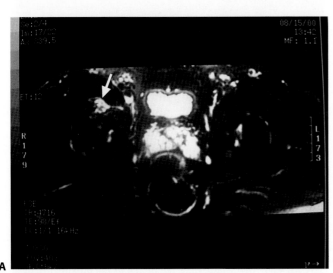

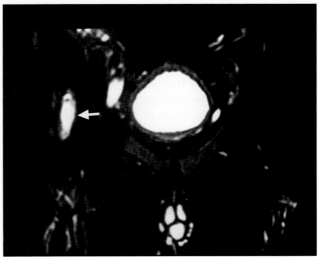

FIGURE 4.21. Iliopsoas bursitis. (A) Axial T2-weighted fat-suppressed image reveals an increased amount of fluid in the iliopsoas bursa (arrow) along the posterior margin of the iliopsoas tendon and muscle. (B) Coronal T2-weighted fat-suppressed image demonstrates the longitudinal orientation of the distended iliopsoas bursa (arrow).

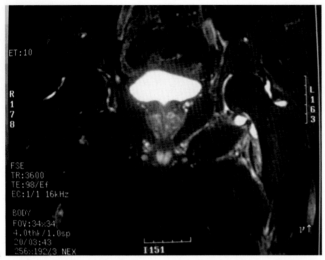

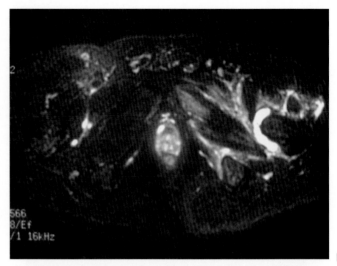

A

B

FIGURE 4.22. Septic arthritis. (A) Coronal T2-weighted fat-suppressed image demonstrates a large joint effusion and increased signal or edema in the paraarticular soft tissues. (B) Axial T2-weighted fat-suppressed image shows a large effusion and marked edema in the paraarticular muscles (adductor muscle group, iliopsoas muscle, and rectus femoris muscle).

or septic effusion. If there is high clinical suspicion for septic arthritis of the hip, or if MRI demonstrates a joint effusion associated with edema in the paraarticular soft tissues in the absence of trauma or known inflammatory arthritis, aspiration is warranted. Abnormal edema or enhancement of osseous structures in the setting of septic arthritis raises the possibility of concurrent osteomyelitis, but is not indicative of such as this can also reflect a reactive process.[70] Bone biopsy in such cases may be necessary to exclude osteomyelitis.

Tumors

Benign and malignant tumors of the proximal femur, acetabulum sacrum, or innominate bone can present as hip pain. In adults, metastatic disease is the most common tumor associated with the pelvis and hip (Figure 4.23). In younger adults and adolescents, osteoid osteomas of the femoral neck can manifest clinically as hip pain (Figure 4.24) and can present challenging management issues, particularly if located along the medial femoral neck. Recently, percutaneous radiofrequency treatment[71] has been advocated for osteoid osteomas and offers a less invasive alternative to surgical excision of the lesion.

Proliferative Synovitis

Synovial osteochondromatosis and pigmented villonodular synovitis are two proliferative forms of synovitis occasionally encountered in the hip. Synovial osteochondromatosis is an intraarticular condition (typically monarticular) that can be seen from childhood on and is characterized by the development of soft tissue nodules from synovial metaplasia that often calcify or ossify. These nodules often become free intraarticular loose bodies and can extend into neighboring soft tissues including bursa and tendon sheaths. Plain radiographs demonstrate multiple small similar-sized calcified or ossified intraarticular loose bodies. Extension of the process into neighboring bone can result in erosions or cystic lesions. MR demonstrates multiple intraarticular nodules (Figure 4.25). The signal intensity of the nodules is dependent on their composition.[72] Noncalcified soft tissue nodules typically demonstrate low signal on T1-weighted images and high signal on T2-weighted images. Calcified nodules typically demonstrate low signal on both T1- and T2-weighted images whereas ossified nodules demonstrate high signal on T1-weighted images.

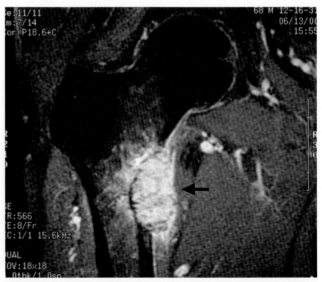

FIGURE 4.23. Metastatic lung carcinoma in the proximal right femur. Coronal T1-weighted fat-suppressed image with contrast reveals a heterogenous mass (arrow) epicentered in the cortex and subcortical bone with elevation of the periosteum.

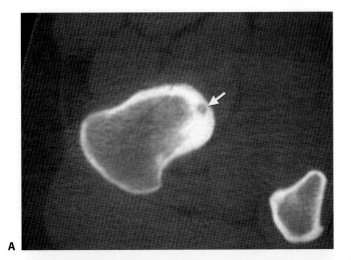

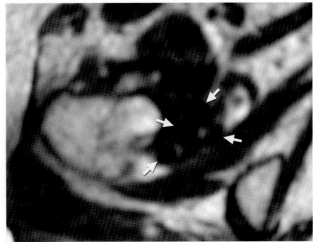

FIGURE 4.25. Synovial osteochondromatosis. Axial T1-weighted image from a low-field-strength scanner demonstrates multiple small low-signal loose bodies (arrows) in the medial joint.

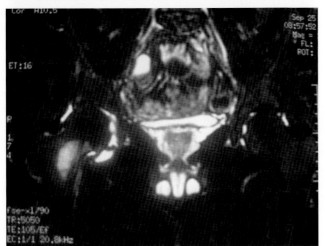

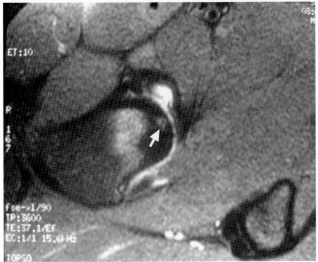

FIGURE 4.24. Intraarticular osteoid osteoma. (A) Axial CT scan demonstrates a small intracortical nidus (arrow) surrounded by increased sclerosis. (B) Coronal T2-weighted fat-suppressed image reveals a semicircular focus of marrow edema in the medial aspect of the femoral neck. (C) Axial proton density fat-suppressed image demonstrates the small nidus (arrow) surrounded by marrow edema in the medial femoral neck.

Pigmented villonodular synovitis primarily occurs in adults and is typically a monoarticular process that is characterized by masslike proliferation of the synovium with associated elements of chronic or acute hemorrhage. Often, the disorder is associated with secondary erosive change in underlying bone or bone cyst formation. In the hip, erosive changes typically occur at the junction of the femoral head and neck (Figure 4.26) or acetabulum.[72] Plain radiographs may demonstrate a joint effusion or paraarticular mass and erosive or cystic changes in the proximal femur or acetabulum. MR typically reveals paraarticular soft tissue masses that are commonly associated with bone erosions (Figure 4.26) and contain hemosiderin (decreased signal on T1- and T2-weighted images).

SUMMARY

Diagnostic imaging plays an important role in the evaluation of adult hip pain. The plain radiograph remains the initial imaging modality in the workup of adult hip pain. The need for secondary imaging of the hip and choice of imaging modality is dependent on the clinical presentation, results of the plain radiograph series, and clinical question to be answered. CT is primarily used in the setting of acute trauma to better demonstrate fracture patterns and to detect intraarticular fragments and associated articular surface fractures. MRI has become the secondary imaging modality of choice in evaluating hip pain for most other clinical presentations and is particularly helpful in detecting marrow-based abnormalities, demonstrating intraarticular and extraarticular pathology, and revealing occult soft tissue and bony injuries in the elderly. MR arthrography is useful in the detection of

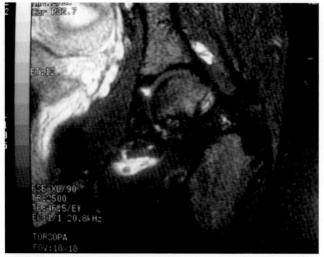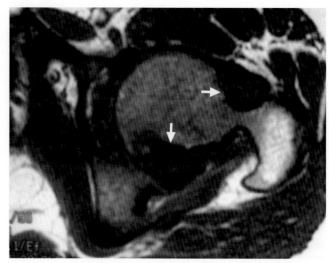

FIGURE 4.26. Pigmented villonodular synovitis. (A) Coronal proton density fat-suppressed image shows nodular thickening of the synovium and a moderate-size effusion. (B) Axial T1-weighted image reveals soft tissue masses eroding into the anterior and posterior aspect of the femoral neck (arrows).

labral injuries and may demonstrate additional intraarticular pathology not seen on conventional MRI including chondral damage, loose bodies, and injuries of the ligamentum teres.

References

1. Conway WF, Totty WG, McEnery KW: CT and MR imaging of the hip. Radiology 1996;198:297–307.
2. Gabriel H, Fitzgerald SW, Myers MT, et al: MR imaging of hip disorders. RadioGraphics 1994;14:763–781.
3. Lang P, Genant HK, Jergesen HE, et al: Imaging of the hip joint. Clin Orthop Relat Res 1992;274:135–153.
4. Czerny C, Hofmann S, Neuhold A, et al: Lesions of the acetabular labrum: Accuracy of MR imaging and MR arthrography in detection and staging. Radiology 1996;200:225–230.
5. Czerny C, Hofmann S, Urban M, et al: MR arthrography of the adult acetabular capsular-labral complex: Correlation with surgery and anatomy. AJR Am J Roentgenol 1999;173:345–349.
6. Grainger AJ, Elliott JM, Campbell RSD, et al: Direct MR arthrography: a review of current use. Clin Radiol 2000;55:170–171.
7. Haims A, Katz LD, Busconi B: MR arthrography of the hip. Radiol Clin North Am 1998;36:691–702.
8. Hodler J, Yu JS, Goodwin D, et al: MR arthrography of the hip: Improved imaging of the acetabular labrum with histologic correlation in cadavers. AJR Am J Roentgenol 1995;165:887–891.
9. Leunig M, Werlen S, Ungersbrock A, et al: Evaluation of the acetabular labrum by MR arthrography. J Bone Joint Surg [Br] 1997;79:230–234.
10. Palmer WE: MR arthrography of the hip. Semin Musculoskel Radiol 1998;12:349–361.
11. Palmer WE: MR arthrography: is it worthwhile? Top Magn Reson Imaging 1996;8:24–43.
12. Petersilge CA, Haque MA, Petersilge WJ, et al: Acetabular labral tears: evaluation with MR arthrography. Radiology 1996;200:231–235.
13. Petersilge CA: Current concepts of MR arthrography of the hip. Semin Ultrasound CT MRI 1997;18:291–301.
14. Plotz GMJ, Brossman J, Schunke M, et al: Magnetic resonance arthrography of the acetabular labrum. J Bone Joint Surg [Br] 2000;82:426–432.
15. Sadro C: Current concepts in magnetic resonance imaging of the adult hip and pelvis. Semin Roentgenol 2000;35:231–248.
16. Petersilge CA: MR arthrography for evaluation of the acetabular labrum.Skeletal Radiol 2001;30:423–430.
17. Erb RE: Current concepts in imaging the adult hip. Clin Sports Med 2001;20:661–696.
18. Sartoris DJ, Resnick D: Plain film radiography: routine and specialized techniques and projections. In: Resnick D, Niwayama G (eds). Diagnosis of Bone and Joint Disorders, 2nd ed, vol 1. Philadelphia: Saunders, 1988:38.
19. Rogers LF: The hip and femoral shaft. In: Rogers LF (ed). Radiology of Skeletal Trauma, 2nd ed, vol 2. New York: Churchill Livingstone, 1992:1113.
20. Judet R, Judet J, Letournel E: Fractures of the acetabulum: classification and surgical approaches to open reduction. J Bone Joint Surg 1964;46A:1615–1646.
21. Nance EP: Investigation of the symptomatic hip: imaging techniques. In: Byrd JWT ed). Operative Hip Arthroscopy. New York: Thieme, 1998:45.
22. Calkins MS, Zych G, Latta L, et al: Computed tomography evaluation of stability in posterior fracture dislocation of the hip. Clin Orthop Related Res 1988;227:152–163.
23. Chung CB, Robertson JE, Cho GJ, et al: Gluteus medius tendon tears and avulsive injuries in elderly women: imaging findings in six patients. AJR Am J Roentgenol 1999;173:351–353.
24. Kneeland JB. MR imaging of sports injuries of the hip. MRI Clin North Am 1999;7:105–115.
25. Kozlov DB, Sonin AH: Iliopsoas bursitis: diagnosis by MRI. J Comput Assist Tomogr 1998;22:625–628.
26. Pritchard RS, Shah HR, Nelson CL, et al: MR and CT appearance of iliopsoas bursal distention secondary to diseased hips. J Comput Assist Tomogr 1990;14:797–800.
27. Moss SG, Schweitzer ME, Jacobson, et al: Hip joint fluid: detection and distribution at MR imaging and US with cadaveric correlation. Radiology 1998;208:43–48.
28. Mitchell DG, Rao VM, Dalinka MK, et al: Femoral head avascular necrosis: correlation of MR imaging, radiographic staging, radionuclide imaging, and clinical findings. Radiology 1987;162:709–715.
29. Vande Berg BE, Malghem JJ, Labaisse MA, et al: MR imaging of avascular necrosis and transient marrow edema of the femoral head. RadioGraphics 1993;13:501–520.
30. Shin AY, Morin WD, Gorman JD, et al: The superiority of mag-

netic resonance imaging in differentiating the cause of hip pain in endurance athletes. Am J Sports Med 1996;24:168–176.

31. Slocum KA, Gorman JD, Puckett ML, et al: Resolution of abnormal MR signal intensity in patients with stress fractures of the femoral neck. AJR Am J Roentgenol 1997; 168:1295–1299.

32. Bogost GA, Lizerbram EK, Crues JV III: MR imaging in evaluation of suspected hip fracture: frequency of unsuspected bone and soft-tissue injury. Radiology 1995;197:263–267.

33. Evans PD, Wilson C, Lyons K: Comparison of MRI with bone scanning for suspected hip fracture in elderly patients. J Bone Joint Surg [Br] 1994;76:158–159.

34. May DA, Purins JL, Smith DK: MR imaging of occult traumatic fractures and muscular injuries of the hip and pelvis in elderly patients. AJR Am J Roentgenol 1996;166:1075–1078.

35. Pandey R, McNally E, Ali A, et al: The role of MRI in the diagnosis of occult hip fractures. Injury 1998;29:61–63.

36. Beltran J, Caudill JL, Herman LA, et al: Rheumatoid arthritis: MR imaging manifestations. Radiology 1987;165:153–157.

37. Hodler J, Trudell D, Pathria MN, et al: Width of the articular cartilage of the hip: quantification by using fat-suppression spin-echo MR imaging in cadavers. AJR Am J Roentgenol 1992;159:351–355.

38. Plotz GM, Bressman J, von Knoch M, et al. Magnetic resonance arthrography of the acetabular labrum:value of radial reconstructions. Arch Orthop Trauma Surg 2001;121:450–457.

39. Mettler FA, Guiberteau MJ: Skeletal system. In: Mettler FA, Guiberteau MJ (eds). Essentials of Nuclear Medicine Imaging, 3rd ed. Philadelphia: Saunders, 1991;209–236.

40. Ghelman B, Freiberger RH: The adult hip. In: Freiberger RH, Kaye JJ (eds). Arthrography. New York: Appleton-Century-Crofts, 1979:189.

41. Newberg AH: Anesthetic and corticosteroid joint injections: a primer. Semin Musculoskel Radiol 1998:2:415–420.

42. Harper MC, Schaberg JE, Allen WC: Primary iliopsoas bursography in the diagnosis of disorders of the hip. Clin Orthop Relat Res 1987;221:238–241.

43. Cardinal E, Buckwalter KA, Capello WN, et al: US of the snapping iliopsoas tendon. Radiology 1996;198:521–522.

44. Jacobson T, Allen WC: Surgical correction of the snapping iliopsoas tendon. Am J Sports Med 1990;18:470–474.

45. Beltran J, Knight CT, Zueler WA, et al: Core decompression for avascular necrosis of the femoral head: correlation between long-term results and preoperative MR staging. Radiology 1990;175:533–536.

46. Iida S, Harada Y, Shimizu K, et al: Correlation between bone marrow edema and collapse of the femoral head in steroid-induced osteonecrosis. AJR Am J Roentgenol 2000;174:735–743.

47. Shimizu K, Moriya H, Akita T, et al: Prediction of collapse with magnetic resonance imaging of avascular necrosis of the femoral head. J Bone Joint Surg 1994;76A:215–223.

48. Mont MA, Hungerford DS: Non-traumatic avascular necrosis of the femoral head. J Bone Joint Surg 1996;77A:459–474.

49. Steinberg ME, Brighton CT, Hayken GD, et al: Early results in the treatment of avascular necrosis of the femoral head with electrical stimulation. Orthop Clin N Am 1984;15:163-175.

50. Turner DA, Templeton AC, Selzer PM, et al: Femoral capital osteonecrosis: MR finding of diffuse marrow abnormalities without focal lesion. Radiology 1989;171:135–140.

51. Hayes CW, Conway WF, Daniel WW: MR imaging of bone marrow edema pattern: transient osteoporosis, transient bone marrow edema syndrome, or osteonecrosis. RadioGraphics 1993;13:1001–1011.

52. Resnick D. Degenerative disease of extraspinal locations. In: Resnick D (ed). Diagnosis of Bone and Joint Disorders, 4th ed, vol 2. Philadelphia: Saunders, 2002:1331.

53. Nakanishi K, Tanaka H, Nishii T, et al: MR evaluation of the articular cartilage of the femoral head during traction. Acta Radiol 1999;40:60–63.

54. Cotten A, Boutry N, Demondion X, et al: Acetabular labrum: MRI in asymptomatic volunteers. J Comput Assist Tomogr 1998;22:1–7.

55. Lecouvet FE, Vande Berg BC, Melghem J, et al: MR imaging of the acetabular labrum: variations in 200 asymptomatic hips. AJR Am J Roentgenol 1996;167:1025–1028.

56. Santori N, Villar RN: Arthroscopic anatomy of the hip. In: Byrd JWT (ed). Operative Hip Arthroscopy. New York: Thieme, 1998:93–104.

57. Byrd JWT: Labral lesions: an elusive source of hip pain: case reports and review of the literature. Arthroscopy 1996;12: 603–612.

58. Ikeda T, Awaya G, Suzuki S, et al: Torn acetabular labrum in young patients. Arthroscopic diagnosis and management. J Bone Joint Surg 1988;70:13–16.

59. Lage LA, Patel JV, Villar RN: The acetabular labral tear: an arthroscopic classification. Arthroscopy 1996;12:269–272.

60. Magee T, Hinson G: Association of paralabral cysts with acetabular disorders. AJR Am J Roentgenol 2000;174: 1381–1384.

61. Gray AJR, Villar RN: The ligamentum teres of the hip: an arthroscopic classification of its pathology. Arthroscopy 1997;13: 575–578.

62. Potter HG, Montgomery KD, Heise CW, et al: MR imaging of acetabular fractures: value in detecting femoral head injury, intraarticular fragments, and sciatic nerve injury. AJR Am J Roentgenol 1993;163:881–886.

63. Schultz E, Miller TT, Boruchov SD, et al: Incomplete intertrochanteric fractures: Imaging features and clinical management. Radiology 1999;211:237–240.

64. Kingzett-Taylor A, Tirman PFJ, Feller J, et al: Tendinosis and tears of gluteus medius and minimus muscles as a cause of hip pain: MR imaging findings. AJR Am J Roentgenol 1999;173: 1123–1126.

65. Curtiss PH, Kincaid WE: Transitory demineralization of the hip in pregnancy. A report of three cases. J Bone Joint Surg 1959;41A:1327–1333.

66. Guerra JJ, Steinberg ME: Distinguishing transient osteoporosis from avascular necrosis of the hip. J Bone Joint Surg [Am] 1995;77:616–624.

67. Potter H, Moran M, Schneider R, et al: Magnetic resonance imaging in diagnosis of transient osteoporosis of the hip. Clin Orthop Relat Res 1992;280:223–229.

68. Harper MC, Schaberg JE, Allen WC: Primary iliopsoas bursography in the diagnosis of disorders of the hip. Clin Orthop Relat Res 1987;221:238–241.

69. Varma DGK, Richli WR, Charnsangavej C, et al: MR appearance of the distended iliopsoas bursa. AJR Am J Roentgenol 1991;156:1025–1028.

70. Lee SK, Suh KJ, Kim YW, et al: Septic arthritis versus transient synovitis at MR imaging: preliminary assessment with signal intensity alterations in bone marrow. Radiology 1999;211:459–465.

71. Torriani M, Rosenthal DI. Percutaneous radiofrequency treatment of osteoid osteoma. Pediatr Radiol 2002;32:615–618.

72. Resnick D. Tumors and tumor-like lesions of soft tissues. In: Resnick D (ed). Diagnosis of Bone and Joint Disorders, 4th ed, vol 4. Philadelphia: Saunders, 2002:4204–4252.

Extraarticular Sources of Hip Pain

Steve A. Mora, Bert R. Mandelbaum,
Levente J. Szalai, Nicholas D. Potter,
Archit Naik, Jeff Ryan, and William C. Meyers

The task of diagnosing and managing extraarticular causes for hip and groin pain represents one of the greatest challenges in sports medicine. The differential diagnosis for hip and groin pain is broad and includes intraarticular hip disorders, acute and chronic muscular tears, pubic symphysis disorders, snapping hip syndrome, peripheral nerve entrapment, and abdominal wall abnormalities. Nonmusculoskeletal etiologies should also be considered: these include urologic disease, gynecologic disease, gastrointestinal problems, infections, and tumors. Also complicating the clinical picture is the nature of groin symptoms, which may be vague, confusing, and generalized around the hip joint, thigh, and abdomen regions. The ambiguous constellation of symptoms can be partly explained by a complex pain referral pattern around the groin and the hip region. These problems are unfortunately frequently misdiagnosed and appropriate treatment often delayed. It is evident that the evaluation of these problems, especially if chronic in nature, may be extremely demanding. Therefore, to avoid misguided treatment strategies and to ultimately ensure treatment success, a diagnostic approach that is methodical and organized must be followed.

This chapter takes a comprehensive look at four infrequently encountered extraarticular disorders of the hip and groin area that can clinically mimic intraarticular hip pathology: osteitis pubis, piriformis muscle syndrome, obturator nerve entrapment, and athletic pubalgia.

We shall discuss the subject of extraarticular sources of hip pain in two sections.

I. Steve A. Mora, Bert R. Mandelbaum: Osteitis Pubis, Piriformis Syndrome, Obturator Nerve Entrapment

II. William C. Meyers, Levente J. Szalai, Nicholas D. Potter, Archit Naik, Jeff Ryan: Athletic Pubalgia

I. OSTEITIS PUBIS, PIRIFORMIS SYNDROME, OBDURATOR NERVE ENTRAPMENT
STEVE A. MORA AND BERT R. MANDELBAUM

OSTEITIS PUBIS

Description

Osteitis pubis is a painful, inflammatory, noninfectious condition of the bone, periosteum, cartilage, and ligamentous structures around the pubic symphysis.[1–5] It is considered the most common inflammatory condition of the pubic symphysis.[5] It is not a rare condition, as proven by the large number of patient series published since its first description in 1923.[6] The first description within the English literature was by Beer in 1924.[7] Most of the early literature on this subject emerged from the field of urology. The first descriptions of osteitis pubis revealed its close association with urologic, gynecologic, and obstetric procedures and complications related to pelvic surgery.[1,8] It is a diagnosis seen in almost every patient population, permitting most medical specialists some familiarity with the diagnosis; nonetheless, it remains poorly understood. Various clinical forms of osteitis pubis are believed to exist.[2,8,9] No single etiologic factor has been identified as the cause for osteitis pubis. Athletic osteitis pubis is probably associated with overstress or microtrauma of the pubic symphysis and its surrounding structures.[10,11] Pelvic instability and muscular imbalance may also play an important etiologic role.[4,12–14] In the athlete, Spinelli[15] in 1932 was the first to describe athletic osteitis pubis in fencers. Osteitis pubis has also been reported in ice hockey, wrestling, Olympic walking, rugby, tennis, running, football, diving, and basketball. Athletic osteitis pubis may evolve into a chronic, painful, disabling condition causing significant amounts of lost playing time. The symptoms may manifest acutely, such as after a forceful kick or an injurious fall, or may present slowly and insidiously.[16] With adherence to nonoperative therapeutic measures, it is, the majority of times, a self-limiting condition.[1] However, surgical measures are thought to improve the small number of cases that become unresponsive to conservative means.[4,8] Since osteitis pubis was described 79 years ago, confusion exists regarding its precise pathogenesis, and the optimal treatments often elude us.

Etiology

A review of the pertinent anatomy and biomechanics is important in understanding this vague entity called osteitis pubis. Joints are classified into three basic types: synarthrosis, which are fibrous and rigid; diarthrosis, which are synovial and freely movable; and amphiarthroses, which are slightly movable.[3] The pubic symphysis is located between the two pubic bones. Articular hyaline cartilage lines the two joint surfaces, which are separated by a thick intrapubic fibrocartilaginous disk. The disk has a transverse anterior width of 5 to 6 mm, anteroposterior width of 10 to 15 mm, and a central raphe.[17] The joint lacks a well-developed synovial lining, making it less susceptible to pathologic inflammatory changes such as those seen with ankylosing spondylitis and Reiter's syndrome.[3] The pelvic architecture is essentially a continuous bony ring with three interspersed semirigid joints, two sacroiliac joints and one pubic symphysis, designed to dissipate undue forces. The thick inferior arcuate pubic ligament rigidly bridges both the inferior pubic rami and provides the symphysis pubis joint with the majority of its stability. Together with the anterior pubic ligament, posterior pubic ligament, and the suprapubic ligament, motion within the pubic symphysis is limited to less than 2 mm in healthy subjects.[13,18] The muscles attaching at or near the pubic symphysis include the pyramidalis and rectus abdominis superiorly, the adductor and gracilis anteroinferiorly, and the obturator and levator ani posteriorly. Sensory nerve innervation comes via the branches from the pudendal and genitofemoral nerves.

Published case reports and retrospective record reviews have been used to postulate an infectious, inflammatory, or traumatic cause of this condition.[3–5,9,10,14,19–21] One may think in terms of four primary clinical types: (a) noninfectious osteitis pubis associated with urologic procedures, gynecologic procedures, and pregnancy; (b) infectious osteitis pubis associated with local or distant infection; (c) sports-related or athletic osteitis pubis; and (d) degenerative/rheumatologic osteitis pubis. Because of the various clinical forms, the clinical history, incidence, sexual predisposition, and the age of onset in the literature varies considerably.

Athletic osteitis pubis is associated with activities requiring repetitive kicking or hip abduction/adduction motions, such as soccer, hockey, and Australian rules football.[9,22] The true pathogenesis of this disorder remains obscure. A number of theories have been proposed, including trauma to the pubis symphysis periosteum, abnormal pelvic biomechanics,[4,23] low-grade indolent infections,[24] inflammatory causes,[1] reflex sympathetic dystrophy, avascular necrosis of the interpubic disk of fibrocartilage,[25] and venous thrombosis of the pubic veins.[5,26] The two strongest arguments against an infectious etiology are the fact that osteitis pubis is a self-limiting condition and surgical specimens have failed to grow organisms.[2,8,23] Additionally, histologic analysis of material obtained from surgical specimens has been consistent with nonspecific chronic inflammatory tissue.[23]

In athletes, the etiology is thought to be associated with muscle imbalance between the abdominal and adductor muscles, pelvis instability, and chronic overuse stress injury.[4,5,10,14,20] Coventry et al.[8] emphasized that external trauma did not play a significant role in their review of 45 cases of osteitis pubis. Muscle imbalance between the abdominal wall musculature and hip adductor muscles has been suggested as a major etiologic factor in athletes.[14,20] The muscles implicated include the rectus abdominis, gracilis, and adductors longus.[5,10] An imbalance between abdominal and adductor muscle groups disrupts the balance of forces around the symphysis pubis, which acts as the central pivot point, leading to chronic microtrauma.[20] As a consequence of the repetitive trauma, blood supply to the injured muscle attachments may be impaired, intensifying the injury and exceeding the capacity of tissue to heal and remodel.[20,27]

Abnormal biomechanics of the pubic symphysis and the sacroiliac joints is the second possible etiologic factor in athletes.[4,22,23] Abnormal vertical motion of the pubic symphysis has been documented in patients with osteitis pubis. In one radiographic review, all patients with osteitis pubis had greater than 2 mm of mobility at the pubic symphysis.[18] Williams et al.[23] postulated that repeated vertical shear stresses and microtrauma resulted in a clinical syndrome consisting of osteitis pubis and coexisting vertical pubic instability greater than 2 mm in a group of competitive rugby football players. All their subjects with recalcitrant osteitis pubis and pelvis instability returned to sports after undergoing arthrodesis of the pubic symphysis joint.

Abnormal motion at the pubic symphysis may be brought about by abnormalities in the sacroiliac or the hip joints. Large increases in rotational and translational motion within the pubic symphysis have been experimentally created in a cadaveric study by fusing the sacroiliac joints.[28] Major and Helms[10] demonstrated clinically and radiographically the coexistence of sacroiliac joint abnormalities in a subgroup of athletes with osteitis pubis. Harris and Murray[4] also found chronic stress lesions in the sacroiliac joint in more than 50% of their subjects. The role of such abnormalities is not clearly understood. Whether the sacroiliac joint plays an etiologic role or is a manifestation of osteitis pubis remains to be determined.

Last, radiographic studies of athletes with osteitis pubis have demonstrated that the underlying pathophysiology may be a chronic stress injury to the pubic bone.[10,11] A prospective, blinded magnetic resonance imaging (MRI) study by Verrall et al.[11] found a high incidence (77%) of increased signal intensity in symptomatic Australian rules football players. The increased signal intensity in the pubic symphysis was characteristic for bone marrow edema caused by a stress injury to the bone. They went on to list other etiologies capable of producing such bone marrow changes including osteomyelitis, infiltrating neoplasm, and direct trauma. These authors proposed that a tension stress injury from chronic stresses across the pubic symphysis was the most likely explanation for their observations. The idea that osteitis pubis is caused by a stress injury, akin to a stress fracture, is a reasonable one as the pubic symphysis is exposed to large amounts of shear stresses during sports activities. This possibility requires further research.

Clinical Presentation

Osteitis pubis is not only a diagnostic problem but also a therapeutic dilemma often requiring a multidisciplinary approach. Making the diagnosis of osteitis pubis is not particularly difficult when the radiographs corroborate the diagnosis. However, the physician is faced with a difficult diagnostic challenge when an athlete presents with groin pain and nondiagnostic radiographs, especially if the symptoms are chronic. In this particular clinical setting, a referral to a general surgeon to rule out an inguinal hernia, spermatic cord problems, abdominal wall defects, and other urologic conditions is warranted. And, in the female athlete, a gynecologist referral to evaluate for conditions such as ovarian cysts, endometriosis, and pelvic inflammatory disease is appropriate.

Fricker et al.[9] reviewed the records of 59 patients with osteitis pubis who presented in their sports clinic. Women averaged 35.5 years of age and men 30.3 years. The sports most frequently involved in this large series were running, soccer, ice hockey, and tennis. The most frequent symptom was pubic and adductor pain. Men also presented with lower abdominal, hip, perineal, or scrotal pain. The pain varies in intensity and duration. The onset may be either acute or insidious. Frequently, the injured athlete is unable to recall an inciting traumatic event. Osteitis pubis can prove difficult to diagnose because the pain symptoms may be ambiguous and generalized around the hip, thigh, and abdomen. This ambiguous constellation of symptoms can probably be explained by the richly innervated pubic symphysis and its complex pain referral patterns.[17]

The athlete's symptom is aggravated by activities that require sudden hip flexion or abduction/adduction such as running, kicking, single-leg pivoting, and jumping. Symptoms may be aggravated with abdominal stress including coughing, sneezing, and defecating.[5] Physical examination findings are localized to the pubic symphysis and surrounding area. Invariably, there is exquisite tenderness to deep palpation of the pubic symphysis and over the adductor muscle origins.[4,8,9] Patients may have decreased hip rotation unilaterally or bilaterally, which may be a result of restricted abduction of the thighs and adductor spasms.[9,17] In severe cases patients may exhibit a *waddling gait* due to pain and tightness of the adductor muscles.[2] A provocative test is reproducing symptoms with resistive adduction with the hips and knees flexed 90 degrees.[14] Coventry and William[2] described two provocative maneuvers: (a) the rocking cross-leg test in which the examiner bears down on the crossed knee while holding down the opposite iliac crest; and (b) the lateral pelvis compression test, done with the patient on his or her side and the examiner pressing the presenting wing.

Laboratory analysis adds little diagnostic value except for ruling out the presence of other pathologic processes such as infection and malignancies. Radiographic changes lag behind clinical symptoms by 2 or 3 weeks, so that early on in the disease process, plain radiographs will be of no diagnostic value.[1,29] The reported radiographic incidence in soccer players is 14% to 28%.[30] Radiographs do not correlate with the clinical severity of the disease.[4,9,17,31] Harris and Murray[4] have defined radiographic changes associated with osteitis pubis in athletes. These findings include marginal irregularity, symmetric bone resorption, widening of the symphysis, reactive sclerosis along the rami, and sacroiliac joint irregularities[2] (Figure 5.1). Cortical avulsions at the site of the adductor tendon insertion may also be seen.[10,16] In patients with pelvis instability, clicking of the symphysis[4] and radiographic abnormalities of the sacroiliac joints may also be present.[9,10] To assess for pubic symphysis instability, flamingo views (single-leg standing anteroposterior radiographs taken while standing on each lower extremity) can be used. Abnormal flamingo views indicating instability demonstrate pubic vertical motion greater than 2 mm.[13,18]

The diagnosis of osteitis pubis can be assisted with further studies such as a technetium-99m isotope bone scan.[29] Positive findings for osteitis pubis show increased uptake at the pubic symphysis on the delayed views, indicating increased bone turnover. MR plays an important role in the evaluation of groin pain in the athlete. MRI is useful for evaluating the surrounding soft tissue structures and bone marrow edema and is especially good for ruling out occult her-

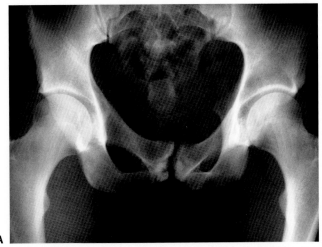
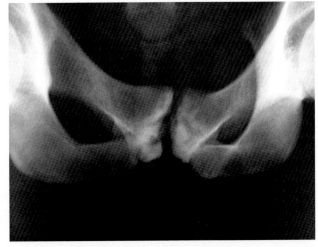

A   B

FIGURE 5.1. Anteroposterior pelvic radiograph and magnified view of a professional soccer player with osteitis pubis. The pubic symphysis shows marginal irregularity, symmetric bone resorption, widening of the symphysis, reactive sclerosis along the rami, and a cortical avulsion.

nias or abdominal muscle avulsion injuries. The role of the CT scan as a diagnostic tool is limited. Rather, the CT scan is useful for identifying other conditions presenting with groin pain such as pelvic and hip stress fractures and bony avulsion fractures. CT-guided aspirations also play an important role for the diagnosis of pubis osteomyelitis.

Differential Diagnosis

It is important to remember that groin pain may be caused by a variety of orthopedic and nonorthopedic problems. It is, therefore, important to be mindful of the comprehensive differential diagnosis and not deemphasize medical disorders. The evaluation begins with a thorough past medical history and a review of systems. In cases that are not straightforward, a history of infections, rheumatologic problems, and gynecologic and urologic problems should be sought. It is also important to be aware of spine conditions such as spinal stenosis, discogenic pain, and herniated nucleus pulposus presenting with referred pain to the groin.

The differential diagnosis of etiologies around the groin area include stress fractures, acute or chronic strain of muscles around the groin area, sports hernia, athletic pubalgia, intraarticular problems, nerve entrapment syndromes, and snapping hip. The differential diagnosis of a stress fracture should be on the top of the list when evaluating an athlete with pain symptoms. If the possibility of a pelvis or femoral neck, nondisplaced fracture is suspected, a bone scan, CT scan, or a MRI is invaluable for confirming the diagnosis.

The most common cause of groin pain in kicking athletes is chronic inflammation of partial tears of the adductor longus muscle.[22,32] Adductor longus muscle and gracilis muscle injuries present with pain at the pubic symphysis sometimes indistinct from osteitis pubis. Small cortical avulsions of calcifications may give the appearance of pubis symphysis involvement.

Provocative maneuvers of the adductors, radiographs, and MRI help define these injuries. Athletic pubalgia (weakening or tearing of the abdominal wall without a hernia) and a true inguinal hernia usually present with chronic groin pain above the symphysis pubis and over the rectus abdominis and spermatic cord (Table 5.1). Characteristically, patients have exertional pain and point tenderness over the conjoined tendon. The pain is aggravated by coughing and by attempting a push-up maneuver. Herniography and MRI have been reported to be useful for diagnosing nonpalpable hernias and insufficiencies of the pelvic floor.[19,33,34] Groin pain of neural origin may be caused by entrapment of genital nerve branches by the inguinal ligament.[35] The ilioinguinal nerve, iliohypogastric nerve, lateral femoral cutaneous nerve, genitofemoral nerve and, most recently, the obturator nerve may be implicated.[36,37] Labral tears of the hip joint are intraarticular lesions that may cause sharp catching hip pain worsened with flexion and rotation movements of the hip. An intraarticular injection of local anesthetic eliminates the pain, thereby narrowing the differential diagnosis to intraarticular causes. Other painful intraarticular lesions include chondral delaminations and osteochondral loose bodies. Snapping hip syndrome is a condition that causes palpable or audible clicking or snapping as the symptomatic hip flexes and extends. One known cause of snapping hip syndrome is an impingement of the iliopsoas when its tendon catches on the pelvic brim or iliopectineal eminence.

If pubic symphysis destruction is present on plain radiography, the most important diagnosis to rule out is osteomyelitis (Table 5.2). A delay in diagnosis and treatment may lead to serious infection and or sepsis complications.[21,38] The radiographic appearance of infection is often indistinct from that of osteitis pubis. Suppurative osteomyelitis may be more unilateral and may be manifested by sequestra and other evidence of

TABLE 5.1. Salient Clinical Features Between Three Common Conditions Occurring in Kicking Athletes.

	Abdominal wall defect (pubalgia)	Athletic pubalgia	Primary osteitis pubis
Symptoms	Exertional symptoms (coughing, sneezing, defecating, sit-ups) kicking	Insidious onset; continuous pain, aggravated or ameliorated by exertion	Usually sudden onset and time-limited after kicking, cutting, pivoting maneuvers
Pathoanatomic zone	II	III	IV
Physical examination	Pain with resisted sit-ups or thigh adduction; no bulge + tenderness	Point tenderness over the pubic symphysis	Tenderness at musculotendinous unit; pain exacerbated with resisted adduction
Plain radiographs	Negative or may show osteitis pubis	Marginal irregularity, sclerosis, widening of pubic symphysis	Pubic symphysis calcifications or small avulsion fragments off adductor insertion
MRI	May show tears of abdominal wall structures	Bone marrow edema, cystic changes	Edema of adductor tendon and its insertion or negative MRI
Special tests	MRI to rule out other causes	±Bone scan positive	
Conservative treatment	Physical therapy or prolonged deep massage	Rest, physical therapy, corticosteroid injections, graduated activities	Rest, physical therapy, graduated activities
Surgery	Pelvic floor repir with or without adductor release	Pubic symphysis wedge resection, plate arthrodesis, adductor release with pubic bone drilling; pelvic floor procedures and adductor releases	Adductor tenotomy pubic symphysis drilling

bone destruction. Tuberculosis septic arthritis runs a more chronic course and is generally less painful than suppurative osteomyelitis.[2] Typical is associated constitutional symptoms include fever, chills, and malaise. If an infection is suspected, the workup should include a PPD (purified protein derivative) test, laboratory studies (blood cultures, CBC, ESR, CRP), and a CT-guided needle biopsy of the pubic symphysis obtained before beginning empiric antibiotic therapy.[3] Inflammatory diseases such as ankylosing spondylitis and Reiter's syndrome may also manifest, although infrequently, with pubic symphysis destructions. Metabolic diseases capable of producing osseous irregularities and bone resorption of the pubic symphysis include renal osteodystrophy and hyperparathyroidism. Osteoarthritic degeneration of the pubic symphysis associated with normal physiologic aging has been well detailed.[39] Last, benign and malignant skeletal tumors are rare but must be considered in cases of chronic unresponsive pain with radiographic changes of the pubic symphysis. The destructive changes will not only involve the pubic symphysis but also extend into the pubic rami. The MRI and CT scan help define the bony and soft tissue structures around these lesions effectively. In addition, abnormal serum alkaline phosphate and calcium levels suggest a neoplastic process.

Treatment

The treatment of athletic osteitis pubis can be tremendously challenging. Treatment begins with immediate patient education, activity modification, and rest. A drawn-out clinical course is frequently seen,

TABLE 5.2. Salient Clinical Features Between Osteomyelitis Pubis and Athletic Osteitis Pubis.

	Osteomyelitis	Osteitis pubis
Basic features	Infectious	Inflammatory/microtrauma/instability
Cultures	Positive (Staphylococcus aureus most common)	No organism
Treatment	Antibiotics, rest, debridement surgery	Rest, NSAIDS, steroid injections, surgery
Causes	Direct vs. indirect inoculation	Overuse, microtrauma, pubic symphysis instability
Clinical features	Fever, tenderness, waddling gait, painful adduction and abduction	Tenderness, waddling gait, painful adduction and abduction
Investigations	X-ray, MRI, bone scan, CT-guided biopsy	X-ray, MRI, bone scan

ultimately challenging the physician, patient, trainers, and coaching staff. The importance of rest and cross-training cannot be overemphasized. The symptoms last from several weeks to months.[2,17,23,31] Fricker et al.[9] reported full recovery averaged 9.5 months in men and 7.0 months in women after conservative treatment. A study by Holt et al.[17] found that patients returned to full activities within 16 weeks after conservative treatment. The mainstay of treatment for athletic osteitis pubis remains nonoperative.[2,4,8,17] The full spectrum of conservative measures has been documented and includes rest, physical therapy, ultrasonography, nonsteroidal anti-inflammatory medication, oral glucocorticoids, bracing, radiation therapy, anticoagulation, and corticosteroid injections into the pubic symphysis.[1,2,4,17,26] The effectiveness of the majority of these treatments has not been validated scientifically. In the athlete, the first line of treatment should be reducing the activity level. Choosing nonpainful and nonimpact exercises is central in the treatment. Shock-absorbing footwear may also diminish the shear forces across the symphysis pubis. Stretching exercises of the trunk and lower extremity should be done, paying particular attention to hip range of motion and adductor stretching and strengthening.[31] A study by Harris and Murray[4] of 37 athletic patients found that spontaneous remission was the most likely outcome and that rest from physical exertion was the most effective treatment. The ideal physical therapy program has not been clearly determined for osteitis pubis. For patients with chronic adductor-related groin pain, active physiotherapy training with a training program aimed at improving strength and coordination of the muscles acting on the pelvis, in particular the abdominal musculature and the adductor muscles, has been proven the most effective[40] (Figure 5.2). Studies evaluating the effectiveness of intraarticular pubic symphysis steroids are limited. Holt et al.[17] suggested that a quicker return to full sports activities could be accomplished with early judicious use of intraarticular corticosteroid injections in a study evaluating 12 intercollegiate athletes. Three of 8 athletes returned to play within 3 weeks of the injection and 3 more athletes within 16 weeks after a repeated injection. The authors recommended a treatment algorithm that began with conservative treatment and then an intraarticular injection of 4 mg dexamethasone, 1 mL 1% lidocaine, and 1 mL bupivacaine if the symptoms persisted after 7 to 10 days of treatment. The injection was done by prepping and draping a shaved area over the pubic symphysis. Fluoroscopic guidance was not used. The pubic symphysis was palpated and then penetrated with the needle. The needle is then gently advanced until a characteristic *pop* is appreciated. The 3-mL anesthetic mixture freely flows into the joint at this point. The authors warned that advancing the

needle more than 1 inch may cause injury to the spermatic cord or lead to penetration of the bladder. This study reported encouraging results; however, the addition of a control group composed of noninjected patients would have strengthened their results.

Surgical procedures such as partial wedge resections of the symphysis pubis and arthrodesis, with and without hardware, should be reserved for those patients with recalcitrant osteitis pubis and who are disabled by their symptoms.[2,4,8,23] Harris and Murray[4] found that surgery was rarely indicated but when necessary their arthrodesis of choice was one using a bone block. These investigators, however, did not publish their surgical data. Wedge resection of the symphysis has also been recommended for treatment of recalcitrant osteitis pubis (Figure 5.3). Some investigators believe that removal of the superior bony pubic symphysis wedge preserves the strong inferior arcuate ligaments, thereby preventing future instability.[2,8] Coventry and William[2] noted rapid resolution of symptoms in 2 patients who underwent a trapezoidal wedge resection and concluded that surgical measures may shorten the clinical course of recalcitrant osteitis pubis. Grace et al.[8] published their work on 10 patients who underwent a similar wedge resection after completing at least 6 months of conservative treatment. At an average postoperative follow-up of 92 months, 7 of the 10 patients were very satisfied with their results, but 3 were not. Interestingly, 2 of these 3 patients had pelvic instability. The authors concluded wedge resection of the symphysis pubis is useful as a first-line surgical procedure because of its short operative time, reliability, and low complication risk. Williams et al.[23] evaluated the benefits of pubic symphysis bone grafting supplemented by compression plating in a group of rugby players with pelvic instability (Figure 5.4). These patients had undergone at least 13 months of conservative treatment and were all found to have pelvic instability seen on flamingo views (>2 mm vertical motion). At a mean follow-up of 52.4 months, all patients were free of symptoms, and follow-up flamingo views confirmed a successful arthrodesis without residual pubic symphysis instability. The authors concluded their technique yielded an excellent arthrodesis and offered a low complication rate. The caveat in this study was that a bone block graft arthrodesis, without the supplementation of a compression plate, was prone to fusion mass stress fractures and, therefore, did not provide the necessary durability. Additionally, these authors echoed other authors' concerns that pubic symphysis wedge resection did indeed predispose patients to late pelvis instability, and hence they discourage its use.[41] We have had some success treating primary osteitis pubis with athletic pubalgia procedures.

Most of the literature regarding surgical management of osteitis pubis has focused exclusively on bony

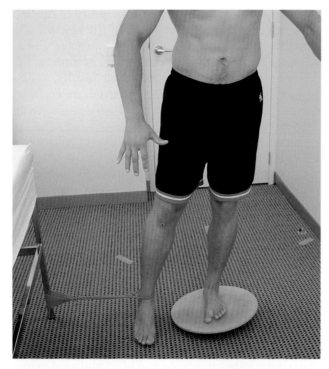
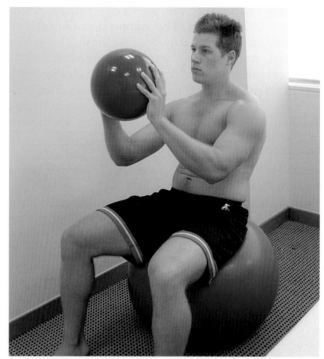
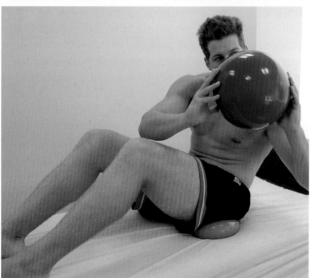
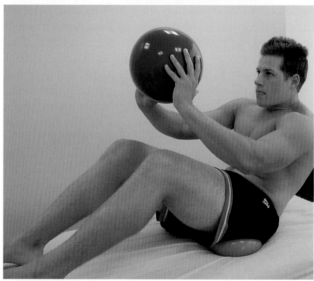

FIGURE 5.2. Strengthening and flexibility exercises aimed at eliminating the muscle imbalance between the abdominal musculature and the hip adductors. (Courtesy of Dr. Ross G. Davidson.)

procedures. The available reports on soft tissue procedures are limited to case reports or small retrospective reviews. A case report by Wiley[16] reported favorable results after surgically excising cortical avulsion of the gracilis tendon at the pubic symphysis. Miguel[14] presented his results of adductor muscle release off the pubis bone with adjunctive drilling into the symphyseal bone. Thirty-three (68%) of 48 athletes (mostly soccer players) who underwent this procedure returned to an acceptable level of sports and 6 (12%) were failures.

In summary, groin pain has a broad differential diagnosis including orthopedic and medically related causes. Once the differential diagnosis is narrowed and

the clinician is certain that urologic, gynecologic, and surgical causes are not the root cause, a focused and methodical management approach can be undertaken. To improve our diagnostic precision and to clearly define the pain complaint, we have instituted a zone-specific approach to this problem (Figure 5.5, Table 5.3). The abdominal, pubic, and thigh areas of the hip are separated into pathoanatomic zones (I, II, III, and IV). By focusing on the specific symptomatic zone, we are able to narrow the differential diagnosis and treatment strategy effectively. The workup would include a referral to a general surgeon, a herniography, and/or MRI to evaluate for the possibility of a posterior abdominal wall defect. The limitation to this approach

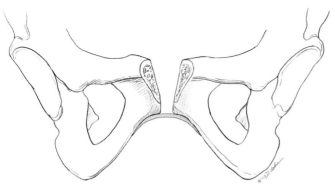

FIGURE 5.3. Partial wedge resection of the pubic symphysis for the treatment of recalcitrant osteitis pubis. A trapezoidal wedge of pubic symphysis bone is excised while sparring the strong inferior arcuate ligament. Theoretically, sparring the arcuate ligament prevents postsurgical pelvic instability.

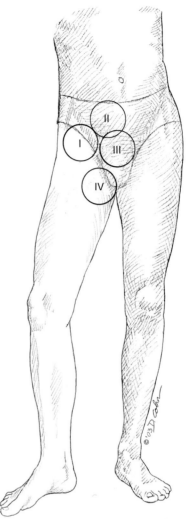

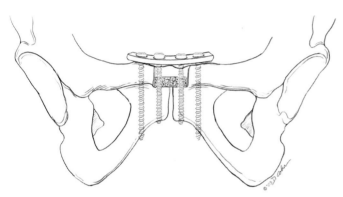

FIGURE 5.4. Pubic symphysis compression plate arthrodesis and inlaid tricortical bone graft for the treatment of recalcitrant osteitis pubis.

FIGURE 5.5. *Groin pain* pathoanatomic clinical zones: Zone I, over hip joint; zone II, inferior edge of rectus abdominis/conjoined tendon/inguinal ring; zone III, directly over bony prominence of pubic symphysis; zone IV, over the insertion and musculotendinous junction of the hip adductors.

TABLE 5.3. Groin Pain Pathoanatomic Zones and Their Respective Differential Diagnosis.

Zone I (hip joint region)	Zone II (suprapubic region)	Zone III (pubic region)	Zone IV (adductor region)
Labral tears, osteochondral loose bodies, and articular cartilage defects of the hip joint	Athletic pubalgia	Osteitis pubis	Adductor/gracilis tears
Snapping hip syndrome	Athletic pubalgia of the abdominal wall musculature and conjoined tendon (a.k.a. pubalgia, Gilmore's groin)	Pubic symphysis instability	Iliopsoas tendon tears and avulsions
Rectus femoris avulsions	Nerve entrapment (ilioinguinal, iliohypogastric, genitofemoral nerves)	Pubis osteomyelitis	Nerve entrapment (obturator and pudendal nerves)
Stress fractures of the femoral neck or rami		Stress fracture of the pubic rami	
Cutaneous nerve entrapment (lateral femoral cutaneous nerve)		Nerve entrapment (ilioinguinal, iliohypogastric, genitofemoral nerve)	

lies in the ability of the patient to localize the pain symptoms. As previously stated, groin pain can be generalized and not always localized to any one zone. Nonetheless, the zone-specific approach can serve as a useful tool to ensure a comprehensive, focused, and thorough diagnostic and management approach for the workup of groin pain in the athlete.

In our practice, osteitis pubis is treated initially with a conservative program focusing on relative rest, anti-inflammatory medication, and physical therapy. Activities that excessively load the pelvis, such as running, jumping, and pivoting sports, should be avoided. A supervised *active* physiotherapy program aimed at conditioning, stretching, and strengthening the abdominal and adductor musculature is heavily emphasized. The majority of our cases respond to this initial treatment but, in recalcitrant cases, intraarticular pubic symphysis steroid injections are considered. The time and number of the injections is purely arbitrary and depends on the patient's needs and the surgeon's style. We will readily inject the pubic symphysis 8 weeks after initiation of the initial phase of treatment if there has been poor and unacceptable clinical progress. Surgery is reserved for patients with refractory disabling symptoms who have failed an extended course of observation, activity modification, physical therapy, and injections. Prior to considering surgery, the patient is referred to a general surgeon specialized in athletic pubalgia. Only if the patient is not deemed a candidate for herniorrhaphy and anterior abdominal wall re-attachment will pubic symphysis stabilization be considered. We prefer the compression plate arthrodesis and bone grafting due to its theoretical durability, decreased chance of failing and less chance for the development of posterior pelvis instability. Adductor release serves as an adjunctive procedure and is always done. We favor platting/bone graft arthrodesis in patients with documented instability of the pubic symphysis confirmed by the flamingo views. An adductor release serves as an adjunctive procedure and is always done.

PIRIFORMIS SYNDROME

Description

The piriformis syndrome is characterized by nondiscogenic, extrapelvic, sciatic nerve compression in the area of the greater sciatic notch. The symptoms include pain and dysesthesias isolated to the buttock region, radiating to the hip or posterior thigh, and/or occurring distally as radicular pain.[42] The symptoms of piriformis syndrome are thought to be caused by entrapment of one or more divisions of the sciatic nerve by the piriformis muscle.[43,44] The original description of this condition dates back to 1928 when Yeoman[45] first described the possibility of a pathologic relationship between the sciatic nerve and the piriformis mus-

cle. Edwards[46] described it as "neuritis of branches of the sciatic nerve, caused by pressure of an injured or irritated piriformis muscle." Freiberg and Vinke[43] were the first to describe the classic findings of Lasegue's sign and tenderness at the sciatic notch over the piriformis muscle. The common peroneal division of the sciatic nerve is thought to be more frequently affected. Anatomic variants of the sciatic nerve as it courses along the piriformis muscle are thought to be contributory factors; however, this association is not grounded in diagnostic studies or surgical observation.[47] Historically, diagnostic studies have not been reliable; therefore, the diagnosis was made strictly on clinical grounds. This fact has severely compromised the credibility of this entity as a valid diagnosis. A fundamental problem lies in the fact that the piriformis muscle has not been proven as the singular structure compressing the sciatic nerve in this syndrome; therefore, the nomenclature *piriformis syndrome* is possibly inaccurate. Any of a number of lesions around the greater sciatic notch may injure or cause dysfunction to the sciatic nerve. This condition is analogous to carpal tunnel syndrome, which is a similar peripheral entrapment neuropathy of the median nerve with an array of causes. Similar to the sciatic nerve, entrapment of the superior and inferior gluteal nerves, posterior femoral cutaneous nerve, and the pudendal nerve can cause symptoms indistinguishable from the piriformis syndrome. It is also theoretically possible that the obturator internus–gamelli complex is an alternate cause of neural compression.[48] The nomenclature is therefore vague, confusing, and possibly erroneous. A new definition, *deep gluteal syndrome*, has emerged in the sports medicine literature. McCrory[48] has recommended adopting this new nomenclature to better reflect the complex and elusive nature of this condition.

Etiology

Compression of the sciatic nerve around the piriformis muscle can be caused one of a number of reasons. The sciatic nerve, like other peripheral nerves, is prone to injury and dysfunction if it is compressed by any of the surrounding tissues along its path. It is reasonable to infer that sciatic pain may be caused by compression anywhere along the nerve's length, from the spinal root level to the popliteal fossa. At the level of the piriformis muscle the sciatic nerve is particularly prone to injury because of its proximity to a vast array of structures including vessels, muscle, fascia, and bony structures, which at any time may become pathologic factors. Any disease affecting the structures that surround the sciatic nerve and its branches, such as aneurysm, tumors, infections, and hypertrophic conditions, may potentially affect the sciatic nerve function. The piriformis muscle syndrome has been reported after inferior and superior gluteal artery aneurysms,[42] after prolonged surgery in the sitting position,[49] after total hip replacements,[50] and secondary to space-occupying lesions.[51,52] Trauma has also been reported as an important etiological factor.[12,53–55]. This observation may be because the sciatic nerve lies within the gluteal area, a region prone to trauma from falls or direct injurious forces. Trauma to the muscles leads to irritation, inflammation, spasm, adhesion, and hypertrophy of the muscle. These traumatic changes may lead to dysfunction of the sciatic nerve and its branches. In a large series by Benson,[12] patients treated surgically had a definite history of an injurious force over their gluteal area. Intraoperative findings in this group of patients revealed piriformis muscle adhesions causing compression of the sciatic nerve.

Hypertrophy or aberrant fibrous bands of the piriformis muscle could theoretically compress the sciatic nerve or any branch within the muscle belly.[53,56] Hypertrophy may be due to increased strain on the hip abductors such as from abnormal gait mechanics or increased lumbar lordosis.[44] Other possible causes for piriformis muscle hypertrophy may include repetitive exercise-induced trauma and from chronic low-energy trauma as a result of sitting on a hard surface for extended periods.

Aberrant anatomy of the sciatic nerve and the piriformis muscle is speculated to play a role in the genesis of piriformis muscle syndrome.[52] Beaton and Anson[47] studied the anatomic variations of the relationship of the sciatic nerve to the piriformis muscle in cadaveric dissection. Typically, the sciatic nerve exits the greater sciatic foramen, passing below the belly of the piriformis (Figure 5.6). In 15% of autopsy cases, the nerve actually passes through the belly of the muscle.[47] Many other variations in the anatomy exist, including bipartite piriformis muscle belly, divisions of the sciatic nerve into its peroneal and tibial divisions occurring superior or within the piriformis muscle, and a piriformis muscle completely anterior to the sciatic nerve.[47,52,57] These anomalies can be seen in asymptomatic individuals and are rarely observed in most surgeries for exploration and decompression of the piriformis muscle.[58–61] Therefore, surgical release of the piriformis muscle in patients with anatomic anomalies and no other objective evidence is not recommended, and an alternative diagnosis should be first sought.

Any mass, tumor, or other space-occupying lesions can have neurologic manifestations when they compress adjacent neurologic structures. Space-occupying lesions known to have manifested as piriformis muscle syndrome include tumors, aneurysms/pseudoaneurysms, persistent sciatic artery, vena comitantes, large tortuous veins, abscesses, and myositis ossificans.[42,51–53]

Clinical Presentation

Knowledge of the anatomy of the sciatic nerve and it relationship to the piriformis muscle and gluteal ves-

sels is fundamental to understand the clinical picture of entrapment of the nerve. The piriformis muscle originates along the ventrolateral surface of the sacrum, where its origin interdigitates with the sacral nerve roots S2, S3, and S4, and continues to run laterally through the greater sciatic notch to exit the pelvis. It then inserts along with both gamelli and the obturator internus tendon into the piriformis fossa of the superior/posterior aspect of the greater trochanter. Collectively, this cluster of muscles forms the short external rotators of the hip. Thus, the piriformis muscle is an external rotator of the extended hip and an abductor when it is flexed. Nerve branches from L5, S1, and S2 innervate the piriformis muscle. The sciatic nerve is formed by the L4, L5, S1, S2, and S3 sacral roots. It exits the pelvis to enter the gluteal region through the greater sciatic notch. At the distal edge of the notch, the nerve is found deep to the piriformis muscle and above the gamelli and obturator internus muscle. The superior and inferior gluteal nerves and arteries are found directly superior and inferior to the piriformis, respectively.

Clues for diagnosing piriformis muscle syndrome can be gained through a detailed and focused clinical examination. Interestingly, the clinical presentation does vary widely between published case reports; therefore, no single examination or criterion is available to confirm the diagnosis. Piriformis muscle syndrome should be suspected in cases of sciatica or posterior gluteal/thigh pain and nondiagnostic MRI of the spine. The symptoms of piriformis muscle syndrome are nonspecific and include pain and dysesthesias occurring in the gluteal region radiating to the hip or posterior thigh, and sometimes in a radicular pain pattern down the leg. The athlete may experience cramping, burning, or aching in the buttock or posterior thigh, making the symptoms indistinct from a hamstring tear or intraarticular hip problems. Robinson,[55] who coined the term *piriformis muscle syndrome*, described a sausage-shaped tender mass over the area of the piriformis muscle as one of the key features of the syndrome. The physical examination also shows tenderness and reproduction of the radicular pain with deep palpation of the piriformis muscle. On rectal or pelvic examination, palpation of the piriformis and sciatic notch may reproduce and aggravate the symptoms. The radicular pain may also be reproduced by passively raising the straightened leg, Lasegue's sign. Frequently, flexion, adduction, and internal rotation (FAIR) of the hip exacerbate the symptoms. Freiberg's sign[58] (pain on passive internal rotation of the hip in neutral extension) and Pace's sign (weakness and pain on resisted abduction–external rotation of the thigh) may be present.[53,54] The neurologic examination can show abnormalities such as abnormal reflexes or motor weakness[42]; however, deficits are rare. There may also be evidence of superior gluteal nerve (weakness of the gluteus medius and minimus muscles), inferior

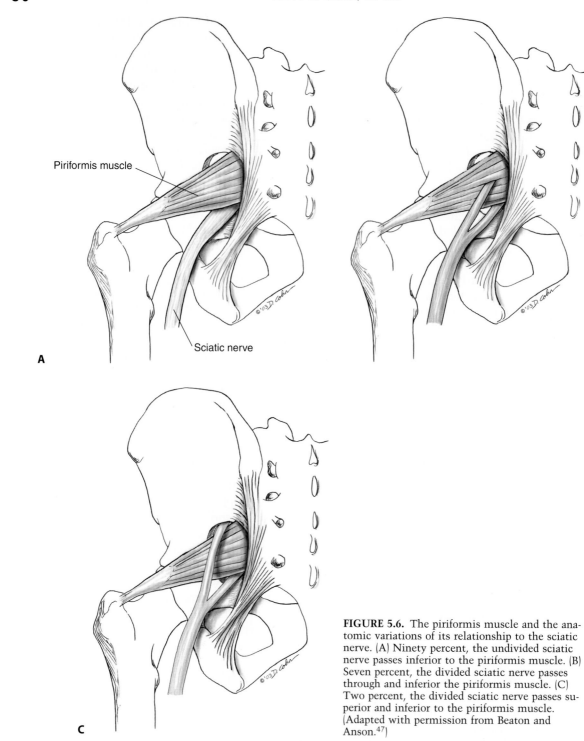

FIGURE 5.6. The piriformis muscle and the anatomic variations of its relationship to the sciatic nerve. (A) Ninety percent, the undivided sciatic nerve passes inferior to the piriformis muscle. (B) Seven percent, the divided sciatic nerve passes through and inferior the piriformis muscle. (C) Two percent, the divided sciatic nerve passes superior and inferior to the piriformis muscle. (Adapted with permission from Beaton and Anson.[47])

gluteal nerve (weakness of the gluteus maximus), pudendal nerve (peroneal sensory loss), and posterior femoral cutaneous nerve involvement.[48]

Historically, imaging studies have been irrelevant. Pelvic CT scan and MRI are used primarily for detecting pathologic lesions such as space-occupying lesion, hematoma, muscle/tendon tears, and intraarticular hip problems. Occasionally, the MRI or CT scan may identify abnormalities, such as hypertrophy of the piriformis muscle, adding support to the clinical diagnosis.[52,62,63] The MRI has been useful for identi-

fying anomalies of the piriformis muscle and variations of the sciatic nerve, but these findings have not proven to have clinical relevance.[44] Nuclear medicine scintigraphy may occasionally show increased uptake within the piriformis muscle but, similar to the CT scan and MRI, it has limited diagnostic benefits.[64–66]

More recently, however, electrodiagnostic testing has provided reliable objective signs.[53,64,65,67] Specialized electrodiagnostic studies seem to be the only diagnostic test able to objectively document functional impingement of the sciatic nerve by the piriformis muscle.[64,65,67] Fishman and Zybert[65] studied the prolongation of the H-reflex on 918 patients who met the criteria for piriformis syndrome. The criteria were(a) positive Lasegue's sign at 45 degrees; (b) tenderness at the sciatic notch; (c) increased pain within the distribution of the sciatic nerve with the leg in the flexion, adduction, and internal rotation (FAIR) position; and (d) electrodiagnostic tests excluding the existence of neuropathy and myopathy. They were able to document a statistically significant difference of H-reflex conductions when the affected limb was placed in the provocative (FAIR) position. Sensitivity and specificity of the FAIR test were found to be 88% and 83%, respectively. These same authors found 79% of their patients experienced 50% reduction in subjective symptoms when treated conservatively with therapy focused on reducing mechanical impingement and injections. The 28 patients who required surgery were found to have a significant improvement with the FAIR test. The FAIR test was also found to be a better predictor of successful treatment, be it physical therapy or surgery.

Last, to aid in the diagnosis and treatment, local anesthetic and steroid injections into the piriformis muscle may provide temporary relief of the symptoms.[42,54,66] When the piriformis muscle is involved, dramatic pain relief usually follows within 10 minutes of injection, supporting the diagnosis.

Differential Diagnosis

The diagnosis of piriformis syndrome remains one of exclusion. Common orthopedic and nonorthopedic etiologies should be put on the top of a differential diagnosis. In patients with atypical presentations or recalcitrant symptoms, it is also important to consider less common problems such as tumors. The differential diagnosis for patients presenting with vague gluteal and posterior thigh pain should be comprehensive. This concept cannot be overstressed in the evaluation and management of these difficult problems.

Because athletes frequently expose themselves to trauma and overstress injuries, muscular injuries and stress fractures should be an important part of the differential diagnosis. Hamstring injuries frequently present with pain in the same distribution as the piriformis muscle syndrome, but the symptoms are usually localized to the tear and readily diagnosed with an MRI. The piriformis muscle is located directly posterior to the hip joint; therefore, symptoms can also be indistinguishable from labral, chondral lesions, and loose bodies of the hip joint. Trochanteric bursitis is another common disorder causing posterior thigh pain. Both intraarticular hip problems and greater trochanteric bursitis may be diagnosed with selective anesthetic injections. In patients who present with radiculitis, more common causes such as lumbar stenosis, central spinal stenosis, lateral recess stenosis, herniated nucleus pulposus, and discogenic pain should be investigated with appropriate imaging studies.

Degenerative arthritis of the hip or the sacroiliac joint may present with gluteal/posterior thigh pain and should be evaluated using imaging studies and differential injections of anesthetic. A number of peripheral nerves around the sciatic notch are prone to injury and capable of producing similar symptoms. Entrapment of the superior gluteal nerve may cause aching, claudication-type buttock pain, weakness of abduction of the affected hip, a waddling gait, and tenderness to palpation in the area of the buttock superolateral to the greater sciatic notch.[68]

Additionally, masses such as hematomas, aneurysms/pseudoaneurysms, neoplasms, and abscesses in the gluteal or posterior thigh area are capable of pressing and injuring adjacent structures including the sciatic nerve. An MRI and CT scan of the pelvis and hip region in such instances are essential for diagnosing such entrapping lesions.

Treatment

Once the diagnosis of piriformis muscle syndrome is reached, several treatment options are available. The correct treatment is one that ideally addresses the impingement lesion in a safe and reliable manner. If the etiology is thought to be impingement from an inflamed, hypertrophied, or contracted piriformis muscle, then the treatment algorithm should begin with rest, antiinflammatory medication, muscle relaxants, and a physical therapy program aimed at stretching the piriformis muscle. Applying physical therapy modalities such as ultrasound treatment, electrical stimulation, and Fluori-Methane spray (dichlorodifluoromethane and trichloromonofluoromethane spray) may also be helpful.[69] The goal of this treatment strategy is to reduce the inflammation and contracture of the piriformis muscle. The stretching maneuvers include placing the lower extremity in the FAIR position. The patient is instructed to bring the knee into the chest and across the midline while in the supine position and in the standing position (Figure 5.7). These exercises are continued in sequential progression until maximal stretching intensity and duration is achieved. These exercises should also be executed after a piriformis muscle surgical release to prevent the reformation of contractures or adhesions. Concurrently, it is also important to address and correct abnormal biomechanical factors such as leg length discrepancies or hip flexor contractures. In cases in which the clinical progress is unacceptable or the diagnosis is unclear, a piriformis muscle anesthetic or corticosteroid injection may be beneficial for confirming the diagnosis and as a treatment adjunct. The injections can be done with or without fluoroscopic and electromyographic guidance.[54,70] Often, anatomic land-

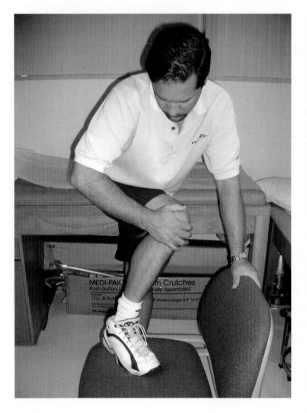

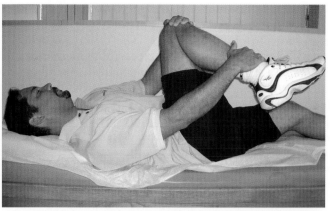

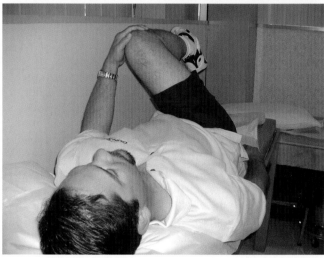

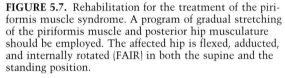

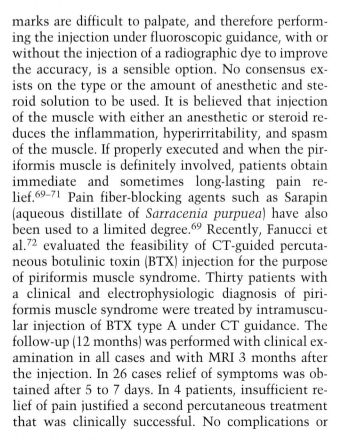

FIGURE 5.7. Rehabilitation for the treatment of the piriformis muscle syndrome. A program of gradual stretching of the piriformis muscle and posterior hip musculature should be employed. The affected hip is flexed, adducted, and internally rotated (FAIR) in both the supine and the standing position.

marks are difficult to palpate, and therefore performing the injection under fluoroscopic guidance, with or without the injection of a radiographic dye to improve the accuracy, is a sensible option. No consensus exists on the type or the amount of anesthetic and steroid solution to be used. It is believed that injection of the muscle with either an anesthetic or steroid reduces the inflammation, hyperirritability, and spasm of the muscle. If properly executed and when the piriformis muscle is definitely involved, patients obtain immediate and sometimes long-lasting pain relief.[69–71] Pain fiber-blocking agents such as Sarapin (aqueous distillate of *Sarracenia purpuea*) have also been used to a limited degree.[69] Recently, Fanucci et al.[72] evaluated the feasibility of CT-guided percutaneous botulinic toxin (BTX) injection for the purpose of piriformis muscle syndrome. Thirty patients with a clinical and electrophysiologic diagnosis of piriformis muscle syndrome were treated by intramuscular injection of BTX type A under CT guidance. The follow-up (12 months) was performed with clinical examination in all cases and with MRI 3 months after the injection. In 26 cases relief of symptoms was obtained after 5 to 7 days. In 4 patients, insufficient relief of pain justified a second percutaneous treatment that was clinically successful. No complications or

side effects were recorded after BTX injection. The MR examination showed a signal intensity change of the treated muscle in 7 patients, whereas in the remaining 2 cases imaged only an atrophy of the treated muscle was detected. The authors concluded that CT-guided BTX injection in the piriformis muscle is a promising and feasible technique that obtains an excellent local therapeutic effect without the risk of imprecise inoculation. Mullin and de Rosayro[71] described caudal epidural injections as an alternate route for anesthetic/steroid introduction. Caudal injections are straightforward and do not place the sciatic nerve at risk from an inadvertent needle injury or anesthetic infiltration. Anesthetic solutions deposited into the caudal space would be expected to diffuse along the nerve root sleeves and along the proximal part of the sciatic nerve. The afferent innervation of the piriformis muscle is also blocked using this method. The reports describing these conservative treatment options have been solely limited to small case reports and limited retrospective reviews. Prospective and controlled studies will ultimately determine their true effectiveness.

The length of time spent on conservative treatment should be individually based. Conservative options should have been fully optimized to the extent of performing up to three intramuscular or caudal injections.[44,69] Surgical exploration and release of all impinging structures is recommended in recalcitrant cases. If the point of entrapment is the piriformis muscle, its surgical release has been proven effective.[12,52,53,56,59,61] Operative treatment consists of sectioning the muscle at its tendinous origin, release of fibrous bands or compressing vessels, and external sciatic neurolysis. The functional loss after a piriformis muscle release is minimal because there are supplementary strong external rotators of the hip remaining. The impinging lesion may not be the piriformis muscle; therefore, it is important to do a methodical exploration of the area. Symptoms usually resolve rapidly after an adequate decompression. Proper patient selection is thought to be critical for a successful outcome. Therefore, before contemplating surgery, the surgeon should review the diagnostic steps leading to the diagnosis and, if necessary, additional or repeat investigations can be performed before embarking on surgery. Surgical exploration and decompression of the piriformis muscle carries potential risks including significant injury to vascular and neural structures. Recently, Benson and Schutzer[12] performed operative release of the piriformis and sciatic nerve neurolysis on 14 patients with posttraumatic piriformis muscle syndrome. Complications included a wound seroma and an infected hematoma. At an average of 2.3 months all their patients were employed, and at a minimum of 2 years postoperatively there were 11 excellent and 4 good results. Hughes et al.[53] also reported on 5 cases treated successfully with surgery. Their technique included obtaining a generous exposure of the posterior gluteal area, ligation of aberrant vessels, and release and resection of the piriformis muscle overlying the sciatic nerve. The authors believed a neurolysis was not necessary. Four of the 5 patients had immediate relief of their symptoms, and all had significant long-lasting improvement.

Summary

In summary, it cannot be overemphasized that successful treatment of this syndrome depends on an accurate diagnosis and knowledge of the exact point of entrapment. The treatment algorithm begins with conservative treatment emphasizing rest, stretching, physical therapy modalities, antispasm medication, and antiinflammatory agents. If necessary, biomechanical factors such as gait abnormalities or leg length discrepancies are addressed. If the patient ceases to make progress or plateaus, the next step should include a piriformis muscle anesthetic/steroid injection and further continuation of previous therapeutic measures. If the injection is found to be diagnostic, repeating the injections up to three times is reasonable. Surgical exploration of the sciatic nerve

and release of the piriformis muscle is effective for recalcitrant cases. The key point to remember during surgery is to explore the length of the sciatic nerve path so that all impinging lesions are thoroughly addressed.

OBTURATOR NERVE ENTRAPMENT

Description

Chronic groin pain is a difficult problem to evaluate. The differential diagnosis for groin symptoms is broad and may include gynecologic, urologic, and colorectal diseases. Moreover, neuropathies of the cutaneous nerves around the hip have been highlighted as etiologic factors for groin pain.[35,37] Nonetheless, the information on this topic is sparse, partly because these injuries are rare. The literature on groin pain of neural origin has mainly focused on the genitofemoral, lateral femoral cutaneous, ilioinguinal, and iliohypogastric nerves.[37] The obturator nerve, in contrast to the other four cutaneous nerves around the groin, lies protected deep within the pelvis and the medial thigh. The cases documenting injury to the obturator nerve have been limited to isolated case reports of neuropathy due to unusual entrapping lesions or as a consequence of surgical complications. Obturator nerve entrapment has been identified as an unusual cause of groin pain in athletes.[36] The neuropathy is possibly caused by an entrapping fascial or vascular structure that is relieved with surgical decompression.

Etiology

Understanding the anatomy of the obturator nerve and its relationship with the adductor muscles is helpful for understanding the syndrome and for surgical planning. The classic description of the anatomic course of the obturator nerve comes from *Gray's Anatomy*.[73] The obturator nerve forms from the convergence to the ventral divisions of the ventral rami of L2, L3, and L4 spinal nerves within the psoas major muscle. The nerve then descends through the psoas muscle to emerge from its medial border at the pelvic brim. The nerve then curves downward and forward around the wall of the pelvic cavity and travels through the obturator foramen, after which it divides into anterior and posterior branches. The anterior branch enters the thigh over the obturator externus muscle and the posterior branch through the fibers of that same muscle. The anterior branch innervates the adductor longus, gracilis, and adductor brevis muscles. It also gives an articular branch to the hip joint near its origin. It divides into numerous named and unnamed branches, including the cutaneous branches to the subsartorial plexus, vascular branches to the femoral artery, communicating branches to the femoral cutaneous nerves, accessory obturator nerve, and directly to the skin of the medial thigh. The posterior division continues to innervate the obturator externus, adductor magnus, the adductor brevis (if it has not received supply from the anterior division) and gives an articular branch to the knee joint. Its supply to the adductors is variable; therefore, care must be taken when dissecting around the obturator foramen, especially superiorly because it descends over the ramus to join the anterior division.[74]

Obturator neuropathy is an uncommon mononeuropathy usually associated with a well-defined event or an invasive procedure.[75] There have been several isolated case reports of obturator nerve injury due to compressive causes and entrapment. Obturator nerve injury has been reported after retroperitoneal hemorrhage, after fractures of the pelvis, invading pelvic tumors, endometriosis, and after aneurysms of the hypogastric artery and obturator hernias.[76–79] It has also been described after procedures such as total hip replacement, forceps vaginal delivery, urologic surgery, and prolonged positioning in the lithotomy position.[80–83] The insult to the obturator nerve in these isolated cases is apparent from the clinical history and description. The etiology of obturator neuropathy without such external insults is much more uncertain. Until recently there have been no athletic or sports-related cases reported. Bradshaw and colleagues[36] reported their observations on 32 surgical cases of obturator neuropathy in athletes. In addition to making surgical observations, they also performed six cadaveric dissections. The salient points made were (a) entrapment of the obturator nerve occurs at the level of the obturator foramen and the proximal thigh rather than in the obturator tunnel; (b) definition of a unique fascial arrangement surrounding the adductor longus and the pectineus muscle that is probably central in the pathogenesis of this condition (Figure 5.8); and (c) the results of positive radionucleotide tests attesting to the presence of inflammatory changes along the adductors, which may also have a contributory effect. Last, the authors point out that the biomechanical differences seen in male anatomy, such as higher iliac bones, smaller pelvic inlet, and a narrower subpubic angle, alter the vector of the obturator nerve and perhaps predispose it to injury.

Harvey and Bell[74] proceeded to map out the details of the fascial planes surrounding the obturator nerve. Their cadaveric study illustrated fascial and vascular anatomy and specifically looked at the fascia surrounding the vascular pedicles and its relationship to the anterior branch of the obturator nerve. The fascial thickening around the vascular pedicle derived from the medial circumflex femoral artery was thought to be most capable of impinging. Their findings seemed to correlate with the surgical findings of Harvey and Bell.[74] Other authors

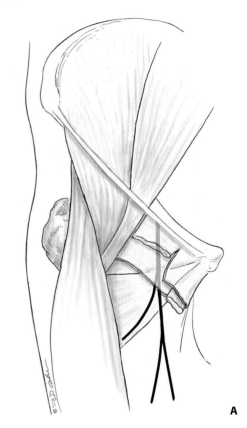

A

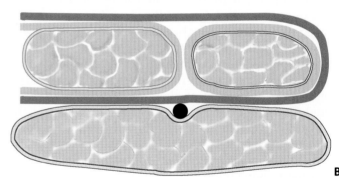

B

FIGURE 5.8. (A, B) Entrapment of the obturator nerve by surrounding muscle fascia. (Adapted with permission from Bradshaw et al.[36])

have also studied the potential sites for obturator nerve entrapment. In 1991, Peri[84] described three critical zones of entrapment for the obturator nerve, including (a) the obturator canal; (b) the interval between the pectineus and the obturator externus muscle and between the adductor longus and the adductor brevis; and (c) the interval between the obturator externus and adductor magnus and the adductor magnus and the adductor brevis where the posterior branch is involved. This study involved 40 dissections in total; however, the descriptions provided lacked useful anatomic detail. To date, the work of Harvey and Bell[74] has provided the clearest anatomic description of the path and the possible sites of obturator nerve impingement.

Clinical Presentation

Patients with obturator neuropathy usually present with insidious onset pain centered over the origin of the adductors at the pubic symphysis. The pain may be indistinguishable from chronic adductor strains, but is usually more posterior in the perineum. The symptoms can include paresthesias, sensory loss, or deep ache pain. It is often difficult to precisely localize the pain, making the diagnosis difficult. The symptoms and signs are frequently exercise induced. The symptoms are analogues to claudication; the pain worsens with exercise and is relieved with rest.

All 29 patients of Bradshaw et al.[36] had medial thigh pain and adductor weakness. The most important specific signs in this study were adductor muscle weakness, adductor spasm, and paresthesias over the medial aspect of the distal thigh. In a retrospective review of 22 cases of obturator neuropathy, the most common symptom was medial thigh or groin pain.[75] Adductor weakness and sensory loss occurred infrequently. When weakness is encountered, it is not in the form of a complete palsy. Complete adductor weakness is not present as the adductor magnus receives dual innervation from both the obturator and the tibial portion of the sciatic nerve. It is important to remember the physical examination findings may be more pronounced after a period of exercise.[36] In cases of suspected obturator nerve impingement, hip extension stretch maneuvers, pectineal muscle stretch (this is performed by the patient first actively externally rotating the limb so that the foot is nearly 80 to 90 degrees outwardly, and then the foot is firmly planted and the trunk twisted in the opposite direction of the foot, thereby creating a passive external rotation moment on the hip and causing the pectineal muscle to stretch), or resisted hip internally rotation will provoke pain.[36,85] Plain radiographs are nondiagnostic. Radionucleotide studies may show delayed phase increased uptake of the pubic rami on the affected side.[36] The needle electromyography (EMG) findings provide the objective findings of acute or chronic denervation only in the short and long adductors. Paraspinal muscle sampling at L2, L3, L4, and in other muscles supplied (iliopsoas and quadriceps) by these nerve roots is normal.[86] Local anesthetic injections are useful for confirming the diagnosis. To improve the accuracy of the injection, the obturator foramen is located with fluoroscopic assistance and injected with a local anesthetic agent. A successful nerve block is confirmed by the production of cutaneous anesthesia over the medial thigh.

Additional diagnostic studies are useful for evaluating and ruling out more common causes for groin pain. A CT scan and MRI may demonstrate muscle atrophy in long-standing cases of obturator neuropathy but, more importantly, these tests are useful for identifying intrapelvic masses capable of compressing the obturator nerve.

Differential Diagnosis

The differential diagnosis has been discussed in the section on Osteitis Pubis.

Treatment

No consensus exists as to what comprises the best treatment options for this condition. The temporal profile of the lesion appears to be an important consideration. Patients with acute-onset lesions, such as from trauma, are thought to improve with conservative measures.[75] Patients with minimal EMG findings may also be given a trial of conservative treatment.[36] Conservative measures include rest, stretching, nerve desensitization, local nerve blocks, ultrasound, interferential treatment, steroid injections, transcutaneous nerve stimulators, and neuropathic pain medication.[31,37,87] Physical therapy should focus on adductor muscle stretching, adductor and pelvic muscle strengthening, and groin stretches. Corticosteroid infiltration of the nerve at the level of the obturator foramina may be carried out with the use of fluoroscopic guidance. Chronic or recalcitrant cases are best treated with surgical decompression of the obturator nerve.[36,87] The key points for a successful surgical procedure include ligating vessels branching off the medial femoral circumflex artery, decompressing the length of the nerve, and bluntly dilating the obturator foramen. The outcome following surgery in athletes is good based on the little information published. All 29 patients surgically managed with obturator nerve decompression by Bradshaw et al.[36] did universally well. This group of athletes resumed to full sports activities within 3 to 6 weeks of the surgery. EMG analysis performed at 6 weeks and 12 months postoperatively showed a normal recording in all patients. These findings corroborate previously published results on successful decompression of nerves around the hip and groin.[37,88]

Summary

Obturator nerve entrapment is a previously unreported cause for hip and groin pain in the athlete. The pathophysiology is one of focal nerve entrapment by fascial or vascular structures. The etiology of these lesions is unclear. This entity is not readily discernible from more common disorders, such as chronic adductor strains, intraarticular hip problems, and abdominal wall defects. The surgeon should be aware of subtleties of the clinical presentation such as symptomatology that increases with exercise and diminishes with rest. Local anesthetic injections and EMG studies are the confirmatory tests. A sensible trial of nonoperative treatment should be instituted, especially for acute cases or those with minimal EMG changes. The outcome of surgical decompression is good based on the sparse data available.

II. ATHLETIC PUBALGIA
*WILLIAM C. MEYERS, LEVENTE J. SZALAI,
NICHOLAS D. POTTER, ARCHIT NAIK, AND
JEFF RYAN*

ATHLETIC PUBALGIA

In this section we list others of the more commonly seen entities causing hip pain in athletes. More detail is provided on the entity called *athletic pubalgia*, a chronic inguinal or pubic area pain that occurs in high-performance athletes. Athletic pubalgia is the most common *fixable* problem in this group of athletes. Please refer to some of our other recent articles for other details about these syndromes. The present section, to a large degree, represents an update on these articles,[89–92] in addition to adding considerably more concerning rehabilitation.

For years, lower abdominal/groin pain has ended the careers of many gifted athletes. These injuries in Major League Soccer, the National Hockey League, the National Football League, and other sports organizations during the past few years have heightened the awareness of this problem. However, the pathophysiologic processes involved in these presumptive injuries have been poorly understood. In 1992 we reported success with an operation for a particular pattern of inguinal pain in a limited number of athletes.[32] We found that a distinct syndrome of lower abdominal/adductor pain in male athletes appeared correctable by a procedure designed to strengthen the anterior pelvic floor. The operation we developed was based on some concepts first suggested by the work of a Yugoslavian surgeon named Nesovic (personal communication). This success led to a much larger experience.[90] The experience now numbers about 1800 patients. The location and pattern of pain and the operative success suggest the cause to be a combination of abdominal hyperextension and thigh hyperabduction, with the pivot joint being the pubic symphysis. We have also improved our knowledge in diagnosing this injury, differentiating it from other injuries, and managing the associated symptoms more effectively.

Definitions and Epidemiology

Many people are afflicted with groin pain, including athletes and nonathletes alike. The differential diagnosis in these patients is extremely important. In this chapter, we confine our comments primarily to abdominal/groin pain in athletes. The term *athlete* refers to a patient actively or recently participating in competitive athletic activity as a livelihood or integral way of life. The term *athletic pubalgia* refers to chronic inguinal or pubic area pain in athletes, which is noted solely on exertion and not explainable preoperatively by demonstrable hernia or other medical diagnoses.

The incidence of athletic pubalgia in various sports is listed in decreasing order: soccer, hockey, football, track and field, baseball, basketball, racquet sports, and swimming. It can be inferred that this type of injury occurs most commonly during the autumn sports. Also, more than 90% of the patients that we have diagnosed with athletic pubalgia have been male. Most female patients are found to have other causes for their pain, such as endometriosis.[93] The precise explanation for the difference in gender incidence is not known. Two possible hypotheses for the higher incidence in male patients are (1) a relatively low participation (until recently) of women in highly competitive sports and (2) a difference in pelvic anatomy. Our thought is that the latter hypothesis is much more likely.

Data from eight athletic trainers in Major League Soccer and the National Hockey League estimate that 9% of players on a given team suffer or will suffer from a syndrome consistent with athletic pubalgia. Another 12% of players have some minor degree of chronic discomfort, which is not disabling. Up to 18% of players had some type of *groin pull* in the past but with subsequent recovery.[32] In another uncontrolled survey of one professional team, 4% of players over a 5-year period retired because of groin pain. This problem was the leading cause of injury-related retirement for that team.[94]

The previously mentioned survey suggests that groin problems are extremely common in high-performance athletes. Roughly half the patients recover from acute injuries without significant sequelae. The remaining half of the patients can be divided into two groups, one in which the chronic pain is minor and the other group in which the pain is severe enough to require significant medical or surgical attention.[30]

For the most part, patients afflicted with this injury are high-performance athletes. However, performance athletes and nonathletes do have a similar potential for this syndrome. Over a 10-year period we have seen this syndrome in only a small number of nonathletes. This small number represents less than 10% of cases that were evaluated for the suspicion of athletic pubalgia.

In contrast with the 95% success rate of pelvic floor repairs in the athletes, successful repair occurred in less than half of the nonathletes who underwent similar operations. The operated nonathletes also had more diffuse symptoms and were more likely to be involved with legal claims and workmen's compensation.

Other Terminology Used to Describe Athletic Pubalgia

Various other terms have been used in the literature to describe what seems to be the same syndrome we have called athletic pubalgia. Those terms include Gilmore's groin, hockey groin syndrome, sportsman's hernia, osteitis pubis, snapping hip syndrome, gracilis syndrome, hockey goalie/baseball pitcher syndrome, and a variety of muscle strains, tendonopathies, and bursitises.

Dr. Gilmore used the term *Gilmore's groin* in his initial study published in 1992, involving 65 professional soccer players in the United Kingdom between 1980 and 1987.[95] Gilmore's groin was described as a condition consisting of three pathologic findings: a torn external oblique aponeurosis, torn conjoined tendon, and dehiscence between the torn conjoined tendon and the inguinal ligament. Gilmore thought this entity stemmed from hip hyperextension and rotation, as occurs in the soccer kicking motion. The onset predominantly idiopathic, which leads one to believe that repeated microtrauma is the major destructive force. A common sign on physical examination is a dilation of the superficial inguinal ring. However, Gilmore stated that the latter finding was not evident in 25% of his patients.

When we describe the syndrome of *athletic pubalgia,* we are referring to a syndrome that we believe is virtually identical to the syndrome that Gilmore describes.

Pelvic Anatomy

A complete description of the anatomy of the pelvis is beyond the scope of this chapter; however, a thorough understanding of the anatomy is essential to diagnose and treat groin injuries and groin and hip pain. For the purpose of our discussion, we describe the pelvis as a girdle,[96] with two pairs of innominate bones, plus the sacrum and the coccyx. The innominate bone is composed of the ileum, the ischium, and the pubis, which also forms a portion of the acetabulum. In the normal state, there is little motion across the joints of the pelvis. However, when considering the highly dynamic pelvis of a performance athlete, it is useful to conceptualize the pelvis as being composed of many tiny joints. The normally static joints of the pelvis can be stretched in the athlete and this, in turn, can result in excessive motion at various sites within the pelvis.

Several important structures insert onto the pelvis and its anterior attachment, the pubic symphysis. These structures include the rectus abdominis, external oblique, internal oblique, and transversus abdominis.[97] Structures that insert along the inferior as-

pect of the symphysis include the adductor muscles, pectineus, gracilis, obturator internus, quadratus femoris, and gluteus muscles. A series of ligamentous arches also exist between the pelvic bones, further stabilizing the joint.

In addition to previously mentioned stabilizing pelvic muscles and ligaments, there are a number of bursae of the anterior pelvis. Although the psoas inserts principally onto the femur, its bursa is rather large and complexly shaped so that it may even touch the anterior pelvic joint. There are also potentially clinically significant bursae behind the symphysis and near the lesser and greater trochanter of the femur.

Athletes exert high-velocity forces across the joints, muscles, tendons, and ligaments of the pelvis. With these considerable forces, damage can occur to any part of the athlete's pelvis, manifesting itself as groin pain.

Etiology

Most patients describe a hyperextension injury in association with hyperabduction of the thigh. The pivot point seems to be the anterior pelvis and pubic symphysis. The location of pain suggests that the injury involves both the rectus abdominis and adductor muscles. In athletic pubalgia, the rectus tendon insertion on the pubis seems to be the primary site of pathology. However, other tendinous insertion sites on the pubic bone may also be involved (Figure 5.9). Because of the injuries of the tendinous insertion sites on the pubis, we can assume that we are dealing with a subtly unstable pelvis.

The location and progression of pain in these athletes suggest a disruption of the pivot apparatus and a redistribution of forces to other musculotendinous attachments during extremes of exercise. The accompanying inflammation includes osteitis, tendonitis, or bursitis, which can all contribute to the groin pain. The pain resulting from the inflammation can be temporarily alleviated by injections or antiinflammatory drugs. Deep massage therapy is another temporarily effective therapy. However, the lack of permanent relief by the previously stated methods suggests that the inflammation is not the primary problem and that stabilization of the anterior pelvis is necessary.[98]

By definition, pubalgia is **not** due to an occult hernia. Furthermore, the pattern of symptoms in athletic pubalgia patients, operative findings, and results of our studies all suggest that the lower abdominal pain and inguinal pain in these patients are not caused by an occult hernia. Although some patients were found to have occult hernias at the time of surgery, the hernias were usually found on the opposite side of the principal symptoms.[65]

The principal complaint of hernia patients is usually a bulge with superior and lateral inguinal pain, consistent with the location of the internal ring. The

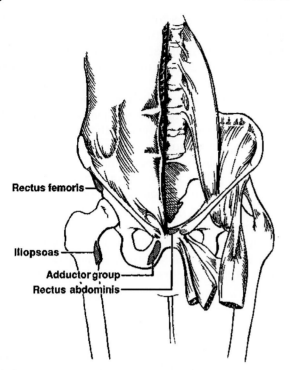

FIGURE 5.9. Insertion sites for muscles that commonly sustain strain injuries resulting in groin pain. (With permission of DC Taylor, WC Meyers, JA Moylan, et al. Abdominal musculature abnormalities as a cause of groin pain in athletes. Am J Sports Med 19:239–242, 1991.[32])

pain in most pubalgia patients is near the pubis, far from the internal ring. In more than 80% of pubalgia cases, the pain is also associated with adduction of the hip against resistance. Progression of the pain often involves the adductors, perineal region, and eventually the opposite side. The combination of a distinct injury, localized pain, and progression suggests an initial injury with subsequent involvement of other structures adjacent to the injury. Athletic pubalgia most likely is not a result of multiple different injuries, particularly because most of these patients often describe a single inciting injury.

Diagnosis

The syndrome of athletic pubalgia is common in high-performance athletes. The syndrome's features include disabling lower abdominal and inguinal pain at extremes of exertion. The pain progresses over months to years and involves the adductor longus tendons and the contralateral inguinal or adductor regions. The diagnosis of this syndrome is generally empiric.

Most patients remember a distinct injury during exertion. Usually, the abdominal pain involves the inguinal canal near the insertion of the rectus muscle on the pubis.[32,99,100] The pain causes most patients to stop competing in sports.

In general, the pain is minimal at rest and begins unilaterally, but becomes bilateral within months or years if the injury is untreated. Two-thirds of the pa-

tients describe the pain with resisted adduction of the hip, which can occasionally be more prominent than the abdominal findings. The pain may also be fleeting, appearing and disappearing on one or the other side, or involve both abdominal and adductor components. Less than 25% of patients have significant, vague symptoms attributable to the anatomic location of the posterior perineum. Interestingly, involvement of the posterior perineum is associated with a decreased likelihood of successful repair.

When examining a patient suspected of having athletic pubalgia, the physical examination must be directed to obtain key findings. Most patients exhibit pain with adduction of the hip against resistance[30] and pain with resisted sit-ups. Twenty-five percent of patients have pubic or peripubic tenderness. One-third have some degree of subjective tenderness along the adductor tendons near the pubis. Superior inguinal or real abdominal tenderness is uncommon. By definition, no patients have hernias.

A common finding that mistakenly dissuades one from making the diagnosis of athletic pubalgia is an MRI or bone scan result of osteitis pubis. When we first started doing pelvic floor repairs in the late 1980s, we avoided operating on anyone with an MRI or bone scan diagnosis of osteitis pubis. However, after a Swedish group[101] had success with pelvic floor repairs in patients diagnosed with osteitis pubis, we also performed pelvic floor repairs on our patients who were previously denied the operation. Our patients subsequently did well, and, therefore, a diagnosis of osteitis pubis is not a contraindication for a pelvic floor repair. From the previously stated results, we can also conclude that CT and bone scans generally have no added value over MRI even if they show osteitis.

On the other hand, a distinct population of patients exists who have severe primary osteitis. They have continuous severe pain and tenderness at rest or exercise. This group of patients will not likely be helped by a pelvic floor repair.

The absence of an MRI finding should not prevent one from making the diagnosis of pubalgia. In fact, most patients on whom we have operated do not exhibit MRI findings of rectus muscle disruption. Most patients do well with pelvic floor repair in the absence of definitive MRI findings. Only 12% of patients had MRI findings that clearly indicated a problem at the rectus insertion site. The relatively small incidence of a specific diagnosis by imaging studies suggests that the problem may be an attenuation of the muscle or tendon due to repeated microtrauma.[30]

Nonspecific MRI findings, on the other hand, occur frequently and localize to the side or sides of injury in more than 90% of patients. The nonspecific findings include focal osteitis and nonspecific abdominal wall, perineal, or adductor findings. They also include asymmetry, distinct inflammation, cortical irregularity, distinct fluid accumulation, irregularity of the rectus abdominis, atrophic changes, small pelvic avulsion fractures, or disruption of the pectineus muscle. It is possible that these nonspecific MRI findings may assist the surgeon in decision making, because the MRI can often predict the side or sides of injury. In addition, the MRI has been noted in its demonstration of other severe problems as per the differential diagnosis.[33]

A history of an inguinal hernia repair, either in childhood or adulthood, without evidence of a recurrent hernia should also not dissuade one from making the diagnosis of pubalgia. A previously successful hernia repair does little to rule out athletic pubalgia. The cause of the syndrome is pelvic instability, not occult hernia; the term *sports hernia* is a misnomer.

A patient who experiences pain symptoms without exertion most likely does not have athletic pubalgia. A certain amount of mild discomfort is certainly acceptable, but severe pain in the absence of exertion is a tip-off that the patient probably does not have the diagnosis of athletic pubalgia. Most patients with this syndrome clearly have pain only with extremes of exertion. With chronicity, the pain begins to interfere with some activities of daily living. Some pain may persist after activity, but almost never is the pain particularly severe at rest. The nonathlete who complains of constant pain almost certainly does not have the diagnosis, even if the symptoms and signs are in the right locations.

Lateral pain in the inguinal region also points toward a diagnosis other than pubalgia. If the pain is clearly lateral to the adductors, one should suspect intrinsic hip disease or a variety of other pelvic disorders.

True testicular pain or epididymal pain should also be ruled out before making a diagnosis of pubalgia. Upper scrotal pain can be in the distribution of the ilioinguinal nerve, which can easily be involved in the inflammatory process. Pain and tenderness along the lateral edge of the pubic symphysis is consistent with the problem of pubalgia, but true testicular or epididymal pain generally is not. Pain with sexual activity is consistent with the syndrome of pubalgia so long as simple exertion is causing the pain; pain with ejaculation only is not consistent with the syndrome.

Management Considerations

Key questions concerning the surgical management of these patients include the following. Does the patient have symptoms that qualify him or her for the syndrome? How disabling is the syndrome? Can the patient be treated nonoperatively? Can the patient be treated medically on a temporary basis to allow the athlete to finish the season? Should one perform an adductor release? What operations are likely to work? And what is the role of nonoperative therapy?

To answer these questions, definitions and presumptions need to be addressed. *Nonoperative therapy* refers to trials of prolonged rest, rehabilitation, oral or injected steroids, or deep massage. The disabling pain has led to a curtailment or cessation of competitive athletic participation and diminution in his or her athletic ability. *Acute* injury refers to pain that has resolved or is clearly better within 2 weeks. *Recurrent acute* refers to evaluation within 2 weeks of a repeat groin injury after complete recovery from an initial episode. *Chronic* refers to the persistence of pain after 6 weeks without evidence of improvement at the time of evaluation.

Again, our data strongly suggest that the principal mechanism of athletic pubalgia is a disruption or attenuation of the rectus muscle insertion on the pubis. This disruption results in instability of the anterior pubis that is manifested by a rearrangement of focus to other musculotendinous attachments of the pubis. Therefore, the best repair would be a broad surgical reattachment at the inferolateral edge of the rectus muscle with its fascial investments to the pubis and adjacent anterior ligaments. This is the operation we most commonly use for athletic pubalgia, and in most cases, this repair significantly ameliorates or eliminates the adductor symptoms.

On a rare occasion, adductor symptoms may persist after pelvic floor repair and become particularly bothersome. This observation suggests that the adductor symptoms are most likely caused by a secondary chronic inflammatory process involving the superior edge of the inferior pubic ramus. This jagged edge rubs on the adjacent soft tissues within the adductor compartment, causing inflammation and pain. The weakening of the anterior abdomen causes a kind of compartment syndrome.

To alleviate the pain associated with this compartment syndrome, an adductor release is performed. An anterior and lateral release of the epimysium of the adductor fascia is performed to expand this compartment. The epimysium is the layer of connective tissue that encloses the entire muscle. During an epimysial release, the edema in the groin is noted to be released. This kind of fascial release is often successful.

Treatment Algorithms

We propose the attached algorithms for the treatment of patients diagnosed with athletic pubalgia. Algorithm 1 (Figure 5.10) describes groin injury treatment during the season, whereas algorithm 2 (Figure 5.11) concentrates on treatment between seasons. Generally, only treat the chronic or persistent acute recurrent problems surgically. Direct steroid injection into symptomatic bursa or other soft tissue sites may give enough temporary relief for patients to continue their season.[100] When the process continues over several

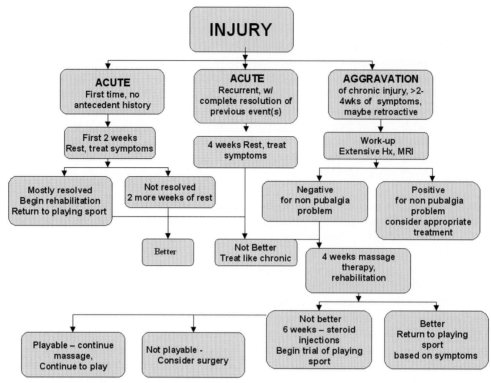

FIGURE 5.10. Algorithm for groin injury treatment during the season.

months and the athlete cannot return to previously expected activity because of pain, an operation should be considered. Deep massage therapy has a role in patients with equivocal symptoms or others in whom surgery for one reason or another is not favored. The effectiveness of deep massage cannot be explained.

Results of Repairs and Releases

A success rate of 95% can be expected from surgical treatment in well-selected patients. This success was initially observed in 200 patients over a 3-year follow-up. The series has now been extended to over 2500 patients. We suggest operating only on the symptomatic side or sides. On the other hand, several patients with particularly severe MRI findings on the opposite side but without symptoms have also undergone bilateral repair with similar success rates.

Our data also clearly indicate that many standard hernia repairs are inadequate in treating athletic pubalgia. In particular, laparoscopic hernia repair does **not** appear to be the correct solution for this problem. The laparoscopic repair emphasizes a *tension-free* mesh insertion that does not stabilize the anterior pelvis. We have now seen over 300 patients who had unsuccessful laparoscopic or open "hernia repair" and subsequently had successful pubalgia surgery.

The generally poor outcomes of the laparoscopic repair and other hernia operations provide additional evidence that the mechanism of athletic pubalgia is

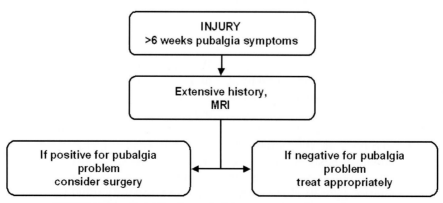

FIGURE 5.11. Algorithm for groin injury treatment between seasons.

not due to an occult hernia. However, a few patients have done well after hernia repairs. The small success rates seem likely due to general fibrosis, which accompanies all operations and inadvertently stabilizes the anterior pelvis. The Cooper's ligament or McVay repair for inguinal hernia seems more likely to treat the problem but also stretches the anterior abdominal musculature down to the more posterior attachments of the anterior pelvis. Therefore, this operation may not provide optimal anterior stabilization. We have seen inconsistent results with the McVay approach; thus, we recommend performing a rectus reattachment and adductor release to treat athletic pubalgia.

Postsurgical Athletic Pubalgia Rehabilitation

Although there are a variety of pathologies and differential diagnoses for groin pain among athletes, the majority involves some kind of muscle imbalance and pelvic instability. In many cases conservative physical therapy is able to correct these abnormalities and the athlete may return to competition with minimal game exposures missed. However, a select group of athletes sustain injuries that frequently recur or do not altogether subside with conservative treatment and result in a significant reduction of athletic competition. These athletes find the only viable opportunity to prolong their career is surgery. After surgery there must then exist a protocol to guide the physical therapy process, which protects and reinforces the repair. The following is a protocol guideline designed for postsurgical athletic pubalgia rehabilitation. However, it is constructed on the basis of the physiological tissue injury cycle, and its focus aims to restore muscular balance and pelvic kinematic symmetry. Thus, it may be thought of as a means to normalize any lower abdominal and pelvic dysfunction in a progressive manner for the goal of returning the athlete to high-performance competition.

The main goals of the athletic pubalgia repair are to reapproximate any damaged tissue and to regain normal muscular balance within the lower abdominal and adductor region. Thus, the goals of postsurgical physical therapy should be to provide an environment conducive to efficient tissue healing, further establish muscular balance within the lower abdominal and adductor region, and incorporate sport-specific progressive therapeutic exercise into the rehabilitation process to enhance the return of the athlete to their sport.

The two areas of concern in establishing muscular balance are the adductor and abdominal regions. The released adductor longus should be dealt with in a manner that promotes functional healing which entails the collagen lying down in a parallel, elastic, and elongated fashion. The abdominal region must be handled with great care by the therapist. The repaired rectus abdominis should be allowed to form a mature scar before being stressed with progressive functional training. The end result should produce an adductor region that has more laxity and an abdominal region that is more taut compared with preoperative conditions. Together these readjusted reciprocal muscles about the pelvis should be able to regain normal kinematics in sport. This *normalized* pelvic posture must then be stabilized through training of the deep abdominals such as the transverse abdominis and lumbar multifidus. With this base of normal kinematics established, the only thing left to do is prepare the athlete for return to sport, which involves training the athlete in all aspects of their respective sport. This principle of *sport specifics* should be kept in mind by the therapist and implemented where possible throughout the rehabilitation process, as it will prepare the athlete intrinsically from the standpoints of the musculoskeletal system and neuromuscular system, as well as with the psychologic aspects.

Preoperative Therapy

Before the operation, as far in advance as possible, the athlete should be educated on the proper techniques of core stabilization exercises. These exercises consist of drawing in the umbilicus and holding it. Then, progression into extremity movements while holding this drawn-in-umbilicus posture is performed. These exercises activate the deep abdominal muscles, specifically the transverse abdominis and obliques, which concurrently activate the multifidus, which together function to stabilize the pelvis and lumbar spine. The time period for this presurgical rehabilitation may vary as the time period from diagnosis to surgery may vary from days to months.

Postoperative Therapy

While we routinely try to get athletes back to full performance within 6 to 7 weeks after surgery, we describe here an off-season, 3-month rehabilitation process.

Phase I, Weeks 1 to 4 (Rest, Stand, Walk)

Weeks 1 through 4 make up phase I of the postoperative rehabilitation program. At this time, the patient is going to rest mainly, refrain from any strenuous activity, and work on maintaining normal upright posture, avoiding any ranges of pain.

Phase II, Weeks 5 to 7 (Core Stabilization and Pool Therapy)

Around week 5 the patient enters phase II. This phase is characterized by core stabilization and pool therapy exercises. At this time the most basic core stabilization exercises, which were learned preoperatively, should be implemented. By week 7 the athlete should progress

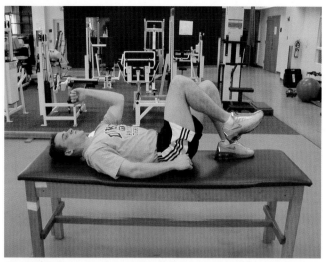

FIGURE 5.12. Supine marching. Begun early in phase II, this entails performing reciprocal arm and leg marching movements while maintaining the drawn-in umbilicus posture to create a focused contraction of the transversus abdominis muscle, which stabilizes the pelvis and lower back during a dynamic activity.

from supine marching (Figure 5.12) with reciprocal arm movements into a running motion simulation (Figure 5.13) with both feet off the ground, flexing opposite hip/knee and shoulder simultaneously. This is a continuum of the core stabilization progression and is training the trunk to stabilize under a stressful functional activity, as it must when returning to sports.

During week 5 it is also beneficial to begin very light stretching of the adductors. The objective here is to make sure the fibroblasts lay down in a parallel elastic arrangement to maintain flexibility and minimize scar shortening, in addition to achieving healing of the muscle in the lengthened state. Then, by week 6 the patient should begin light quadriceps and hip flexor stretching, while focusing on keeping a neutral pelvis. Any abdominal pain should be avoided.

The second directive of phase II focuses on pool therapy where the athlete may work in functional patterns. Pool walking is the first step, initiated at week 5. Later in the second month the patient progresses by increasing the distance and speed of the pool walking, so that pool running is achieved by week 7. At this time multidirectional activities, such as cariocas and side-slides, may also be incorporated in the pool. This strengthens all muscles involved in gait and initiates stress to the healing tissue in a manner that it will experience once returning to sport. Thus, the tissue will begin to heal, with both the ability to accommodate movement and at the same time to limit excessive motion during activity. Also at this time mini-squats, heel raises, and standing hip abduction/adduction/flexion/extension should be performed in the pool. On land the patient may begin elliptical running and straight leg raises (SLRs) in flexion/extension/abduction.

PHASE III, WEEKS 8 TO 10 (PROGRESSIONAL STRENGTHENING, ENDURANCE, AGILITY)

By week 8 the athlete should be advancing into phase III, which is characterized by progressive strengthening, endurance, and agility activities. This is a period in which the athlete's rehabilitation becomes more dynamic, intense, and functionally driven. This phase tests and strengthens all components of the musculoskeletal (including the new repair) and neuromuscular systems. The athlete is now well into the remodeling stage, and these exercises force the remodeling tissues to progressively develop to withstand repeated stress such as occurs during athletic competition.

WEEK 8

Week 8 exercises have been set up to give the patient some variability in exercises and also some choice in which exercises to do on each desired day (Table 5.4, Figures 5.14, 5.15, 5.16). It is constructed so each day the athlete will get abdominal and core stability training both statically and dynamically, cardiovascular work on a machine and, independently, lower extremity strengthening and balance training. By category, the patient is developing stability (category A), endurance (category B), strength (category C), and proprioception (category D). Categories A, B, and C may be mixed to the patient's predilection; however, category D should be performed last so we can first fatigue the musculoskeletal system to create an environment in which we could then tax and get as much gain out of the neuromuscular system as possible.

WEEK 9

The setup in week 9 is a progression toward gaining more sport-specific/functional training (Table 5.5, Fig-

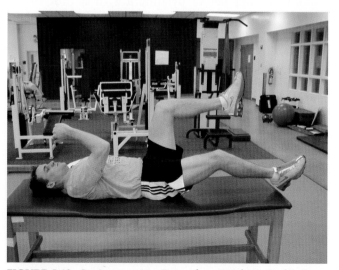

FIGURE 5.13. Supine running. Begun later in phase II, this is an exercise progressed from supine marching, which is done with the same drawn-in umbilicus posture to create a focused contraction of the transversus abdominis muscle, which stabilizes the pelvis and lower back during an even greater dynamic activity.

TABLE 5.4. Rehabilitation Protocol: Phase III, Week 8.[a]

Category A
    Group 1: Core-stabilization exercises (3 sets of 15 repetitions) + (daily sitting)
      Plank exercises (30 sec 2×, in all three directions) (see Figures 5.14, 5.15)
    Group 2: Crunches (20 repetitions 1–2× holding at top 2–3 sec) [stabilize pelvis]
      Push-ups (15–30 repetitions 2–3×)
Category B
    Group 1: Jogging ¹/₂ mile forward; 100 yards backward (straight only)
      Elliptical (30 min)
    Group 2: Pool exercises
      —Increase repetitions and intensity from week 6
        ——In deep well (with noodle floaties)
      —Reciprocal flexion/extension scissor kicking (1 min ×3)
      —Bilateral abduction/adduction (leg portion of jumping-jacks) (1 min ×3)
        Stationary bike (20–30 min)
Category C
    Group 1: Heel raises (increase reps: 2× unilateral, 1× bilateral)
      Minisquats (20–30 repetitions ×2)
    Group 2: Straight leg raises (2–3 sets) flexion/extension/abduction
Category D
    Group 1: Standing on *wobble board* (1 min ×3)
    Group 2: 1 leg standing on mini-tramp (mimic sport) (1 min ×3) (see Figure 5.16)

[a]One group from each of the four categories must be selected for each day, and the opposite group must be completed on the following day. Complete all stretching from week 6 (2× for 30 sec, 2–3 × per day).

ure 5.17). Running and agility work on land (category A) is now 66% of the rehabilitation, while the other 33% involves pool work and isolated strengthening (category B). Abdominal strengthening is a key component to protecting the repair; thus, it is involved 100% of the time. Now that the patient is involved in highly demanding athletic activity, it is important that a day of rest is given to ensure physiologic recovery. All stretching activities from the previous week should be continued.

Week 10
Week 10 is a further progression toward sport-specific training and returning to athletic competition (Table 5.6, Figure 5.18). Now running and sport-specific activity encompass 83% of the rehabilitation time,

while pool therapy and isolated strengthening make up 17%. Abdominal work and stretching are performed on all rehabilitation days, and again the rest day is essential for physiologic recovery of stressed tissues.

During week 10, specific activities that simulate particular aspects of the athlete's sport, such as cutting and changes of direction, should be initiated. This crucial aspect of the rehabilitation progression further tests and strengthens all components of both the musculoskeletal and neuromuscular system.

PHASE IV, WEEKS 11 AND 12 (SPORT SPECIFICS)

Weeks 11 and 12
Around week 11 the athlete enters phase IV of the rehabilitation protocol (Table 5.7, Figure 5.19). At this

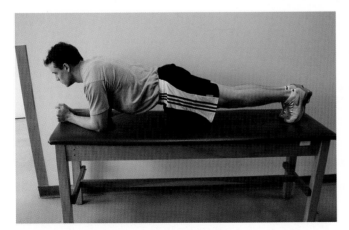

FIGURE 5.14. Plank exercise (prone). Begun in week 8, this exercise isometrically strengthens core stability through targeting all the abdominals. It is essential to maintain a straight and rigid core with a slightly posterior pelvic tilt.

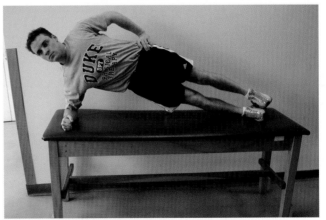

FIGURE 5.15. Plank exercise (side lying). Begun in week 8, this exercise also isometrically strengthens core stability, although in comparison with the prone plank exercise, the side-lying exercise focuses more on the internal and external oblique musculature.

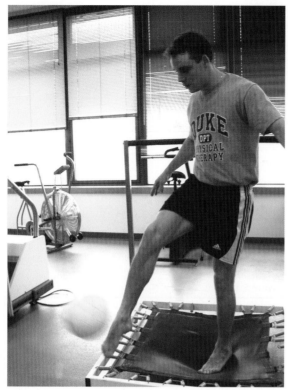

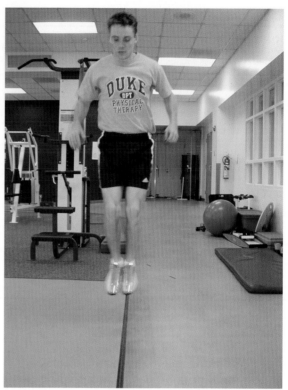

FIGURE 5.16. Mini-tramp (sport-specific activity). Begun in week 8 as part of category D, the athlete mimics a skilled activity specific to his or her respective sport while balancing one legged on a mini-tramp. This activity provides core and extremity strengthening while retraining the athlete's proprioception in a sport-specific manner.

FIGURE 5.17. Plyometrics (two-feet lateral hops). Began in week 9 of phase III, this is the introductory exercise of plyometrics. The athlete performs small, quick, side-to-side hops over a line on the floor. The duration of this exercise may initially be 30 seconds and progress up to 1 minute or more. Plyometrics are useful in training the neuromuscular and musculoskeletal systems for sport.

TABLE 5.5. Rehabilitation Protocol: Phase III, Week 9.[a]

Category A
  Jogging $^1/_2$ to 1 mile as tolerated and with good symmetric form
  Agility drills
    Backward running (30 yards 4×)
    Side-slides (30 yards 4× each direction)
    Cariocas (30 yards 4× each direction)
    Sprinting $^1/_2$ to $^3/_4$ speed ×4 (30–50 yards, with a 25 yard warm-up and slow-down)
    Figure 8's (15 yards × 5 yards, #8) (5 cycles 1–2× at $^1/_2$ to $^3/_4$ speed)
    Lunges (3 sets of 10)
    Plyometrics: Two feet together, small lateral jumps over a line (30–45 sec ×3)
  Abdominals
    Plank sxercises (45 sec 2×, in all three directions)
    Abdominal crunches (30 repetitions 2× holding at top 2–3 sec)
    Begin bilateral leg lowering exercise (10 repetitions 1–2×) (knees flexed to 90 degrees)
Category B
  Pool exercises as done in week 7
  Heel raises on land (increase reps, 2× unilateral, 1× bilateral)
  Minisquats with 5–10 lb dumbbells (30 repetitions 2–3×)
  Straight leg raises (SLR) (2–3 sets) flexion/extension/abduction/adduction (once repetitions of 10–10–15 are achieved, ankle
    weights in 2-lb increments may be added)
  Adduction is now added into the SLRs since abdominal strength has been increased and additional adductor strength is necessary
    for lateral agility movements.
  Abdominals
    Plank exercises (45 sec 2×, in all three directions)
    Abdominal crunches (30 repetitions 2× holding at top 2–3 sec)
    Begin bilateral leg lowering exercise (10 repetitions 1–2×) (knees flexed to 90 degrees)

[a]Two of 3 days category A will be performed, and on the third day category B will be performed. Two cycles of categories A and B equals 6 days; the 7th day is a rest day.

TABLE 5.6. Rehabilitation Protocol: Phase III, Week 10.

Category A[a]
  Jogging 1–1$^1/_4$ miles (with ball of particular sport) as tolerated and with good symmetric form
  Agility drills
    Backward running (50 yards 5×)
    Side-slides (50 yards 5× each direction)
    Cariocas (50 yards 5× each direction)
    Sprinting $^3/_4$ speed (75 yards, with a 25-yard warm-up and slow-down)
    Figure 8's with ball (15 yards × 5 yards, #8) (8 cycles 2× $^3/_4$ speed)
    Lunges (3 sets of 10)
    Polyometrics
    Two feet together, small lateral jumps over a line (45 sec ×2) (see Figure 5.17)
    Two feet together, small forward/backward jumps over a line (45 sec ×2)
    4 square (45 sec ×2)
  Push-ups
    Regular (30 repetitions ×2)
    Plyometric push-ups (15–20 ×2)
  Abdominals
    Plank exercises (45 sec–1 min, 2–3×, in all three directions)
    Abdominal crunches (30 repetitions 3× holding at top 2–3 sec) [may add weight to chest in 5-lb increments for increased resistance]
    Bilateral leg lowering exercise (15 repetitions 2×) (with knees extended)
  Proprioception
    Wobble board with one leg in middle of board (1–2 min ×3 each leg). Actively do a sports activity (kick soccer ball,
      catch/throw a baseball or football, etc.)
    Mini-tramp (2 min ×3 each leg); actively do a sports activity (as wobble board)
Category B[b]
  Hip machine (3 sets weight to tolerance) flexion/extension/abduction/adduction
  Pool exercises as done in week 8 with progression in repetitions and/or sets
  Heel raises on land (increase reps: 2× unilateral, 1× bilateral)
  Minisquats with 10–15 lb dumbbells (30 repetitions 3×)
  Abdominals
    Plank exercises (45 sec–1 min, 2–3×, in all three directions)
    Abdominal crunches (30 repetitions 3× holding at top 2–3 sec); may add weight to chest in 5-lb increments for increased resistance
    Bilateral leg lowering exercise (15 repetitions 2×) (with knees extended) (see Figure 5.18A, B)X

[a]Category A is to be performed 5 days of a 7-day period; category B is to be performed 1 day of the 7 days, and the 7th day is a rest day.
[b]2× per week.

time sport-specific exercise should be the major focus of the training sessions while increasing the running mileage in $^1/_4$-mile increments. The goal at this point is to incorporate all aspects and every motion that oc-curs in the athlete's particular sport into rehabilita-tion before returning to athletic competition.

In addition, a base of exercises should be incorpo-rated to complete the recovery process. Plyometrics

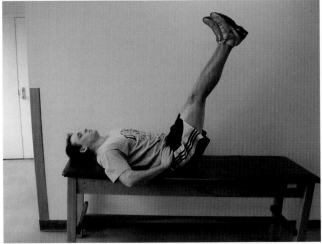

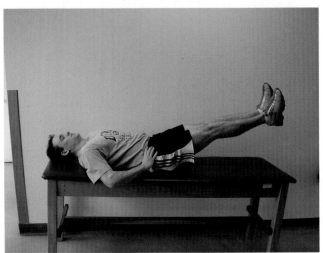

A

B

FIGURE 5.18. Bilateral leg lowering. Begun in week 9, this exer-cise requires a good deal of attention and guidance on behalf of the therapist or athletic trainer. The athlete begins lying in supine with hips flexed to 90 degrees and knees extended (A). Pelvic stabiliza-tion via the drawn in umbilicus should be used and maintained throughout the following movement. From this position, the legs are lowered by eccentric contraction of the hip flexors to a point at which the pelvis begins to tilt anteriorly (B). This anterior tilt sig-nifies the inability of the abdominals to isometrically stabilize the pelvis any further. Immediately at this point the legs are slowly brought back up to 90 degrees of hip flexion. As abdominal strength increases, the athlete should be able to lower his or her legs further toward the floor before allowing an anterior tilt and having to raise them to their starting position.

TABLE 5.7. Rehabilitation Protocol: Phase IV, Weeks 11 and 12.

Plyometrics
    Single-foot small lateral jumps over a line (45 sec ×2 each foot) (see Figure 5.19)
    Single small forward/backward jumps over a line (45 sec ×2 each foot)
    4 square with one foot (45 sec ×2 each foot)
    Large lateral jumps (45 sec 2–3×)
Push-ups
    Regular (30 repetitions ×2)
    Plyometric push-ups (15–20 ×3)
Hip machine should still be done twice per week (3 sets)
Pool exercises can be used sparingly to change up rehabilitation (once every 2 weeks)
Proprioception
    Increase wobble board and mini-tramp difficulty and time in one standing

should be increased, and pool exercises can be used sparingly to change the program. Abdominal exercises should be performed daily. The patient should try to complete them at the site of training intermittently with sport-specific drills to overload the muscles and force them to function under fatigue. Through basic physiologic principles, we know this is how we are going to make them stronger and more effective in a sports-specific manner. The patient should gradually work into this concept to prevent an additional injury from occurring.

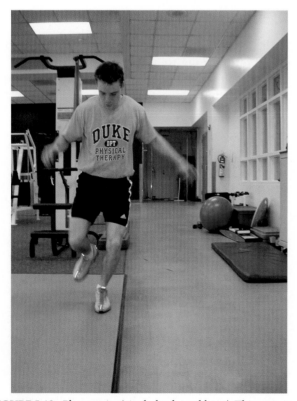

FIGURE 5.19. Plyometrics (single-leg lateral hops). This exercise is performed as a continuum to the two-feet lateral hops. The athlete performs small, quick, side-to-side hops over a line on the floor using only one foot. The duration of the exercise may also begin at 30 seconds and progress to 1 minute or more.

PHASE V, 3 MONTHS (RETURN TO PLAY)

Around the third month postoperatively, the athlete should be progressively returning to practice and, soon after, to competition. The athlete must be completely prepared physically, technically, and psychologically before fully entering athletic competition. This remains the combined responsibility of the health care staff, coach, and athlete to ensure safety and efficiency in returning to sport. It is also important to maintain abdominal and core strengthening even with the return to competition to prevent any future injuries.

OTHER DIFFERENTIAL DIAGNOSES OF EXTRAARTICULAR HIP PAIN

Several other diagnoses must be considered in patients with groin pain, including other musculoskeletal disorders, as well as more severe visceral problems. Problems that we have encountered in patients with inguinal pain include inflammatory bowel disease, prostatitis, aseptic necrosis of the hips, herpes, pelvic inflammatory disease, and rectal or testicular cancer.[101] These other possible diagnoses emphasize the importance of a detailed, careful history and physical examination. Musculoskeletal syndromes commonly considered in the differential diagnosis of lower abdominal or groin pain in the athlete include adductor injuries,[102] piriformis and hamstring syndromes,[65,102–104] *snapping* hip syndrome,[101] iliopsoas tendonitis,[105] iliotibial band syndrome,[102] sacroiliac sprain,[96] osteitis pubis,[16] stress fractures,[106] soft tissue injuries,[101] contusions,[105] bursitis,[107] and myositis ossificans.[96]

Extraarticular Sources of Hip Pain in Women

Athletic pubalgia in female athletes is very rare. Although the exact reason for this is unknown, it is hypothesized that anatomic differences in the pelvis may play a major role. Although athletic pubalgia is a possible cause of groin pain in women, endometriosis-associated lower abdominal or inguinal pain is much more common.

Other sources of groin pain in women have been noted to be ovarian cystic disease, pelvic inflammatory disease, symptomatic Crohn's disease, and menstrually cyclical nonexertional pain that was without a known cause. It has also been suggested that with a direct connection between the uterus and frequent finding of endometriosis embedded in the round ligament that traction has something to do with the accompanying pain. If one of these pathologies is suspected, then laparoscopy is suggested to confirm and correct any abnormality that may be present.

OTHER SOURCES OF HIP PAIN

Although the scope of this chapter is to identify the extraarticular causes of hip pain, for completeness sake, we would like to briefly mention a few intraarticular sources of hip pain. Intraarticular hip pathology may be an important cause of groin or thigh pain. Some of the more important or more frequent diagnoses to consider include synovitis, loose congenital or traumatic bodies, septic or osteoarthritis, avascular necrosis, torn acetabular labrum, or a hypertrophied ligamentum teres.

References

1. Abrams, M Sedlezky I, Stearns DB: Osteitis pubis. N Engl J Med 1949;240:637–641.
2. Coventry MB, William MC: Osteitis pubis: observations based on a study of 45 patients. JAMA 1961;178:898–905.
3. Gamble JG, Simmons SC, Freedman M: The symphysis pubis. Anatomic and pathologic considerations. Clin Orthop 1986;203:261–272.
4. Harris NH, Murray RG: Lesions of the symphysis pubis in athletes. In: Proceedings of the British Orthopaedic Association. J Bone Joint Surg [Br] 1974;56:563–564.
5. Lentz SSV: Osteitis pubis: a review. Obstet Gynecol Surg 1995;50:310–315.
6. Leagueu MB, Rochet WL: Les cellulites perivesicales et pelviennes après certaines cystostomies ou prostatectomies suspubiennes. J Urol Med Chir 1923;15:1–11.
7. Beer E: Periostitis and ostitis of symphysis and rami of pubis following suprapubic cystotomies. J Urol 1928;20:233–236.
8. Grace JN, Sim FH, Shives TC, Coventry MB: Wedge resection of the symphysis pubis for the treatment of osteitis pubis. J Bone Joint Surg [Am] 1989;71:358–364.
9. Fricker P, Taunton J, Ammann W: Osteitis pubis in athletes: infection, inflammatory or injury? Sports Med 1991;12:266–279.
10. Major NM, Helms CA: Pelvic stress injuries: the relationship between osteitis pubis (symphysis pubis stress injury) and sacroiliac abnormalities in athletes. Skeletal Radiol 1997;26:711–717.
11. Verral GM, Slavotinek JP, Fon GT: Incidence of pubic bone marrow oedema in Australian rules football players: relationship to groin pain. Br J Sports Med 2000;35:28–33.
12. Benson ER, Schutzer SF: Posttraumatic piriformis syndrome: diagnosis and results of operative treatment. J Bone Joint Surg [Am] 1999;81:941–949.
13. Chamberlain W: The symphysis pubis in the roentgenol examination of the sacro-iliac joint Am J Roentgenol 1930;24:621–625.
14. Miguel A: Groin pain and adductor muscle release. Presented at the International Football and Sports Medicine Conference, Los Angeles, CA, March 22–24, 2002.
15. Spinelli A: Nuova malattia sportive. La pubialgia degli schemitori. Ortopedia e Traumatologia Dell Apparto Motore 1932;4:111–127.
16. Wiley JJ: Traumatic osteitis pubis: the gracilis syndrome. Am J Sports Med 1983;11:360–363.
17. Holt MA, Keene JS, Graf BK, Helwig DC: Treatment of osteitis pubis in athletes. Results of corticosteroid injections. Am J Sports Med 1995;23:601–606.
18. Walheim G, Olerun S, Ribbe T: Mobility of the pubic symphysis measurements by an electromechanical method. Acta Orthop Scand 1984;55:20–208.
19. Ekberg O, Blomquist P, Olsson S: Positive contrast herniography in adult patients with obscure groin pain. Surgery (St. Louis) 1981;89:532–535.
20. Hanson PG, Angive, Juhl J: Osteitis pubis in sports activities. Physician Sportsmed 1978;10:111–114.
21. Sequeira W, Jones E, Siegal M, Lorenz M, Kallick C: Pyogenic infections of the pubic symphysis. Ann Intern Med 1982;96:60–66.
22. Renstrom P: Pelvic and groin injuries: an overview. Presented at the International Football and Sports Medicine Conference, Los Angeles, CA, March 22–24, 2002.
23. Williams PR, Thomas DP, Downes EM: Osteitis pubis and instability of the pubic symphysis. When nonoperative measures fail. Am J Sports Med 2000;28:350–255.
24. Goldstein AE, Rubin SW: Osteitis pubis following suprapubic prostatectomy. Am J Surg 1947;74:480.
25. Stutter BD: Complications of osteitis pubis including report of case of sequestrum formation giving rise to persistent purulent urethritis. Br J Surg 1954;42;164–172.
26. Watkin NA, Gallegos CR, Moisey CU: Osteitis pubis. A case of successful treatment with anticoagulants. Acta Orthop Scand 1995;66:569–570.
27. Waters P, Millis M: Hip and pelvic injuries in the young athlete. Clin Sports Med 1988;7:513–526.
28. Miller J, Schultz A, Anderson G: Load displacement behavior of the sacroiliac joints. Orthop Res 1987;5:92–101.
29. Briggs RC, Kolbjornsen PH, Southall RC: Clin Nucl Med 1992;17:861–863.
30. Smodlaka VN: Groin pain in soccer players. Physician Sports Med 1980;8:57–61.
31. Lynch SA, Renstrom P: Groin injuries in sports: treatment strategies. Sports Med 1999;28:137–144.
32. Taylor DC, Meyers WC, Moylans JA, Lohnes J, Basset FH, Garrett WE: Abdominal musculature abnormalities as a cause of groin pan in athletes; inguinal hernias and pubalgia. Am J Sports Med 1991;19:239–242.
33. Smedberg SGG, Broome AEA, Gullmo A, Roos H: Herniography in athletes with groin pain. Am J Surg 1985;149:378–382.
34. Gilmore J: Groin pain in the soccer athlete: fact, fiction, and treatment. Clin Sports Med 1998;17:787–793.
35. Akita K, Niga S, Yamato Y, Muneta T, Sato T: Anatomic basis of chronic groin pain with special reference to sports hernia. Surg Radiol Anat 1999;21:1–5.
36. Bradshaw C, McCrory P, Bell S, Brunker P: Obturator nerve entrapment. A cause of groin pain in athletes. Am J Sports Med 1997;25:402–408.
37. Lee CH, Dellon AL: Surgical management of groin pain of neural origin. J Am Coll Surg 2000;191:137–142.
38. Sexton DJ, Heskestad L, Lambeth WR, McCallum R, Levin LS, Corey GR: Postoperative pubic osteomyelitis misdiagnosed as osteitis pubis: report of four cases and review. Clin Infect Dis 1993;17:695–700.

39. Sutro CJ: The pubic bones and their symphysis. Arch Surg 1936;32:823.

40. Holmich P, Uhrskou P, Ulnits L, et al: Effectiveness of active physical training as treatment for long-standing adductor-related groin pain in athletes: randomised trial. Lancet 1999;353(9151):439–443.

41. Moore RS, Stover MD, Matta JM: Late posterior instability of the pelvis after resection of the symphysis pubis for the treatment of osteitis pubis. J Bone Joint Surg [Am] 1998;80:1043–1048.

42. Papadopoulos AM, McGillicuddy JE, Albers JA: Unusual causes of piriformis muscle syndrome. Arch Neurol 1990;47:1144–1146.

43. Freiberg AH, Vinke TH: Sciatica and the sacroiliac joint. J Bone Joint Surg 1934;16:126–139.

44. Rodrigue T, Hardy RW: Diagnosis and treatment of piriformis syndrome. Neurosurg Clin N Am 2001;12:311–319.

45. Yeoman W: The relationship of arthritis of the sacroiliac joint to the sciatica. Lancet 1928;2:1119–1122.

46. Edwards FO: Pyriformis syndrome. In: Yearbook of Selected Osteopathic Papers. Colorado Springs: American Academy of Osteopathy, 1962:39–41.

47. Beaton LE, Anson BJ: The relationship of the sciatic nerve and its subdivision to the piriformis muscle. J Bone Joint Surg 1938;20:686–688.

48. McCrory P: The "piriformis syndrome": myth or reality? Br J Sports Med 2001;35:209–210.

49. Brown JA, Braun MA, Namey TC: Piriformis syndrome in a 10 year old boy as a complication or operation with the patient in the sitting position. Neurosurgery 1988;23:117–119.

50. Uchio Y, Nishikawa U, Ochi M, Shu N, Takata K: Bilateral piriformis syndrome after total hip arthroplasty. Arch Orthop Trauma Surg 1998;117:177–179.

51. Beauchesne RP, Schutzer SF: Myositis ossificans of the piriformis muscle; an unusual cause of piriformis syndrome. J Bone Joint Surg [Am] 1997;79:906–910.

52. Chen WS: Bipartite piriformis muscle: an unusual cause of sciatic nerve entrapment. Pain 1994;58:269–272.

53. Hughes SS, Goldstein MN, Hick DG, Pellegrini VD: Extrapelvic compression of the sciatic nerve. J Bone Joint Surg [Am] 1992;74:1553–1559.

54. Pace JB, Nagle D: Piriformis syndrome. West J Med 1976;124:435–439.

55. Robinson DR: Pyriformis syndrome in relation to sciatic pain. Am J Surg 1947;73:355–358.

56. Vandertop WP, Bosma NJ: The piriformis syndrome. J Bone Joint Surg [Am] 1991;73:1095–1097.

57. Sayson SC, Ducey JP, Maybrey JB, Wesley RL, Vermilion D: Sciatic entrapment neuropathy associated with an anomalous piriformis muscle. Pain 1994;59:149–152.

58. Freiberg AH: Sciatic pain and its relief by operations on the muscle and fascia. Arch Surg 1937;34:337–350.

59. Mizuguchi T: Division of the piriformis muscle for the treatment of sciatica. Arch Surg 1976;111:719–722.

60. Petersilge CA, Yoo JU, Boswell MV, et al: MR examination of the greater sciatic notch of patients with a clinical diagnosis of piriformis syndrome. J Radiology (in press).

61. Solheim LF, Siewers P, Paus B: The piriformis muscle syndrome. Sciatic nerve entrapment treated with section of the piriformis muscle. Acta Orthop Scand 1981;52:73–75.

62. Jankiewicz JJ, Hennrikus WL, Houkom JA: The appearance of the piriformis muscle syndrome in computed tomography and magnetic resonance imaging. Clin Orthop Relat Res 1991;262:2075–2079.

63. Rossi P, Cardinali P, Serrao M, Parisi L, Bianco F, De Bac S: Magnetic resonance imaging findings in piriformis syndrome: a case report. Arch Phys Med Rehabil 2001;82:519–521.

64. Fishman LM, Dombi GW, Michaelsen C, et al: Piriformis syndrome: diagnosis, treatment, and outcome-a 10-year study. Arch Phys Med Rehabil 2002;83:295–301.

65. Fishman LM, Zybert PA: Electrophysiologic evidence of piriformis syndrome. Arch Phys Med Rehabil 1992;73:359–364.

66. Karl RD Jr, Yedivach MA, Hartshome MF, et al: Scintigraphic appearance of the piriformis muscle syndrome Clin Nucl Med 1985;10:361–363.

67. Synek V: Short latency somatosensory evoked potentials in patients with painful dysaesthesias in peripheral nerve lesions. Pain 1987;29:49–58.

68. Rask MR: Superior gluteal nerve entrapment syndrome. Muscle Nerve 1980;3:304–307.

69. Barton PM: Piriformis syndrome: a rational approach to management Pain 1991;47:345–352.

70. Kirkaldy-Willis WH, Hill RJ: A more precise diagnosis for low back pain. Spine 1979;4:102–109.

71. Mullin V, de Rosayro M: Caudal steroid injection for treatment of piriformis syndrome. Anesth Analg 1990;7:705–707.

72. Fanucci E, Masala S, Sodani G, et al: CT-guided injection of botulinic toxin for percutaneous therapy of piriformis muscle syndrome with preliminary MRI results about denervative process. Eur Radiol 2001;11:2543–2548.

73. Gray H: Myology. In: Williams P, Warwick R (eds). Gray's Anatomy, 36th ed. London: Churchill Livingstone, 1990:595–596.

74. Harvey G, Bell S: Obturator neuropathy. An anatomic perspective. Clin Orthop 1999;363:203–211.

75. Sorenson EJ, Chen JJ, Daube JR: Obturator neuropathy: causes and outcomes. Muscle Nerve 2002;25:605–607.

76. Kleiner JB, Thorne RP: Obturator neuropathy caused by an aneurism of the hypogastric artery. J Bone Joint Surg [Am] 1989;71:1408–1409.

77. Kozlowski JM, Beal JM: Obturator hernia: an elusive diagnosis. Arch Surg 1977;112:1001–1002.

78. Redwine DB, Sharpe DR: Endometriosis of the obturator nerve. A case report. J Reprod Med 1990;35:434–435.

79. Rogers LR, Borkowski GP, Albers JW, Levin KH, Barohn RJ, Mitsumoto H: Obturator mononeuropathy caused by pelvic cancer: six cases. Neurology 1993;43:1489–1492.

80. Bischoff C, Schonle PW: Obturator nerve injuries during intra-abdominal surgery. Clin Neurol Neurosurg 1991;93:73–76.

81. Pellegrino MJ, Johnson EW: Bilateral obturator nerve injuries during urologic surgery. Arch Phys Med Rehabil 1988;69:46–47.

82. Siliski JM, Scott RD: Obturator nerve palsy resulting from intra-pelvic extrusion of cement during total hip replacement. Report of four cases. J Bone Joint Surg [Am] 1985;67:1225–1228.

83. Warner MA, Warner DO, Harper CM, Schroeder DR, Maxson PM: Lower extremity neuropathies associated with lithotomy position. Anesthesiology 2000;93:938–942.

84. Peri G: The "critical zones" of entrapment of the nerves of the lower limb. Surg Radiol Anat 1991;13:139–143.

85. Busis N: Femoral and obturator neuropathies. Neurol Clin 1999;17:633–652.

86. Kimura J: Electrodiagnosis in Diseases of Nerve and Muscle. Principles and Practice, 2nd ed. Philadelphia: Davis, 1989:5506–509.

87. Anderson K, Strichland SM, Warren R: Hip and groin injuries in athletes. Am J Sports Med 2001;29:521–533.

88. Harms BA, DeHaas DR, Starling JR: Diagnosing and management of genitofemoral neuralgia. Arch Surg 1984;119:339–341.

89. Meyers WC, Foley DP, Garrett WE Jr, et al: Management of severe lower abdominal or inguinal pain in high-performance athletes. Am J Sports Med 2000;28:2–8.

90. Meyers WC, Foley DP, Mandelbaum BR, et al: Successful management of severe lower abdominal or inguinal pain in high performance athletes. (Submitted manuscript).

91. Meyers WC, Lanfranco A, Castellanos A: Surgical management

of chronic lower abdominal and groin pain in high-performance athletes. Curr Sports Med Rep 2002;I:301–305.

92. Meyers WC, Ricciardi R, Busconi BD, Mandelbaum BR, Waite RJ: Athletic pubalgia and groin pain. In: Principles and Practice of Orthopaedic Sports Medicine. 2000:223–230.

93. Hackney RG: The sports hernia: a cause of chronic groin pain. Br J Sports Med 1993;27:58–62.

94. Pro Hockey Athletic Trainers Meeting, Salt Lake City, UT, June 21–24, 1997.

95. Gross ML, Nasser S, Finerman GAM: Hip and pelvis. In: DeLee JC, Drez DJ (eds). Orthopaedic Sports Medicine. Philadelphia: Saunders, 1994.

96. Anson BJ, Morgan EH, McVay CB: Surgical anatomy of the inguinal region based upon a study of 500 body-halves. Suvremenna Meditsina 1960;111:707–725.

97. Ingoldby CJH: Laparoscopic and conventional repair of groin disruption in sportsmen. Br J Surg 1997;84:213–215.

98. Williams P, Foster ME: Gilmore's groin—or is it? Br J Sports Med 1995;29:206–208.

99. Ashby EC: Chronic obscure groin pain is commonly caused by enthesopathy: 'tennis elbow' of the groin. Br J Surg 1994;81:1632–1634.

100. Renstrom AFH: Tendon and muscle injuries in the groin area. Clin Sports Med 1992;11:815–830.

101. Griffin LH: Sports Medicine. Rosemont, IL: American Academy of Orthopaedic Surgeons, 1994.

102. Puranen J, Orava S: The hamstring syndrome: a new diagnosis of gluteal sciatic pain. Am J Sports Med 1988;16:517–521.

103. Puranen J, Orava S: The hamstring syndrome: a new gluteal sciatica. Ann Chir Gynaecol 1991;80:212–214.

104. Busconi B, McCarthy J: Hip and pelvic injuries in the skeletally immature athlete. Sports Med Arthrosc Rev 1996;4:132–157.

105. Knapp TP, Mandelbaum BR: Stress fractures. In: The U.S. Soccer Sports Medicine Book 327–345.

106. Renstrom P, Peterson L: Groin injuries in athletes. Br J Sports Med 1980;14:30–36.

107. Gilmore OJ: Gilmore's groin—ten years of experience of groin disruption. Sports Med Soft Tissue Trauma 1992;3(3): .

6

Gross Anatomy

J.W. Thomas Byrd

The four distinguishing features of a diarthrodial (synovial) joint are (1) a joint cavity, (2) articular cartilage, (3) synovial membrane producing synovial fluid, and (4) a ligamentous capsule. Ball-and-socket joints demonstrate multiaxial articulations and are one of six types of diarthrodial joints. Hip motion most closely represents the true ball-and-socket configuration. This configuration has significant implications for the technical ability to assess this joint arthroscopically.

Additionally, the hip is the joint most densely encased by its soft tissue envelope, necessitating extra-length arthroscopic instruments. More importantly, it requires significant skills in localization and triangulation techniques to instrument the joint, challenging the surgeon's proprioceptive abilities.

Distraction is usually employed to separate the articular surfaces sufficiently to allow for introduction of the arthroscope and operative instruments. Distraction must overcome the powerful musculature surrounding the hip as well as the dense ligamentous capsule. Adequate relaxation, whether through general or epidural anesthesia, negates the dynamic muscle compressive forces, leaving only minimal static muscle effects. However, the dense capsule, measuring more than 0.5 cm in thickness in some areas, represents a formidable static restraint to distraction, necessitating the magnitude of traction forces often required in hip arthroscopy. With maintained tension, even this dense, relatively noncompliant structure can relax through the process of physiologic creep, often allowing the ability to adequately distract the hip without having to rely on excessive force. Understanding these anatomic and structural principles is important in the ability to perform effective arthroscopy.

The surgeon must be properly oriented and aware of the important extraarticular structures, as with any joint.[1,2] This preparation begins with proper knowledge of the topographic anatomy, which is critical to interpreting the spatial relationship of deep structures.

TOPOGRAPHIC ANATOMY

Palpation of the bony landmarks about the hip is straightforward. It is nonetheless important to appreciate these landmarks and understand their relationship to the deep soft tissue structures. The principal landmarks include the greater trochanter, anterior superior iliac spine, pubic symphysis, iliac crest, posterior iliac spine, and the ischium (Figure 6.1).

Two and perhaps three of these landmarks are critical for proper orientation during arthroscopy (Figure 6.2).[3–5] The principal landmark is the greater trochanter; its superior margin as well as its anterior and posterior borders must be noted. The anterior superior iliac spine is the second important landmark for determining the position of the anterior portal. The surgeon needs to be careful not to compromise the exposure of these areas during draping of the patient.

The pubic symphysis has been used by some authors as a landmark for establishing the position of the anterior portal.[6,7] Palpation and orientation are reproducible, but must be done before draping the patient, as it is difficult to incorporate this area into the operative field.

MUSCULATURE

The hip musculature can be conceptualized as a superficial layer and a deep layer. The fascia lata covers the entire hip region including the three muscles that make up the superficial layer: the tensor fascia lata, sartorius, and gluteus maximus (Figure 6.3). The fascia lata also splits to cover the deep and superficial surface of the tensor fascia lata and gluteus maximus encasing these muscles. The tensor fascia lata and the gluteus maximus insert as a continuation, forming the iliotibial band. The gluteus maximus also partly inserts into the proximal femur at the gluteal tuberosity. This fibromuscular sheath was described by Henry[8] as the "pelvic deltoid," reflecting the fashion in which it covers the hip much as the deltoid muscle covers the shoulder. Interestingly, the gluteus maximus is the largest muscle in the body, and the sartorius, which crosses two joints, although quite weak, is the longest.

The gluteus medius has a transitional relationship between the superficial and deep musculature layers (Figures 6.3, 6.4). Its origin from the iliac crest is relatively superficial and covered by a portion of the

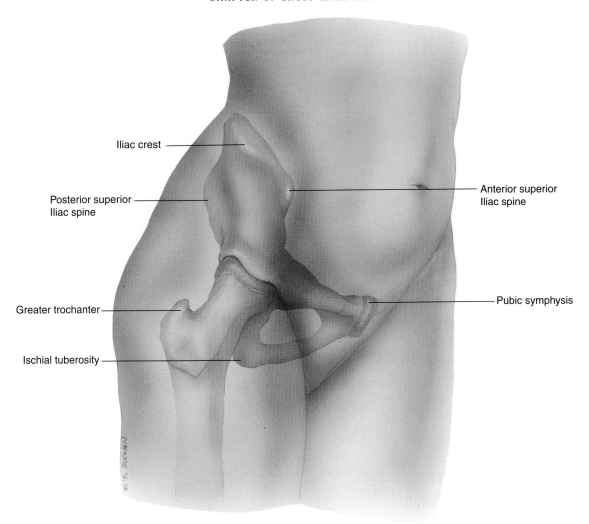

FIGURE 6.1. Palpation requires thorough knowledge of the topographic anatomy.

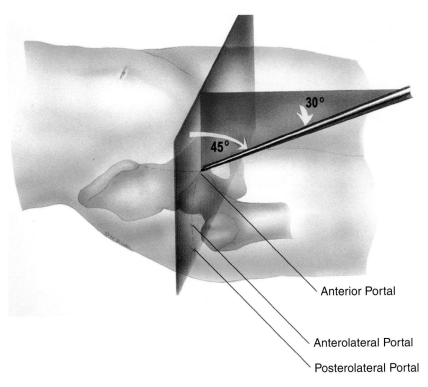

FIGURE 6.2. The lateral two portals (anterolateral and posterolateral) are placed directly over the superior margin of the greater trochanter at its anterior and posterior borders. The anterior portal is positioned at the site of intersection of a sagittal line drawn distally from the anterior superior iliac spine and a transverse line across the tip of the greater trochanter.

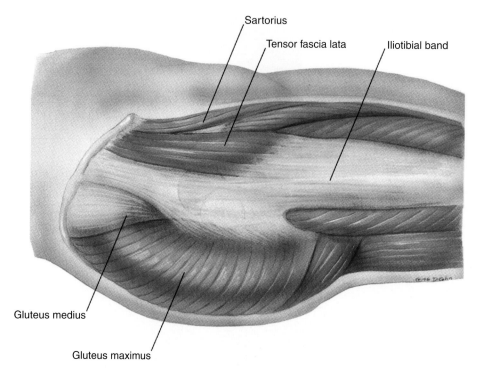

Sartorius

Tensor fascia lata

Iliotibial band

Gluteus medius

Gluteus maximus

FIGURE 6.3. Superficial muscular layer of the hip.

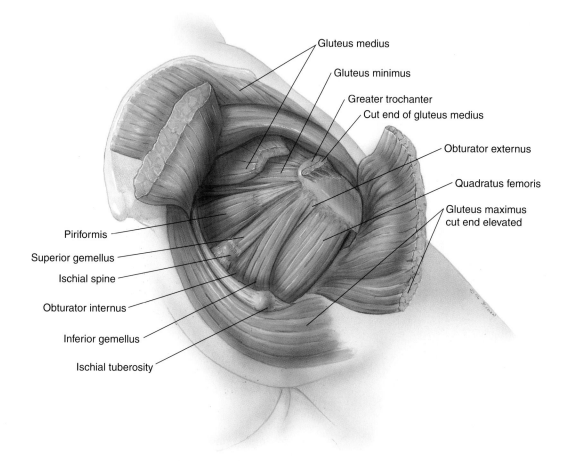

Gluteus medius

Gluteus minimus

Greater trochanter

Cut end of gluteus medius

Obturator externus

Quadratus femoris

Gluteus maximus
cut end elevated

Piriformis

Superior gemellus

Ischial spine

Obturator internus

Inferior gemellus

Ischial tuberosity

FIGURE 6.4. Deep structures (posterior view).

fascia lata, whereas its insertion into the greater trochanter corresponds with the deep muscles.

Posteriorly, the deep muscle layer includes the piriformis, the obturator internus with a common tendinous insertion including the superior and inferior gemelli, the obturator externus, and the quadratus femoris (see Figure 6.4). Laterally, the gluteus minimus lies on the deep surface of the gluteus medius. Anteriorly, the origin of the rectus femoris, including its direct and reflected heads, covers the anterior capsule (Figure 6.5). Just anterior to this is the iliopsoas tendon, formed from the muscles of the iliacus and psoas major inside the pelvis, coursing on the way to its insertion on the lesser trochanter.

Medially, the hip is bordered by the adductor muscle group including the adductor longus, magnus, and brevis, and the gracilis (see Figure 6.5). These muscles are of limited clinical significance for hip arthroscopy except when considering a medial approach to the joint, which has been described as a technical entity, but has thus far found limited clinical application.[9]

NEUROVASCULAR STRUCTURES

The femoral neurovascular structures (nerve, artery, and vein) exit the pelvis under the inguinal ligament halfway between the anterior superior iliac spine and the pubic tubercle (Figure 6.6). They are relatively anterior to the hip joint, with the nerve being the most lateral. These structures lie on the anterior surface of the iliopsoas muscle, and thus the muscle separates the femoral neurovascular structures from the hip.

The lateral femoral cutaneous nerve originates from the lumbar plexus and exits the pelvis under the inguinal ligament close to the anterior superior iliac spine (see Figure 6.6). This nerve is known to be sensitive to external compression (meralgia paresthetica). It is also known to be vulnerable to injury during harvesting of iliac crest bone graft when the harvest site is carried too close to the anterior superior iliac spine and to damage by improperly placed arthroscopic portals.

The lateral circumflex femoral artery arises from the profunda femoris (deep femoral artery) shortly af-

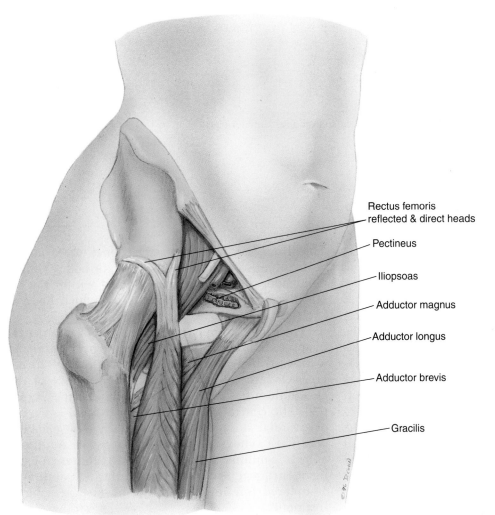

Rectus femoris
reflected & direct heads

Pectineus

Iliopsoas

Adductor magnus

Adductor longus

Adductor brevis

Gracilis

FIGURE 6.5. Deep structures (anterior view).

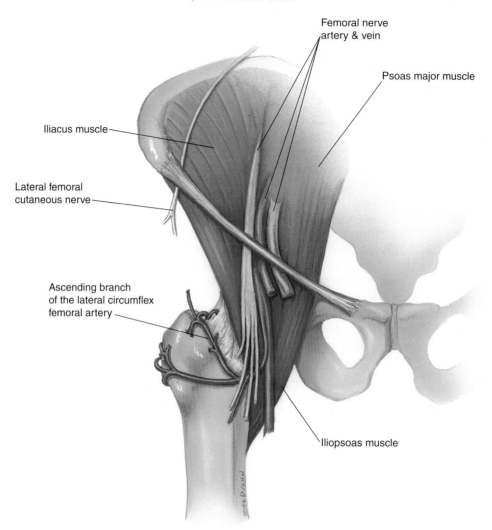

FIGURE 6.6. Neurovascular structures (anterior view).

ter it takes off from the femoral artery (see Figure 6.6). The ascending branch of the lateral circumflex femoral artery has an oblique course along the direction of the intertrochanteric line.

The superior gluteal nerve and artery are the most superior of 10 neurovascular structures that exit through the sciatic notch (Figure 6.7). They course transversely in a posterior to anterior direction between the deep surface of the gluteus medius and the superficial surface of the gluteus minimus, innervating and supplying blood to both. The sciatic nerve exits the notch under the piriformis tendon and then lies posterior to the other short external rotators in a vertical direction as it courses distally (see Figure 6.7).

An intricate vascular anastomosis converges at the lower border of the quadratus femoris consisting of the ascending branch of the first perforating artery, the descending branch of the inferior gluteal artery, and transverse branches of the medial and lateral circumflex femoral arteries (see Figure 6.7).

CAPSULAR AND JOINT ARCHITECTURE

The ilium, ischium, and pubic bones unite at the acetabulum, forming the innominate bone. During childhood, these bones are separated within the acetabulum by the triradiate cartilage, which fuses at skeletal maturity.

The acetabulum has an inclined abduction angle of approximately 35 degrees from the horizontal and a forward flexed position of approximately 20 degrees (Figure 6.8A,C). The articular surface of the acetabulum has a horseshoe or lunate shape (Figure 6.9). The central inferior acetabular fossa is devoid of articular surface. It is occupied by a fat pad covered with synovium called the pulvinar. Additionally, it contains the acetabular attachment of the ligamentum teres. The socket of the acetabulum is completed inferiorly by the transverse acetabular ligament.

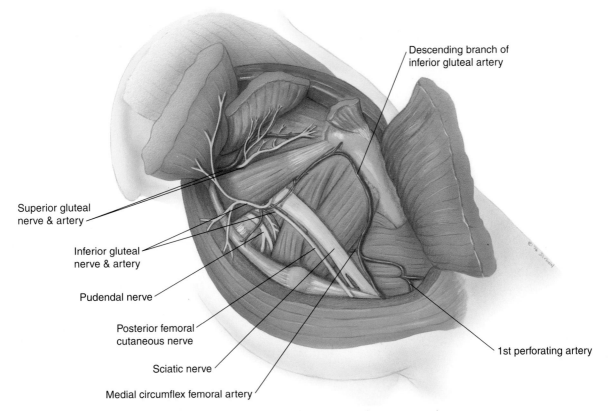

FIGURE 6.7. Neurovascular structures (posterior view).

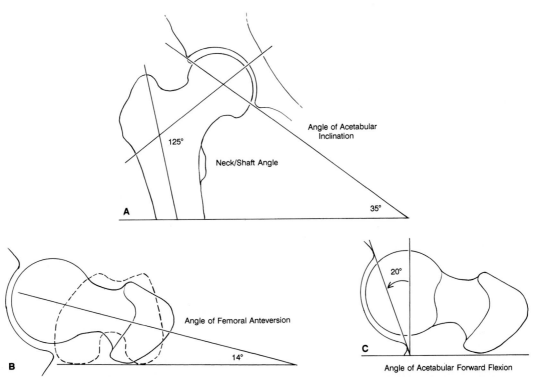

FIGURE 6.8. (A) Acetabular orientation averages 35 degrees of abduction from the horizontal plane. The neck shaft angle formed between the axis of the femoral neck and femoral shaft averages 125 degrees. (B) Femoral anteversion, determined by the angle created between the bicondylar axis of the knee and the axis of the femoral neck in the transverse plane, averages 14 degrees. (C) The acetabulum is also oriented with 20 degrees of forward flexion relative to the sagittal plane.

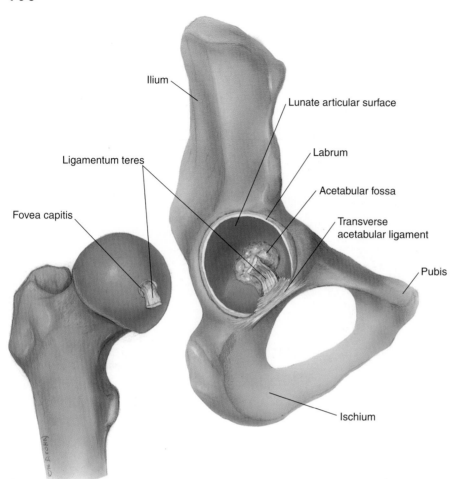

Ilium

Lunate articular surface

Labrum

Acetabular fossa

Transverse
acetabular ligament

Ligamentum teres

Fovea capitis

Pubis

Ischium

FIGURE 6.9. Formed from portions of the ilium, ischium, and pubis, the lunate-shaped articular surface of the acetabulum surrounds the fossa containing the acetabular attachment of the ligamentum teres and fat, both encased in synovium. The labrum effectively deepens the socket and is contiguous with the transverse acetabular ligament inferiorly. The articular surface of the femoral head forms approximately two-thirds of a sphere. Medially, the ligamentum teres attaches at the fovea capitis. The diameter of the femoral neck is only 65% of the diameter of the femoral head, which allows for freer range of motion without marginal impingement.

The labrum is a fibrocartilaginous structure that attaches to the bony rim of the acetabulum, effectively deepening to a socket. The labrum terminates inferiorly at the anterior and posterior margins of the acetabular fossa. It then becomes contiguous with the transverse acetabular ligament, which completes the circumferential ring of the acetabulum. We are learning that the labrum is a nonhomogeneous structure with considerable variation in different areas of the acetabulum (see Chapter 8).

Although variable, the proximal femur has a neck shaft angle that averages 125 degrees, with approximately 14 degrees of femoral neck anteversion (see Figure 6.8A,B). The femoral head has an articular surface that forms approximately two-thirds of a sphere, articulating with the acetabulum (see Figure 6.9). Medially, on the articular portion of the femoral head, is a pit called the fovea capitis, the site of the femoral attachments of the ligamentum teres.

The bony architecture of the hip provides it with significant intrinsic stability. This stability is further enhanced by an intricate complex of capsular ligaments. This complex consists of four distinct ligaments that provide varying contributions to the joint.

The intricate nature and specific design of the capsular ligaments has been well defined by various anatomic studies. However, over time, more will be learned about the ligaments as a better appreciation is gained of the arthroscopic appearance of this anatomy. Perhaps this construct will even be partially redefined.

Anteriorly, the capsule consists primarily of the iliofemoral ligament or ligament of Bigelow (Figure 6.10). It has an inverted Y shape beginning from its iliac attachment on the superior aspect of the acetabulum. It then fans out in a spiraling pattern to its femoral attachment along the intertrochanteric line. It is one of the strongest ligaments in the body, and the spiraling direction of its fibers makes it taut in extension in a *wringing-out* mechanism and relaxed in flexion.

The ischiofemoral ligament reinforces the posterior capsule (Figure 6.11). It too has a spiraling pattern as it courses from its ischial attachment on the posterior acetabular rim to its femoral attachment on the superolateral neck, medial to the base of the greater trochanter.

The pubofemoral ligament, although relatively weak, reinforces the inferior and anterior capsule from

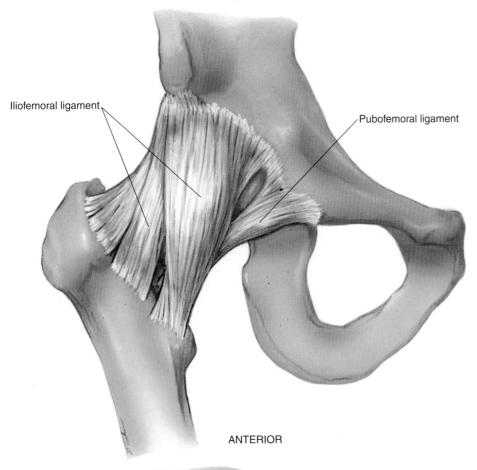

Iliofemoral ligament

Pubofemoral ligament

ANTERIOR

FIGURE 6.10. The iliofemoral ligament (ligament of Bigelow) has the shape of an inverted Y as it spirals from its attachment on the iliac portion of the superior acetabulum to its femoral attachment on the anterior neck. It is quite powerful and becomes taut in extension. The relatively weak pubofemoral ligament reinforces the inferior and anterior capsule, where it blends with the medial edge of the iliofemoral ligament.

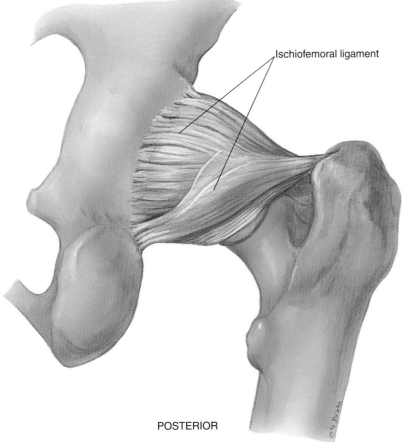

Ischiofemoral ligament

POSTERIOR

FIGURE 6.11. The ischiofemoral ligament reinforces the posterior capsule, spiraling from its attachment on the ischial portion of the posterior acetabulum to the superolateral aspect of the femoral neck.

the pubic part of the acetabular rim where it blends with the medial edge of the iliofemoral ligament (see Figure 6.10). Again, the spiraling nature of this complex tends to screw the femoral head medially into the acetabulum during extension, which has several clinical implications. First, this explains why patients with an irritable hip, whether the result of trauma, disease, or infection, tend to rest with the hip in a slightly flexed position, relaxing the capsule. Second, from a surgical standpoint, it would appear advantageous to perform arthroscopy with the hip flexed, further relaxing the capsule. However, this can create potential concern for portal placement, as discussed in Chapter 7.

The fourth ligament is the ligament of the head of the femur (ligamentum teres) (Figure 6.12). Coursing from its attachment in the acetabular fossa to the fovea of the femoral head, it is intracapsular, yet encased in synovium, making it extrasynovial. Its relatively weak, redundant nature makes it unlikely that this has any significant stabilizing effect on the hip. The size and strength of this ligament are variable, and it is occasionally absent, the significance of which is unknown.

A deep layer of fibers within the ligamentous capsule courses circularly around the neck of the femur, creating the zona orbicularis (see Figure 6.12). This layer may serve as a collar to constrict the capsule and help maintain the femoral head within the acetabulum.

VASCULAR SUPPLY TO THE FEMORAL HEAD

Intraarticular isolation of the femoral head and neck makes it highly dependent on its tenuous vascular supply. Its susceptibility to circulatory compromise is an ongoing source of concern to physicians who treat hip pathology. Ischemic insult followed by avascular necrosis (AVN) of the femoral head, similar to other forms of osteonecrosis, has been clearly linked to certain disease states and types of exposure although it is less clearly associated with others and often purely idiopathic.[10] AVN has been associated with previous trauma including fracture and dislocation and may occur iatrogenically in association with surgical procedures that violate the vascular pattern.

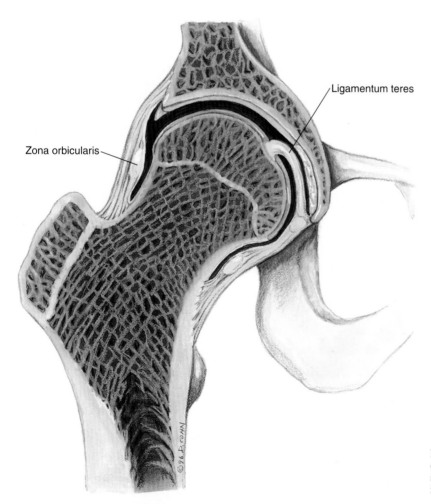

Ligamentum teres

Zona orbicularis

FIGURE 6.12. The ligamentum teres is redundant and weak and contributes little to the capsular stability of the hip. Encased in synovium, it is intracapsular, yet extrasynovial.

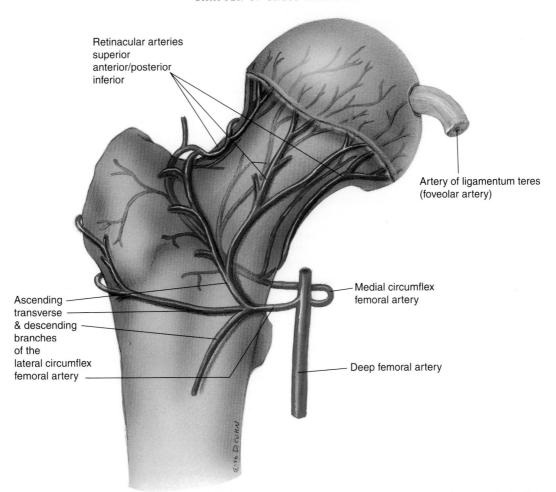

Retinacular arteries
superior
anterior/posterior
inferior

Artery of ligamentum teres
(foveolar artery)

Ascending
transverse
& descending
branches
of the
lateral circumflex
femoral artery

Medial circumflex
femoral artery

Deep femoral artery

FIGURE 6.13. The femoral head receives arterial blood flow from an anastomosis of three sets of arteries: (1) the retinacular vessels, primarily from the medial circumflex femoral artery and, to a lesser extent, the lateral circumflex femoral artery; (2) terminal branches of the medullary artery from the shaft of the femur; and (3) the artery of the ligamentum teres from the posterior division of the obturator artery.

The poorly defined and uncertain nature of AVN is reflected in the myriad surgical procedures that have been described in its management, none of which has proven to be superior, and few of which have even been shown to be truly effective in altering the natural course of the process.[11]

Arterial blood supply to the femoral head is achieved through an anastomosis of three sets of arteries (Figure 6.13). The principal vessels ascend in the synovial retinaculum, which is a reflection of the ligamentous capsule onto the neck of the femur. These vessels arise mainly posterior superiorly and posterior inferiorly from the medial circumflex femoral artery, which is supplemented to a lesser extent from the lateral circumflex femoral artery. These vessels anastomose with the terminal branches of the medullary artery from the shaft of the femur. The third source is the anastomosis within the femoral head from the artery of the ligamentum teres, which arises from a posterior division of the obturator artery. This vessel may persist with advanced age, but in approximately 20% of the population it never develops.

References

1. Anderson JE: Grant's Atlas of Anatomy, 7th ed. Baltimore: Williams & Wilkins, 1978.
2. Hoppenfeld S, deBoer P (eds): Surgical Exposures in Orthopaedics. The Anatomic Approach. Philadelphia: Lippincott, 1984.
3. Byrd JWT: Hip arthroscopy utilizing the supine position. Arthroscopy 1994;10:275–280.
4. Byrd JWT, Pappas JN, Pedley MJ: Hip arthroscopy: an anatomic study of portal placement and relationship to the extra-articular structures. Arthroscopy 1995;11:418–423.
5. Glick JM: Hip arthroscopy using the lateral approach. Instr Course Lect 1988;37:223–231.
6. Johnson L: Hip joint. In: Johnson L (ed). Diagnostic and Surgical Arthroscopy, 3rd ed. St. Louis: Mosby, 1986:1491–1519.
7. Ide T, Akamatsu N, Nakajima I: Arthroscopic surgery of the hip joint. Arthroscopy 1991;7:204–211.
8. Henry AK: Extensile Exposure, 2nd ed. New York: Churchill Livingstone, 1973.
9. Gross RH: Arthroscopy in hip disorders in children. Orthop Rev 1977;6:43–49.
10. Jones JP: Concepts of etiology and early pathogenesis of osteonecrosis. Instr Course Lect 1994;43:499–512.
11. Steinberg ME: Early diagnosis, evaluation and staging of osteonecrosis. Instr Course Lect 1994;43:513–518.

7

Portal Anatomy

J.W. Thomas Byrd

There has been much variation, as well as precision, in the description in the literature of portal placements for hip arthroscopy. The attention given to these detailed descriptions is important for two reasons: (1) accessibility of the joint and (2) avoidance of the major surrounding neurovascular structures.

The tip of the greater trochanter is the common landmark used in describing a variety of lateral portals.[1–3] Equal variation can be found in the description of an anterior portal (Figure 7.1). Eriksson et al.,[4] Frich et al.,[5] and Gross[6] base the portal lateral to the femoral pulse. Ide et al.[7] describe an anterior portal 1 cm lateral and distal to the midpoint of a line between the anterior superior iliac spine and the symphysis pubis. Johnson[8] also describes the symphysis pubis as a landmark, positioning a portal at the site of intersection of a sagittal line drawn distally from the anterior superior iliac spine and a transverse line drawn laterally from the pubic symphysis. Dorfmann et al.,[9] following a cadaveric study, were most comfortable with a portal inserted midway along a line between the anterior superior iliac spine and the superior tip of the greater trochanter. Conversely, Glick et al.[10] describe an anterior portal at the site of intersection of a sagittal line drawn distally from the anterior superior iliac spine and a transverse line across the tip of the greater trochanter. Similarly, Watanabe[11] describes the same approach in his text on arthroscopy of small joints. A medial approach was also described by Gross,[6] applicable in the pediatric population with hip dysplasia.

I use three standard arthroscopy portals (Figure 7.2).[12] Two of these are placed laterally (anterolateral and posterolateral) over the superior margin of the greater trochanter and can effectively enter the hip under direct fluoroscopic control. Positioning of the anterior portal requires more triangulation technique. Herein are described the three standard portals that I use for hip arthroscopy (see Chapter 11) and the specific anatomic relationship of the major structures to these portals (Table 7.1).[13]

All three portals are routinely established for each arthroscopic procedure and usually found to provide adequate accessibility of the joint. If, however, an alternative portal is necessary, knowing the anatomic relationship of the extraarticular structures to these index portals should be helpful in safely establishing supplemental entry sites.

ANTERIOR PORTAL

The anterior portal is established by drawing a sagittal line distally from the anterior superior iliac spine and a tranverse line from the superior margin of the greater trochanter (see Figure 7.2). The intersection of these two lines marks the site of the anterior portal. The portal must be directed approximately 45 degrees cephalad and 30 degrees toward the midline. In the clinical setting, this is performed under fluoroscopic control as well as direct visualization through the arthroscope from the anterolateral portal, which is established first for introduction of the arthroscope.

The anterior portal lies an average of 6.3 cm distal to the anterior superior iliac spine. It penetrates the muscle belly of the sartorius and the rectus femoris before entering through the anterior capsule (Figure 7.3).

Typically, the lateral femoral cutaneous nerve is divided into three or more branches at the level of the anterior portal. The portal passes within several millimeters of one of these branches, usually the most medial branch (Figure 7.4). Consequently, moving the portal more laterally, a maneuver that has occasionally been described for avoidance of the lateral femoral cutaneous nerve, is ineffective. It simply places the portal more within the remaining branches of the nerve. In fact, moving the portal more medially would more effectively avoid the lateral femoral cutaneous nerve, but this maneuver would be ill advised because of the increasingly closer proximity of the femoral nerve.

Because of the multiple branches, the lateral femoral cutaneous nerve is not easily avoided by altering the portal position, but it is protected by using meticulous technique in portal placement. Specifically, it is most vulnerable to a skin incision placed too deeply, lacerating one of the branches.

Passing from the skin to the capsule, the anterior portal runs almost tangential to the axis of the femoral nerve and lies only slightly closer at the level of the capsule with an average minimum distance of 3.2 cm (Figure 7.5).

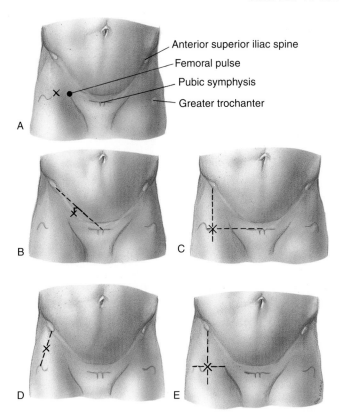

Anterior superior iliac spine

Femoral pulse

Pubic symphysis

Greater trochanter

A

B

C

D

E

FIGURE 7.1. Various descriptions of an anterior portal have been proposed: (A) based lateral to the femoral pulse; (B) 1 cm lateral and distal to the midpoint of a line between the anterior superior iliac spine (ASIS) and symphysis pubis; (C) site of intersection of a sagittal line from the ASIS and a transverse line from the symphysis pubis; (D) midpoint of a line between the ASIS and superior tip of the greater trochanter; (E) intersection of a sagittal line from the ASIS and a transverse line from the tip of the greater trochanter. Note: I strongly discourage consideration of the portal described in B; this does not appear to represent a safe approach to the joint. Also, note that palpation of the femoral pulse as a landmark can be difficult once the surgical field has been sterilely prepared.

Although variable in its relationship, the ascending branch of the lateral circumflex femoral artery is usually approximately 3.7 cm inferior to the anterior portal (Figure 7.6). In some cadaver specimens, a small terminal branch of this vessel has been identified lying within millimeters of the portal at the level of the capsule. The clinical significance of this is uncertain, and there have been no reported cases of excessive bleeding from the anterior position.

ANTEROLATERAL PORTAL

The anterolateral portal lies most centrally in the *safe zone* for arthroscopy and thus is the portal established first for introduction of the arthroscope. It is positioned directly over the superior margin of the greater trochanter at its anterior border (see Figure 7.2). Accounting for the slightly anterior position of the femoral head resulting from femoral neck anteversion, this allows a relatively straight shot into the hip joint under fluoroscopic guidance in the anteroposterior (AP) plane. Care should be taken during portal placement to assure neutral rotation of the hip because excessive internal or external rotation alters the relationship of the greater trochanter with the femoral head.

The anterolateral portal penetrates the gluteus medius before entering the lateral aspect of the cap-

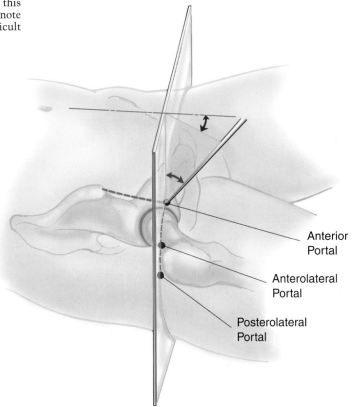

Anterior Portal

Anterolateral Portal

Posterolateral Portal

FIGURE 7.2. The site of the anterior portal coincides with the intersection of a sagittal line drawn distally from the anterior superior iliac spine and a transverse line across the superior margin of the greater trochanter. The direction of this portal courses approximately 45 degrees cephalad and 30 degrees toward the midline. The anterolateral and posterolateral portals are positioned directly over the superior aspect of the trochanter at its anterior and posterior borders. (Courtesy of Smith & Nephew Endoscopy, Andover, MA.)

TABLE 7.1. Distance from Portal to Anatomic Structures Based on an Anatomic Dissection of Portal Placements in Eight Fresh Cadaver Specimens).

Portal	Anatomic structure	Average (cm)	Range (cm)
	Anterior superior iliac spine	6.3	6.0–7.0
	Lateral femoral cutaneous nerve[a]	0.3	0.2–1.0
Anterior	Femoral nerve (level of sartorius)[b]	4.3	3.8–5.0
	Femoral nerve (level of rectus femoris)	3.8	2.7–5.0
	Femoral nerve (level of capsule)	3.7	2.9–5.0
	Ascending branch of lateral circumflex femoral artery	3.7	1.0–6.0
	[c]Terminal branch	0.3	0.2–0.4
Anterolateral	Superior gluteal nerve	4.4	3.2–5.5
Posterolateral	Sciatic nerve	2.9	2.0–4.3

[a]Nerve had divided into three or more branches and measurement was made to the closest branch.

[b]Measurement made at superficial branch of sartorius, rectus femoris, and capsule.

[c]Small terminal branch of ascending branch of lateral circumflex femoral artery identified in three specimens.

Source: From Byrd et al.,[13] with permission of Arthroscopy.

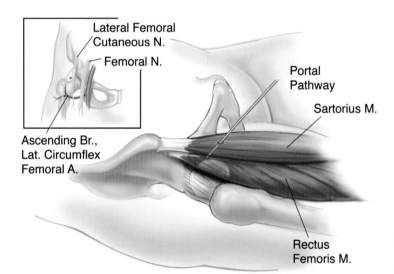

FIGURE 7.3. Anterior portal pathway/relationship to lateral femoral cutaneous nerve, femoral nerve, and lateral circumflex femoral artery. (Courtesy of Smith & Nephew Endoscopy, Andover, MA.)

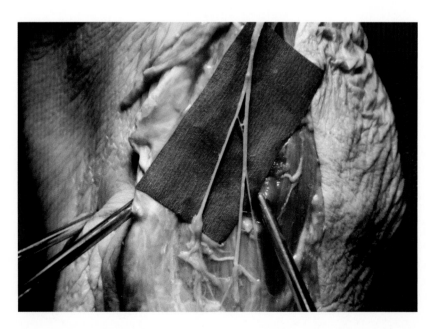

FIGURE 7.4. The relationship of the anterior portal to the multiple branches of the lateral femoral cutaneous nerve is shown. Multiple branches at the level of the portal are characteristic, and the branches always extend lateral to the portal. (Reprinted with permission from Byrd et al.[13])

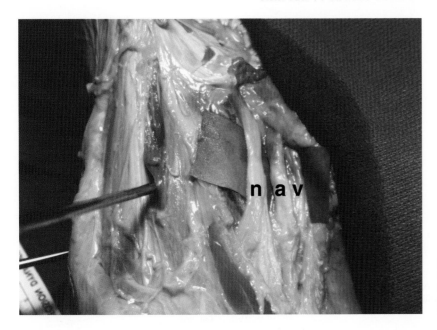

FIGURE 7.5. The femoral nerve (n) lies lateral to the femoral artery (a) and vein (v). The relationship of the anterior portal as it pierces the sartorius is shown. (Reprinted with permission from Byrd et al.[13])

sule at its anterior margin (Figure 7.7). The structure of most significance relative to this portal is the superior gluteal nerve (Figure 7.8). After exiting the sciatic notch, the superior gluteal nerve courses transversely posterior to anterior across the deep surface of the gluteus medius. Its relationship is the same with both the lateral portals, with an average distance of 4.4 cm.

POSTEROLATERAL PORTAL

The posterolateral portal is positioned similar to the anterolateral portal except at the posterior margin of the greater trochanter (see Figure 7.2). Again, it is a relatively straight shot under fluoroscopic control, but

it is facilitated by direct visualization through the arthroscope from the anterolateral portal. Maintaining direct visualization is of greater importance because the posterolateral portal gets closer to major structures, specifically the sciatic nerve.

The posterolateral portal penetrates both the gluteus medius and minimus before entering the lateral capsule at its posterior margin (Figure 7.9). Its course is superior and anterior to the piriformis tendon (Figure 7.10). It lies closest to the sciatic nerve at the level of the capsule. The distance to the lateral edge of the nerve averages 2.9 cm.

Several technical errors or alterations in technique during arthroscopy can place the sciatic nerve at greater risk. First, although hip flexion may relax the capsule, easing distraction, it may potentially draw the

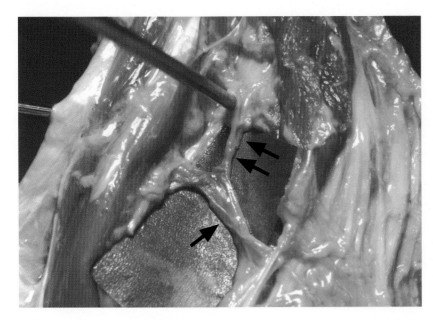

FIGURE 7.6. The ascending branch of the lateral circumflex femoral artery (arrow) has an oblique course distal to the anterior portal seen here at the level of the capsule. This specimen demonstrates a terminal branch (double arrow) coursing vertically adjacent to the portal. (Reprinted with permission from Byrd et al.[13])

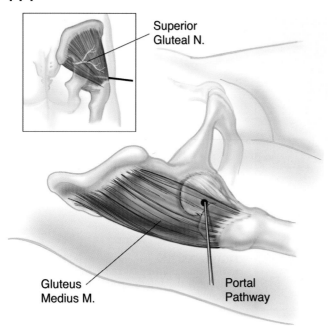

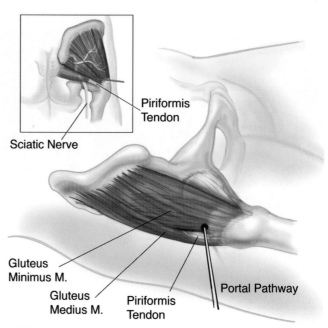

FIGURE 7.7. Anterolateral portal pathway/relationship to superior gluteal nerve. (Courtesy of Smith & Nephew Endoscopy, Andover, MA.)

FIGURE 7.9. Posterolateral portal pathway/relationship to sciatic nerve and superior gluteal nerve. (Courtesy of Smith & Nephew Endoscopy, Andover, MA.)

sciatic nerve closer to the joint, making it more vulnerable to injury. Second, it is important to maintain neutral rotation during portal placement. If the hip is inadvertently externally rotated, this moves the greater trochanter more posterior relative to the femoral head and the hip joint (Figure 7.11). This type of starting position, again, can place the sciatic nerve more at risk for injury. Thus, although slight flexion may relax the capsule, excessive flexion should be avoided. Also, care should be taken to ensure that the hip is in neutral rotation during portal placement. Intraoperative rotation of the hip may facilitate visualiza-

tion of portions of the femoral head but should not be performed until after all portals have been established.

NOMENCLATURE

Special mention should be made of the nomenclature used in describing arthroscopy portals. The anterior portal is not a true anterior approach to the hip. However, it is as far anterior as can safely and reliably be positioned. Thus, for distinction from the various lateral portals, it is referred to as the anterior portal.

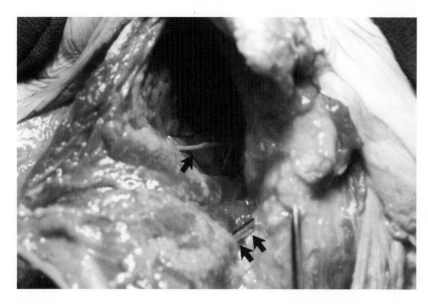

FIGURE 7.8. The superior gluteal nerve (arrow) is shown coursing transversely on the deep surface of the gluteus medius. It passes above the anterolateral portal (double arrows), which is seen between the deep surface of the gluteus medius and the capsule. (Reprinted with permission from Byrd et al.[13])

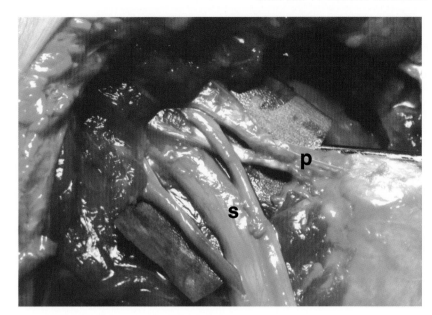

FIGURE 7.10. The relationship of the postero-lateral portal is shown with the piriformis tendon (p) and the sciatic nerve (s). Note the anomaly where the sciatic nerve is formed from three divisions distal to the sciatic notch and the lateralmost division passes through a split muscle belly of the piriformis. (Reprinted with permission from Byrd et al.[13])

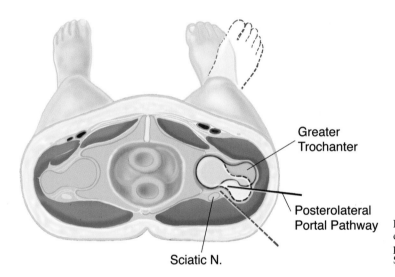

Greater Trochanter

Posterolateral Portal Pathway

Sciatic N.

FIGURE 7.11. Neutral rotation of the operative hip is essential for protection of the sciatic nerve during placement of the posterolateral portal. (Courtesy of Smith & Nephew Endoscopy, Andover, MA.)

Glick et al.[10] refer to the portals placed over the anterior and posterior margins of the superior aspect of the greater trochanter as anterior paratrochanteric and posterior paratrochanteric portals. This nomenclature has also been adopted by McCarthy et al.[14] in their review of hip arthroscopy.

I have used the terms *anterolateral* and *posterolateral* for simplicity and consistency with the terminology commonly used for other joints. Standard portals are usually described in an abbreviated fashion, defining only their relationship to the joint. Portal descriptions in relationship to a topographic landmark are usually reserved for specialty portals or portals that are only occasionally used.

I recommend that, until the nomenclature becomes truly standardized, when referencing literature on hip arthroscopy, it is always important to review the details regarding the description of portal placement. One must not rely solely on the portal name to automatically create an image of which portal is being discussed.

References

1. Blitzer CM: Arthroscopic management of septic arthritis of the hip. Arthroscopy 1993;9:414–416.
2. Klapper R, Silver DM: Hip arthroscopy without traction. Contemp Orthop 1989;18:687–693.
3. Holgersson S, Brattström H, Mogensen B, Lidgren L: Arthroscopy of the hip in juvenile chronic arthritis. J Pediatr Orthop 1981;1:273–278.
4. Eriksson E, Arvidsson I, Arvidsson H: Diagnostic and operative arthroscopy of the hip. Orthopaedics 1986;9:169–176.
5. Frich LH, Lauritzen J, Juhl M: Arthroscopy in diagnosis and treatment of hip disorders. Orthopaedics 1989;12:389–391.

6. Gross RH: Arthroscopy in hip disorders in children. Orthop Rev 1977;6:43–49.

7. Ide T, Akamatsu N, Nakajima I: Arthroscopic surgery of the hip joint. Arthroscopy 1991;7:204–211.

8. Johnson L: Hip joint. In: Johnson L (ed). Diagnostic and Surgical Arthroscopy, 3rd ed. St. Louis. Mosby, 1986:1491–1519.

9. Dorfmann H, Boyer T, Henry P, DeBie P: A simple approach to hip arthroscopy. Arthroscopy 1988;4:141–142.

10. Glick JM, Sampson TG, Gordon RB, Behr JT, Schmidt E: Hip arthroscopy by the lateral approach. Arthroscopy 1987;3:4–12.

11. Watanabe M: Arthroscopy of Small Joints. Tokyo: Ogaku Shoin, 1985.

12. Byrd JWT: Hip arthroscopy utilizing the supine position. Arthroscopy 1994;10:275–280.

13. Byrd JWT, Pappas JN, Pedley MJ: Hip arthroscopy: an anatomic study of portal placement and relationship to the extra-articular structures. Arthroscopy 1995;11:418–423.

14. McCarthy JC, Day B, Busconi B: Hip arthroscopy: applications and technique. J Am Acad Orthop Surg 1995;3:115–122.

8

Arthroscopic Anatomy of the Hip

Richard N. Villar and Nicola Santori

The human hip is a ball-and-socket joint contained within a capsule that runs along the axis of the joint from the rim of acetabulum to the neck of femur. The bony architecture of this joint provides the inherent stability required for erect posture but at the same time impairs access to the joint itself.

The gross anatomy of the hip has been well known since ancient times. Nevertheless, the average orthopedic surgeon is often not confident in this area, especially in the knowledge of the intraarticular structures, because hips operated on in an orthopedic department are mostly degenerating joints. The surgeon may not believe it is important to distinguish anatomic structures that he or she is planning to replace.

Arthroscopy has permitted the identification of new pathologic entities in the hip, allowing a detailed analysis of normal and pathologic anatomy. The chances for successful hip arthroscopy depend primarily on the ability of the surgeon to distinguish what is a normal finding from what is abnormal and causing hip symptoms.

DEVELOPMENT OF THE NORMAL HIP

To understand the biomechanics and the functions of the intraarticular structures, it is important to review some aspects of the development of the hip. Both femur and pelvis are preformed in cartilage. Of the eight ossification centers of the hemipelvis, three form the acetabulum. These are the iliac, ischial, and pubic ossification centers, meeting at the triradiate cartilage. The iliac center appears prenatally at the ninth week of intrauterine life. The ischial and pubic centers appear at the fourth and fifth months, respectively. At birth, the acetabulum is still a cartilaginous cup. Between the ages of 8 and 9 years, ossification of the acetabulum begins. Fusion of the ilium, ischium, and pubis within the acetabulum occurs between the ages of 16 and 18 years.[1]

In the early fetal period, the acetabulum is a deeply set cavity that almost totally encloses the femoral head. As growth proceeds, the shape progressively changes so that at birth it becomes shallower and covers just one-third of a complete sphere. After birth, this process reverses and the cavity steadily deepens once more. The progressive shallowing of the acetabulum allows an increased range of movement at the time of birth.

On the femoral side, the center of ossification for the femoral head appears during the first year of life and is located laterally within the head. Similar to the acetabulum, the head also undergoes a change of shape during development. Its anteroposterior diameter is slightly greater than the transverse up to the age of 3 years. At that point, the head becomes almost a perfect sphere. Then the transverse diameter becomes larger, making the head ovoid. Because of this pattern of development of both sides of the hip, the femoral head is poorly contained at the time of birth.

Soft tissue structures of the hip joint arise from the same undifferentiated mesenchyme and similarly undergo a progressive development. By the 11th week of gestation, the capsule, internally lined with synovial cells, the labrum glenoidale, and the ligamentum teres, is well differentiated. The capsule, initially very thin, becomes progressively pluristratified, gaining thickness and strength. It is generally considered the most important structure contributing to hip stability. Joint, and consequent capsular, laxity may occur in either sex, but is more frequent in female subjects.[2-4] The labrum increases the depth of the acetabular cavity and progressively takes on a fibrocartilaginous structure during development.

Horii and coauthors[5] have evaluated the degrees of coverage of the femoral head, comparing three age groups: A, 6 to 8 years old; B, 9 to 11 years old; and C, 12 to 13 years old and using 10 healthy adults as controls. They found that coverage of the femoral head by the acetabulum in young children was less than in adults at all positions. However, interestingly, the total coverage including the labrum was greater than in adults.

In the lower part of the joint the labrum is normally continuous with the transverse ligament. The ligamentum teres differentiates from the interzone of the embryonic mesenchyme and runs from the femoral head to the medial border of the acetabular fossa behind the transverse ligament. It provides stability and restraint during the early phases of hip development. Furthermore, it gives mechanical support to the artery of the ligamentum teres or foveolar artery. This vessel is an important nutritional source during certain periods of growth. The anatomy of the circulation to the head is not constant during development, but differs significantly at different ages. During fetal life, three groups of vessels supply the hip joint: the lateral epiphyseal, the anterior metaphyseal, and the foveolar artery. From 4 months of infancy onward, the vessels of the ligamentum teres regress. At this stage they play no part in the nutrition of the ossification center; the main supply until the age of 7 years is the lateral epiphyseal vessels. The contribution from the artery of the ligamentum teres increases again in early adolescence (7 to 11 years). It penetrates the ossification center and enlarges toward the rest of the head. For the first time, connection develops between the terminal branches of the lateral epiphyseal artery and the foveolar artery. These are the only two sources of blood supply of the epiphyseal ossification center. The adolescent pattern of blood supply is maintained until approximately 17 years of age when the epiphysis becomes linked with the metaphysis by interconnecting vessels.

ARTHROSCOPIC ANATOMY

Femoral Head

The head forms approximately two-thirds of a sphere and is covered throughout with articular cartilage, except at the fovea. Anteriorly, the articular surface extents to the neck. It faces anterosuperomedially and geometrically resembles part of the surface of an ovoid. Kurrat and Oberlander found maximal thick-

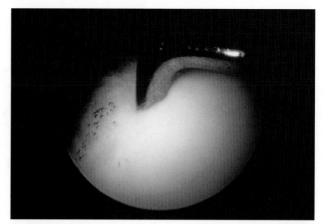

FIGURE 8.2. Softening of the femoral head cartilage with initial fibrillation.

ness of the articular cartilage on the anterolateral portion of the femoral head.[6] Normal hyaline cartilage, as in other joints, has a shining white appearance on direct inspection (Figure 8.1). When using the 70-degree arthroscope, it is possible to visualize approximately 80% of the articular surface. This view is simplified by rotating the leg during the procedure. Anteriorly, the cartilage extends on the femoral neck for a short distance, which is thought to be a reaction to the pressure from the iliopsoas tendon crossing the joint in this region. The spherical shape of the head of the femur does not ease the orientation within the joint. The only fixed landmark on its surface is the insertion of the ligamentum teres on the fovea. This area is located on the anteromedial portion of the head and was previously known as the *bare area*. Because of deformation and magnification, it is not always possible to detect abnormalities of the overall shape of the head. However, damage to the hyaline cartilage is clearly and easily seen. The consistency of the articular surface can also be assessed with a probe and is usually indentable (Figure 8.2).

Acetabulum

The name *acetabulum* comes from the Latin and means *vinegar cup* from the similarity in shape with this article from ancient Rome. To the arthroscopic surgeon it appears horseshoe shaped, encircling the acetabular fossa, the lunate surface. It can be divided into a superior part, an anterior column, and a posterior column. The classic theory says that no evidence of the existence of the triradiate cartilage is considered to remain in the adult hip. At this stage, the anterior one-fifth of the acetabulum is formed by the pubis, the posterosuperior two-fifths by the ilium, and the posteroinferior two-fifths by the ischium. The normal surface appears white, smooth, and glistening. The thickness of the articular cartilage is reported to be maximal on the anterosuperior quadrant.[6] With the

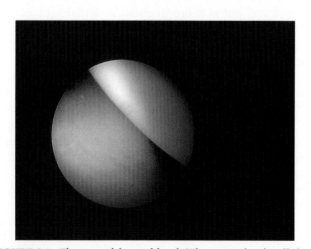

FIGURE 8.1. The normal femoral head. (The copyrights for all the illustrations in this chapter are retained by Dr. Villar.)

70-degree arthroscope, from the lateral approach, it is possible to see consecutively the three zones and most of their articular surfaces.

The horseshoe shape of the acetabulum (Figure 8.3) is a fixed landmark and allows easy orientation within the joint. Peripheral margins of the acetabulum are overlaid by the perimeter of the labrum and cannot always be seen. The inner borders of the articular surface of the acetabulum have a rounded cartilage edge; these form the margins of the acetabular fossa or cotyloid fossa. Sometimes a central osteophyte can be seen in this area (Figure 8.4); it is more often located on the inner margin of the anterior column, although a posterior central osteophyte is also possible.

Adjacent to anterior or posterior apex of the acetabular fossa, within its lunate surface, a silvery stellate crease is frequently seen (Figure 8.5). The significance of this finding is unknown, but in our experience, no correlation with clinical symptoms has been identified. The inexperienced surgeon must be aware of its existence so as not to confuse it with early degenerative changes.

Rarely, a transverse groove running anteriorly from the stellate crease to the anterior margin of the acetabulum is present. It does not have a degenerative appearance and is lined with normal articular cartilage. This groove was identified in a few cases of more than 500 patients undergoing hip arthroscopy over a 5-year period.[7] It is possible that it represents a vestige of the triradiate cartilage.

ARTHROSCOPIC FINDINGS IN THE INITIAL STAGES OF HIP OSTEOARTHRITIS

Early degenerative changes of the hip are not an uncommon arthroscopic finding. Standard radiographic projections have poor diagnostic ability in detecting

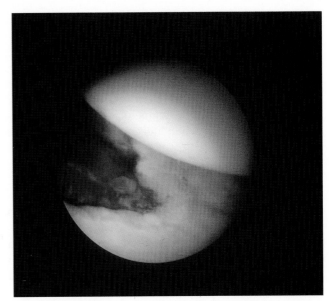

FIGURE 8.4. Acetabular central osteophyte.

precocious chondral damage. In a previous study,[8] we reviewed records and radiographs of 234 hip arthroscopies and compared intraoperative and radiographic findings. Sixty patients (32.2%) of the 186 with normal preoperative radiographs had evidence of osteoarthritis at the time of surgery. This evidence makes initial osteoarthritis the most likely cause of hip symptoms in young patients (average age, 36 years) with normal radiographic findings.

One more interesting finding was the preponderance of female subjects (71% versus 29%) in the group with normal radiographic findings. Quantification of the damage was obtained by dividing the acetabulum and the femoral head in quadrants. Hips with normal radiographic findings but arthroscopic osteoarthritis were found to have less chondral damage (1.9 quadrants) compared with those with radiographically evident osteoarthritis (4.2) quadrants. Hips with normal

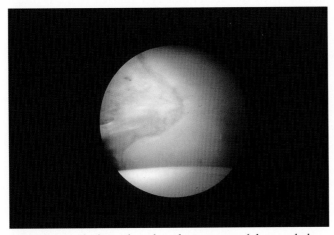

FIGURE 8.3. The horseshoe-shaped appearance of the acetabulum.

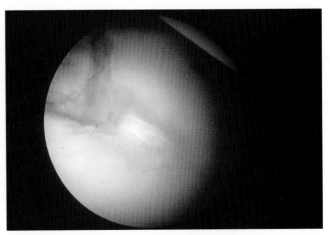

FIGURE 8.5. The stellate crease.

radiographic findings also were more likely to have only one side (60%) of the joint involved.

Hip osteoarthritis appears to begin on one of the two sides of the joint and not as a generalized disease. The hip, due to its peculiar ball-and-socket shape, is poorly studied with a conventional anteroposterior projection. Radiographic signs of osteoarthritis become evident only when degenerative changes are fairly widespread within the joint (4.2 quadrants).

Acetabular Fossa

When good distension of the joint is obtained, this portion of the acetabulum can be safely seen. However, often a *fat pad* lies within the fossa and can expand into the cavity and obscure the view. Usually, the fossa has a flattened superior margin and anterior and posterior borders. From the posteroinferior part of the fossa arises the ligamentum teres. Superiorly, the fossa is lined by dense fibroconnective tissue, lacking a synovial lining. The lower part of the fossa is occupied by adipose tissue; this appears well vascularized and is usually mobile when suction on the outflow is applied. Sometimes the adipose tissue can behave like a pedunculated structure within the joint. It is said to contain numerous proprioceptive nerve endings. When it becomes compressed, it partially extrudes from the acetabular fossa beneath the transverse ligament.

A thickened band of fibrous tissue, the transverse ligament (Figure 8.6), closes the lowest portion of the acetabular fossa. This structure bridges the open end of the horseshoe-shaped acetabulum and can occasionally be probed with a hook. It divides the acetabular fossa from the inferior recess. Close to the transverse ligament, synovial tissue from the inferior recess encroaches on and passes beneath the ligament into the fossa. The inferior recess is a frequent hiding place for loose bodies, although it is unlikely they cause any great harm in such a position.

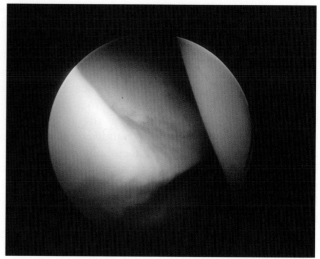

FIGURE 8.7. Acetabular labrum.

Acetabular Labrum

The acetabular labrum (Figure 8.7), or labrum glenoidale, gives permanent stability to the hip joint by deepening the acetabular cavity. The labrum is triangular in cross section with the apex forming the free thin edge. The diameter of this free edge is smaller than its fixed edge and is somewhat less than the maximum diameter of the femoral head. It provides coverage and support to the anterior, superior, and posterior surfaces of the femoral head.

As with the glenoidal labrum in the shoulder, it produces a valve effect that significantly increases the stability of the joint. Takechi and coauthors[4] have measured the intraarticular pressure both inside and outside the labrum in a hemipelvectomy specimen. They found that the pressure within the inner part of the joint, inside the labrum, was almost double that outside the labrum. This explains why it is so difficult to obtain a satisfactory distraction of the hip without injecting saline or air into the joint.[9]

Histologically, the fibrocartilaginous labrum is connected with the acetabular articular cartilage through a 1- to 2-mm zone of transition. A consistent projection of bone extends from the bony acetabulum into the substance of the labrum that is attached via a zone of calcified cartilage with a well-defined tidemark.[10]

At the time of arthroscopy, the labrum appears to overlap the hyaline cartilage around the perimeter of the acetabular cup. It continues downward into the transverse ligament of the acetabulum. This structure is usually regarded as the anatomic extension of the labrum across the notch. Sometimes, at the margins of the acetabular fossa, the labrum does not directly continue into the transverse ligament. In such cases, an area of acetabular articular cartilage intervenes between the two structures. No instability of the labrum seems to be associated with this finding.

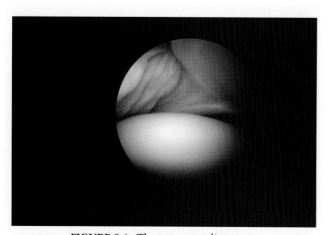

FIGURE 8.6. The transverse ligament.

The labrum is the first structure that the arthroscopic surgeon can damage. To avoid it, proper identification of the joint line must be made. If, on the image intensifier, the guidewire is too close to the bony margin of the cup, it is possible to disrupt the labrum during the insertion of the trochar. In this case, it is better to reposition the guidewire before the introduction of instruments.

Once entered, with a 70-degree arthroscope, it is possible to visualize the majority of the circumference of the labrum and the transverse ligament. In its anterior, superior, and posterior portions, it has a meniscus-like consistency and it is indentable with a probe. In the inferior part, the transverse ligament, it no longer has a fibrocartilaginous structure and consists of strong, flattened fibers, which cross the acetabular fossa. The labrum blends with the margins of the acetabulum, except inferiorly. Here it is usually separated from the hyaline cartilage by a distinct groove, the labral groove (Figure 8.8). Commonly, the labrum is inverted, although it may be everted, and sometimes mobile. In a review of 37 cases operated for labral pathology,[11] 2 cases of unstable acetabular labra have been reported; both were teenaged girls with generalized ligamentous laxity. At the time of arthroscopy, the labrum subluxed during internal and external rotation of the limb. The absence of a trauma in the history of these 2 patients suggests this finding could be a peculiar congenital feature of labral development of ligament laxity.

Average width of the acetabular labrum is reported to be 5.3 mm (SD, 2.6 mm).[12] It enlarges significantly the size of the acetabulum. Tan and coauthors[12] reported an increase of acetabular surface area from 28.8 cm² without the labrum to 36.8 cm² ($P < 0.0001$) with the labrum. The volume of the acetabulum without the labrum is 31.5 cm³; with the labrum, it is 41.1 cm³ ($P < 0.0001$).

Although the labral cross section is almost con-

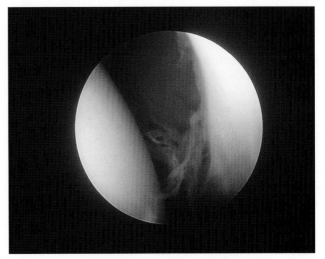

FIGURE 8.9. Perilabral sulcus.

stantly triangular, its thickness varies in different portions. It is larger and thicker in the posterosuperior region and thinner in the anteroinferior region. Hypertrophy of the labrum combined with elongation of the ligamentum teres, and eburnation around the acetabular notch, have been reported in proven cases of hip dysplasia.[13]

On arthroscopic observation, in the young adult, the labrum has an avascular, meniscus-like, elastic appearance, whereas in the elderly it can appear yellow and degenerate. Suzuki and coauthors[14] have described hypervascularity of the labrum as a striking finding in every stage of Legg–Calvé–Perthes disease.

Within the joint, the acetabular labrum divides the peripheral portion lined with synovia from the intraarticular portion. Three distinct gutters are identified outside the articular portion of the joint: the perilabral sulcus (Figure 8.9), the anterior gutter (Figure 8.10), and the posterior gutter.

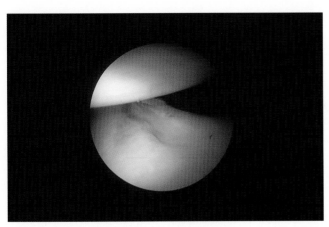

FIGURE 8.8. The labral groove.

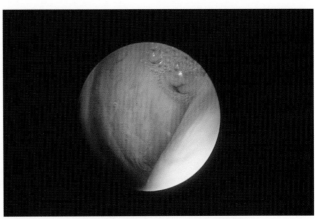

FIGURE 8.10. The anterior gutter.

CLASSIFICATION OF ACETABULAR LABRAL TEARS

Pathologic alterations of the acetabular labrum are a documented cause of discomfort, clicking, and catching of the hip.[11,15–17] Arthroscopy is an excellent method of diagnosis and treatment of this condition. Arthrography, computed tomographic (CT) arthrography, plain CT scanning, and magnetic resonance imaging (MRI) cannot rival the accuracy of direct intraarticular inspection.[15,18–21] Only recently, Petersilge reported excellent results with MR arthrography.[22] although this was not compared with hip arthroscopy.

A classification of labral pathology may be made according to etiology, morphology, and location of the tear.[11]

Etiologic Classification

TRAUMATIC

A clear history of injury to the hip is required. No arthroscopic evidence of degenerative changes of labrum or articular cartilage must be present. The injury mechanism must clearly involve the hip and can be major, such as a car accident with fracture-dislocation, or minor, such as a simple twisting injury of the lower limb. The latter is considered one of the most frequent causes of labral tear in the traumatic group.[15]

Traumatic etiology is reported to account for 30 of the 55 labral tears (54%) in the Fitzgerald series.[15] Lage and coauthors,[11] in their arthroscopic study, found a much lower incidence of trauma (18.9%) in their report on labral ruptures. Such patients usually recall an acute onset of pain, although they do not often remember the specific hip position at the time of injury.

DEGENERATIVE

The white avascular meniscal-like appearance is lost and the labrum looks yellowish and degenerate. Articular damage is frequently present. Cystic changes of the labrum associated with aging have been reported by Ueo and coauthors.[16] This group accounts for 48.6% of the labral tears in the experience of Lage and coauthors.[11]

In a relatively recent publication, Seldes and coauthors[10] studied 55 embalmed and 12 fresh-frozen adult hips with a mean age of 78 years. Of these, 96% (53 of 55) had labral tears, with 74% of the tears located in the anterosuperior quadrant. They concluded that acetabular labrum tear appears to be an acquired condition that is highly prevalent in aging adult hips. Labral tears occur early in the arthritic process of the hip and maybe one of the causes of degenerative hip disease.

IDIOPATHIC

No degenerative change, and no history of previous injury, can be present for a labral tear to be classified in this group. Fitzgerald[15] reported that 25 of 55 of his patients (46%) had no previous history of trauma, but he did not identify those with degenerative changes. Lage and coauthors[11] included 27.1% of their cases in this group.

CONGENITAL

Two cases of unstable subluxing acetabular labra have been recognized by Lage and coauthors.[11] No history of trauma, no acetabular dysplasia, and no morphologic anomalies are the requisites to classify a labrum as congenitally abnormal. Internal and external rotation produces labrum subluxation. Generalized ligamentous laxity, young age, and female sex are apparently associated with this finding.

Acetabular Dysplasia

A labrum rupture in the dysplastic hip is often observed.[20,23] Probably the excessive pressure that is constantly exercised on the acetabular rim and the surrounding soft tissues is responsible for labrum fail-

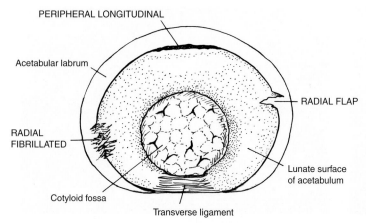

FIGURE 8.11. Morphology of labral tears. Unstable tears are excluded. (From Lage et al.,[11] with permission of Villar.)

ure. Consequently, rupture of the labrum in the dysplastic hip occurs more frequently in the superior region, rather than anteriorly or posteriorly.[19,23]

MORPHOLOGIC CLASSIFICATION

The only morphologic classification of labral tears reported in the literature is that of Lage and coauthors.[11] This scheme includes four groups (Figure 8.11). The incidence of tears within each group is reported in parentheses in the following discussion.

Radial Flap

The radial flap (56.8%) is similar to a meniscal flap (Figure 8.12). The free edge of the labrum is disrupted, and a flap lies free within the joint.

Radial Fibrillated

The radial fibrillated tear (21.6%) is frequently associated with generalized degenerative damage to the hip (Figure 8.13). The free margin appears fibrillated, and the labrum is often yellowish and frail in consistency.

Longitudinal Peripheral

Longitudinal peripheral tears (16.2%) correspond to the meniscal tears in the red peripheral zone and can be of variable length (Figure 8.14). Ikeda and coauthors[17] described this type of rupture in seven cases. Bucket-handle lesions of the labrum would fit into this group, but were never identified by Lage and coauthors,[11] although previously described in the literature.[24,25] Fitzgerald[15] reported that 41 of 49 tears (83.7%) surgically treated in his series were longitudinal separations of the labrum from the acetabulum.

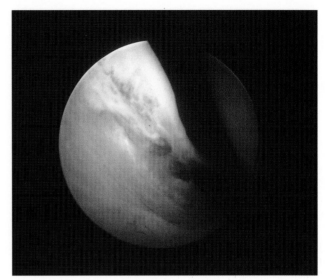

FIGURE 8.13. Labral tear, radial fibrillated. (From Lage et al.,[11] with permission of Villar.)

Unstable

Unstable (5.4%) tears were a reflection of abnormal labral function rather than shape, representing the two subluxing labra classified as being of congenital etiology (Figure 8.15).

LOCATION OF TEARS

Ninety-two percent anterior and 8% posterior tears have been identified by Fitzgerald[15]; 62.2% anterior, 29.7% posterior, and 8.1% superior were recognized by Lage and coauthors.[11] Conversely, Ikeda and coauthors[17] found six posterior labral tears of the seven included in their report.

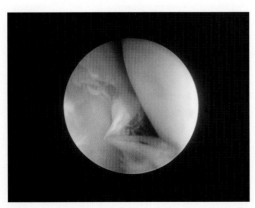

FIGURE 8.12. Labral tear, radial flap. (From Lage et al.,[11] with permission of Villar.)

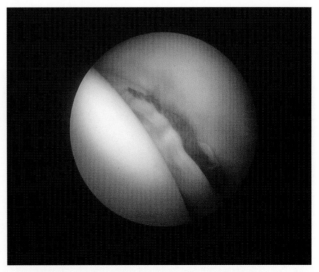

FIGURE 8.14. Labral tear, longitudinal peripheral. (From Lage et al.,[11] with permission of Villar.)

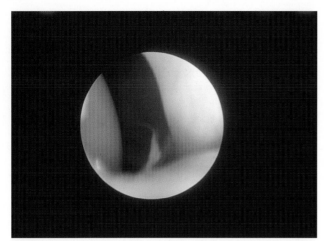

FIGURE 8.15. Unstable subluxing labrum. (From Lage et al.,[11] with permission of Villar.)

Differences in both morphology and location of the rupture reported by different authors[11,15,17] are significant. This variation may be explained partially by the fact that most of the Fitzgerald[15] cases were treated with open surgery, whereas Lage and coauthors[11] always used an arthroscopic technique. The unusually high rate of posterosuperior tears recognized by Ikeda and coauthors[17] has not found support in the literature.[11,15] Tears of the acetabular labrum seem most commonly to be located anteriorly.

LIGAMENTUM TERES

The ligamentum teres (Figure 8.16), or round ligament of the hip, arises from the posteroinferior portion of the acetabular fossa. Occasionally, it originates from both sides of the notch and blends with the transverse ligament. It runs across the notch, reaching the so-

called bare area on the apex of the femoral head (fovea) (Figure 8.17).

The ligament is a triangular flat band surrounded by a thin layer of synovium and, although it is intracapsular, may thus be considered extrasynovial. It encloses the central artery of the femoral head, fatty tissue, and a complicated sensory nerve supply. These structures cannot normally be distinguished arthroscopically, although occasional capillaries may be seen on its surface. Due to the course of this structure, it is not easy to palpate the ligament, at least at the femoral insertion, using a lateral approach; however, this may be accomplished with a curved hook if good distraction is obtained. The synovium around the base of the ligamentum teres extends across the floor of the acetabular fossa. It is in continuity with the synovium that passes beneath the transverse ligament arising from the inferior recess. Sometimes, through the synovium, it is possible to distinguish two different bands at the base of the ligament originating from the anterior and posterior margins of the acetabular notch.

The ligamentum does not constitute a mechanical block to inferior subluxation of any great degree. During hip arthroscopy, even if a high distractive force is applied to open the joint, the ligamentum teres never appears taut. The force used at hip arthroscopy serves to compress rather than distract the ligament. Physiologically, it is tense in adduction and relaxed in abduction.

Many theories exist as to the function of this structure, apart from its role as joint stabilizer. In this respect, if stability were its prime function, it does not act satisfactorily. It cannot, for example, prevent congenital dislocation. When traumatic dislocation of the hip occurs, frequently the proximal attachment of the ligament is torn from the fovea or in its midsubstance.

It is said to act as a windshield wiper, spreading synovial fluid across the articular surface during

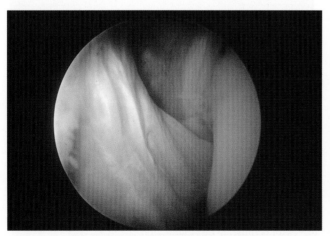

FIGURE 8.16. The ligamentum teres.

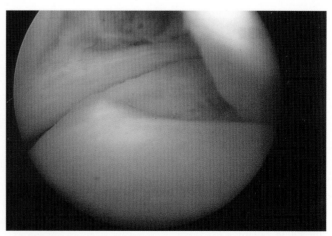

FIGURE 8.17. Foveal insertion of the ligamentum teres.

movement. Certainly, a significant role is to support and protect the central artery of the femoral head. This vessel usually arises from the deeper lateral branch of the obturator artery, although sometimes it originates from the medial circumflex branch of the profunda femoris. It enters the hip joint by passing under the transverse ligament, into the cotyloid fossa, and travels along the ligamentum teres to the fovea capitis where it penetrates into the bone. Wolcott,[26] on anatomic grounds, and Waldenstrom,[27] on clinical grounds, both believed it can sustain the nutrition of the entire head by itself. The caliber of the vessel is variable, being sometimes barely that of a capillary. Often, however, it is a large vessel and supplies a significant part of the head. The frequency of femoral head necrosis after dislocation, with consequent ligamentum teres rupture, may support the importance of this structure. Occasionally, the ligament and the central artery are absent or only the synovial sheath exists.[28]

Ligamentum Teres Damage

It is difficult to depict the pathology of a structure of essentially unknown function. Therefore, to date, little has been published supporting the existence of specific syndromes arising from the ligamentum teres.

As we have described, sometimes the ligament is absent altogether[28] and the patient apparently suffers no remarkable consequences. However, collapse of part of the femoral head is a recognized complication after hip dislocation. Ligamentum teres rupture is assured when such major trauma occurs. Although it is possible that osseous and capsular vessels are injured, the decreased blood flow consequent on central artery disruption is likely to be partially responsible for head collapse. It is possible, although as yet unproven, that the ligamentum may also have a biomechanical function. Whether loss of such a function is also responsible for head collapse is not known.

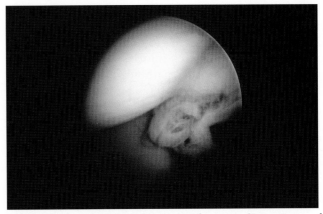

FIGURE 8.19. Ligamentum teres, partial rupture. (From Gray and Villar,[29] with permission of Villar.)

In a retrospective arthroscopic review of ligamentum teres rupture, Gray and Villar[29] identified 20 patients with ligamentum pathology. Three groups of patients were distinguished. Group 1 in their study included 7 patients with complete ligamentum teres rupture (Figure 8.18). In 4, the cause was fracture dislocation, in 2 previous closed reductions of CDH and in 1 a serious twisting injury of the hip. In two cases, at arthroscopy, an osteochondral fragment attached to the disrupted ligament was found. Group 2 included eight cases with partial rupture of the ligament (Figure 8.19). No specific injuries were identified in the previous history of these patents. A long (2 to 12 years) history of hip discomfort, pain, and aching, with occasional clicking, was the justification for arthroscopic surgery. In group 3 (5 cases), a degenerate, frayed ligament, combined with generalized degenerative changes, was identified (Figure 8.20). Arthroscopic de-

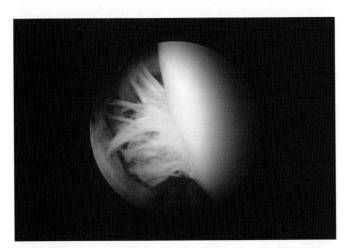

FIGURE 8.18. Ligamentum teres, complete rupture. (From Gray and Villar,[29] with permission of Villar.)

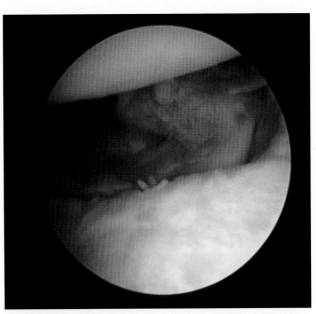

FIGURE 8.20. Ligamentum teres, degenerative, frayed. (From Gray and Villar,[29] with permission of Villar.)

bridement gave unpredictable results in their series. However, the best outcome was obtained in group 1 and, to a lesser extent, in group 3. This is the first series of ligamentum teres injuries reported in the literature. However, other pathologic conditions could be related to ligamentum teres problems.

It is a common finding for the arthroscopic surgeon, after acute dislocation of the hip, that a much wider opening of the joint is possible with mild distraction. This event could perhaps be a warning sign of joint instability and may herald subsequent osteoarthritis.

Fitzgerald[15] reported acute intraarticular hemorrhage of the ligamentum teres as a clinical entity. He suggests that this event must be considered when discussing the differential diagnosis of labral tears. Both conditions can cause what he describes as "mechanical pain" of the hip. We have not arthroscopically identified this entity as a primary cause of hip pain.

Undoubtedly, much still needs to be learned about the importance and incidence of these ligamentum teres lesions. An increased knowledge of both ligamentum function and treatment of damage to it promises to advance the management and understanding of hip pathology.

NECK OF THE FEMUR

The neck of the femur is best seen if the arthroscopy is performed without distracting the joint. This is because, when significant traction is applied, the capsule is stretched and lies close to bone, reducing the space around the femoral neck. Usually the anterior portion of the neck is more accessible, the space being increased by flexing the hip. The anterior gutter is larger because the capsule reaches the inter-

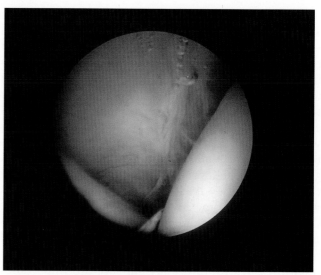

FIGURE 8.22. The zona orbicularis.

trochanteric line, whereas posteriorly its insertion is more proximal, 1 cm above the trochanteric crest. Synovial longitudinal folds reflected upward along the neck of the femur are frequently present. They have a highly vascularized appearance and contain small vessels originating from the medial femoral circumflex artery. If one or more loose bodies are present within the joint, the anterior and posterior gutters close to the femoral neck may well contain them (Figure 8.21).

CAPSULE

The fibrous capsule is a thick and strong structure that encircles the proximal femur and the acetabular cup. Proximally, the capsular insertion is located 5 to 6 mm above the acetabular margin, leaving a little space beyond the acetabular labrum called the *perilabral sulcus*. Inspection of this area is possible with a 70-degree arthroscope, pulling back the cannula to the edge of the joint.

The point of insertion of the fibrous capsule to the femur varies. Anteriorly it is attached to the intertrochanteric line, laterally to the base of the femoral neck, posteriorly 1 cm above the intertrochanteric crest, and medially to the femoral neck near the lesser trochanter. The capsule may be likened to a cylindrical sleeve enclosing the joint and the femoral neck. The capsule is thicker anteriorly than posteriorly and consists of two sets of fibers, circular and longitudinal.

Zona Orbicularis

The circular fibers are named zona orbicularis (Figure 8.22) and are of arthroscopic interest because they form a ring around the neck of the femur. This ring

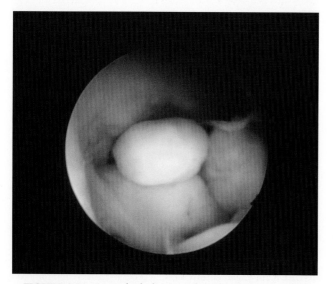

FIGURE 8.21. Loose body lying within the posterior gutter.

has no direct attachment to the bone and is seen arthroscopically as a capsular condensation projecting into the synovial lining, embracing the distracted femoral head. External rotation of the limb during the procedure allows the zona orbicularis to relax, whereas internal rotation tightens it around the femoral neck. The maneuver can be used to differentiate the zona orbicularis from the acetabular labrum.

Capsular Ligaments

The longitudinal fibers are greatest in number and strength but have less arthoscopic interest. Rarely, it is possible to identify the iliofemoral ligament, or ligament of Bigelow. It has a triangular shape, its apex being attached between the anterior inferior iliac spine and the acetabular rim, its base to the intertrochanteric line. Because the central part is thinner, it is often referred to as being Y shaped. Other ligaments reinforcing the capsule are the pubofemoral and the ischiofemoral ligaments. None is usually seen with the arthroscope. The latter has some arthroscopic importance because it thickens the back of the capsule and is perforated using the rare posterior approach.

Retinacula of Weibrecht

Dvorak and coauthors[30] have reported that the Weitbrecht's retinacula can be seen on the posterosuperior aspect of the femoral neck when looking anteriorly from a posterior paratrochanteric portal. This is a flattened band reflecting from the fibrous capsule of the hip joint to the head and neck of the femur, present in 94.8% of male and 92.5% of female subjects. Nutrient arteries for the femoral head run through the retinacula. Noriyasu and coauthors[31] have reported that there are two types of retinacula: a complete band shape and a posterior membranous shape.

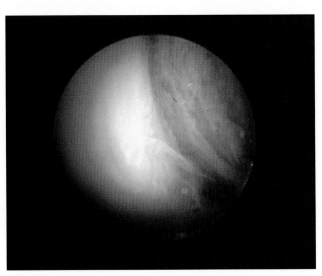

FIGURE 8.23. Normal synovium.

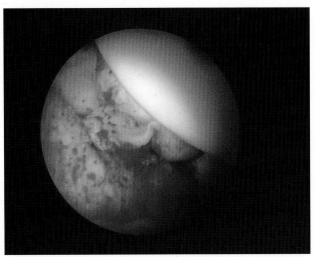

FIGURE 8.24. Hemorrhagic synovium. The result of distraction and irrigation.

Psoas Bursa

A circular aperture between the pubofemoral and iliofemoral ligaments sometimes joins the articular cavity with the subtendinous psoas (iliac) bursa. This structure separates the capsule from the iliopsoas muscle and is lined with synovium.

Synovial Membrane

The inner surface of the capsule is extensively lined with a highly vascularized pink layer of synovial membrane (Figure 8.23). This tissue also covers part of the neck contained within the joint, both surfaces of the acetabular labrum, the ligamentum teres, and the fat within the acetabular fossa. At the femoral attachment of the joint capsule, the synovial membrane is reflected up toward the head as far as the articular margin. The synovium may have a hemorrhagic appearance (Figure 8.24), and an occasional vascular papillary projection of a polypoid nature can be seen. These findings must not be mistaken for a synovitis.

CONCLUSIONS

We have given here a complete and detailed description of the intraarticular structures of the hip. All the illustrations were taken at the time of arthroscopic surgery. No cadaveric images have been included. As in other joints, structures of clinical significance can be assessed better with arthroscopy than with any other technique. Numerous variations of the standard anatomy have been discussed. The understanding of these findings, which remain within the boundaries of the *normal*, is essential for the surgeon who challenges hip arthroscopy.

Indications for surgery are diverse. However, these have not been discussed in this chapter. Primarily, we believe the arthroscopist must distinguish between normal and pathologic findings and then correlate them with clinical symptoms. Only then may he or she plan the operative technique.

References

1. Ponseti IV: Growth and development of the acetabulum in the normal child. J Bone J Surg 1979;60A:575–585.
2. Hisaw FL: Experimental relaxation of the pubic ligaments in the guinea pig. Proc Soc Exp Biol Med 1921;23:661–689.
3. Wilkinson JS: Prime factors in the aetiology of congenital dislocation of the hip. J Bone Joint Surg 1963;45B:268–285.
4. Takechi H, Nagashima H, Ito S: Intra-articular pressure of the hip joint outside and inside the labrum. J Jpn Orthop Assoc 1982;56:529–536.
5. Horii M, Kubo T, Hachiya Y, et al: Development of the acetabulum and the acetabular labrum in the normal child: analysis with radial-sequence magnetic resonance imaging. J Pediatr Orthop 2002;22:222–227.
6. Kurrat HJ, Oberlander W: The thickness of the cartilage in the hip joint. J Anat 1978;126:145–155.
7. Santori N, Villar RN: The iliopubic groove: a possible consequence of incomplete triradiate fusion. Two case reports. J Anat 1997;191:461–463.
8. Santori N, Villar RN: Arthroscopic findings in the initial stages of hip osteoarthritis. Orthopedics 1999;22:405–409.
9. Villar RN: Hip Arthroscopy, vol 5. Oxford: Butterworth-Heinemann, 1992:529–536.
10. Seldes RM, Tan V, Hunt J, et al: Anatomy, histologic features, and vascularity of the adult acetabular labrum. Clin Orthop 2001;382:232–240.
11. Lage AL, Patel JV, Villar RN: The acetabular labral tear: an arthroscopic classification. Arthroscopy 1996;12:269–272.
12. Tan V, Seldes RM, Katz MA, et al: Contribution of acetabular labrum to articulating surface area and femoral head coverage in adult hip joints: an anatomic study in cadavera. Am J Orthop 2001;30:809–812.
13. Glick JM: Hip arthroscopy. In: McGinty JB (ed). Operative Arthroscopy. New York: Raven Press, 1991:663–676.
14. Suzuki S, Kasahara Y, Seto Y, et al: Arthroscopy in nineteen children with Perthés disease: pathologic changes of the synovium and the joint surface. Acta Orthop Scand 1994;65:581–584.
15. Fitzgerald RH: Acetabular labral tears: diagnosis and treatment. Clin Orthop 1995;31:60–68.
16. Ueo T, Suzuki S, Iwasaki R, et al: Rupture of the labra acetabularis as a cause of hip pain detected arthroscopically, and partial limbectomy for successful pain relief. Arthroscopy 1990;6:48–51.
17. Ikeda T, Awaya G, Suzuki S, et al: Torn acetabular labrum in young patients; arthroscopic diagnosis and management. J Bone J Surg [Br] 1988;70:13–16.
18. Nishina T, Saito S, Ozhono K, et al: Chiari pelvic osteotomy for osteoarthritis. The influence of the torn and detached acetabular labrum. J Bone J Surg [Br] 1990;72:765–769.
19. Klaue K, Durnin CW, Ganz R: The acetabular rim syndrome. A clinical presentation of dysplasia of the hip. J Bone J Surg [Br] 1991;73:423–429.
20. Suzuki S, Awaya G, Okada Y, et al: Arthroscopic diagnosis of ruptured acetabular labrum. Acta Orthop Scand 1986;57:513–515.
21. Edward D, Lomas D, Villar RN: Comparison of MRI and hip arthroscopy in diagnosis of disorders of the hip joint. J Bone J Surg [Br] 1994;76(suppl):52.
22. Petersilge CA: MR arthrography for evaluation of the acetabular labrum. Skeletal Radiol 2001;30:423–430.
23. Dorrel JH, Caterall A: The torn acetabular labrum. J Bone J Surg [Br] 1986;68:400–403.
24. Dameron TB Jr: Bucket handle tear of the acetabular labrum accompanying posterior dislocation of the hip. J Bone J Surg [Am] 1959;41:131–134.
25. Ide T, Akamatsu N, Nakajima I: Arthroscopic surgery of the hip joint. Arthroscopy 1991;7:204–211.
26. Wolcott WE: The evolution of the circulation of the developing femoral head and neck. Surg Gynecol Obstet 1943;77:61–82.
27. Waldenstrom H: Necrosis of the femoral head owing to insufficient nutrition from the ligamentum teres. Acta Chir Scand 1934;75:185–196.
28. Gray's Anatomy, 37th ed. New York: Longman, 1989:518–526.
29. Gray AJR, Villar R: The ligamentum teres of the hip: an arthroscopic classification of its pathology. Arthroscopy 1997;13:575–578.
30. Dvorak M, Duncan CP, Day B: Arthroscopic anatomy of the hip. Arthroscopy 1990;6:264–273.
31. Noriyasu S, Suzuki T, Sato E, et al: On the morphology and frequency of Weitbrecht's retinacula in the hip joint. Okajimas Folia Anat Jpn 1993;70:87–90.

9

The Lateral Approach

Thomas G. Sampson

Hip arthroscopy was first done in the supine approach; however, in the early experiences it was fraught with problems and was not predictably successful in entering the joint. History has shown us that Burman was first to arthroscope a series of hips; however, those were all cadavers and mainly in the periarticular capsule.[1] Traction was introduced by Erikkson to enter the true joint.[2] My associate Dr. James M. Glick performed 11 cases between 1977 and 1982 and had difficulty getting in on 2 occasions.[3] Because of my experience with the lateral decubitus positioning and anatomy in total hip replacements, the idea of approaching hip arthroscopy with a similar technique was introduced (Figure 9.1). We dissected a cadaver hip to determine the most direct access to the intraarticular space and developed the anterior peritrochanteric and posterior peritrochanteric trochanteric portals (Figure 9.2). Later, these were referred to as the *anterolateral* and *posterolateral* portals. The first patient on whom we used the lateral approach was a massively obese woman with hip pain who Dr. Glick had previously arthroscoped without success in the supine position. In the lateral decubitus position, the obese portions of her thigh drooped down and away to expose a prominent greater trochanter (Figure 9.3). The neurovascular structures are safely away from the portals and the surgeon is familiar with their location (Figure 9.4). These portals offer direct access into the femoroacetabular joint.

The Chick fracture table was initially used for hip distraction. This apparatus was abandoned because the peroneal post limited hip extension and increased the risk of neuropraxias (Figure 9.5A). Traction was fashioned after our methods for shoulder arthroscopy using a Buck's traction boot, rope, and wall-mounted pulleys (Figure 9.5B). The distraction was limited to the amount of weight used; however, the system was inconvenient and inconsistent in the amount of joint distraction obtained. As a result, two new distractors were developed: the Hip Distraktor (Arthronix, New York, NY), which was the first (Figure 9.6), and the Hip Distractor (OSI Systems, Hawthorne, CA), which attaches to the Jackson table (Figure 9.7). Both systems incorporated a digital tensiometer and a perineal post with more than 9 cm diameter of padding. Joseph

McCarthy developed a distractor without a tensiometer that could fit any operating room table (Figure 9.8).

Initially, the standard arthroscopic instruments were used. However, it became clear that the standard length arthroscopes could not reach the depth of all hips and straight graspers and shavers were inadequate for reaching around the head of the femur and the concavity of the acetabulum.[4] Newer designs with shorter hubs on the arthroscope became available, and curved instruments are still being developed. The Glick Hip Set (Stryker, Kalamazoo, MI) (Figure 9.9) contains long cannulated sheaths and arthroscopes and a variety of long graspers, as well as slotted cannulas for introduction of curved instruments (Figure 9.10). The Dyonics hip set (Smith & Nephew, Andover, MA) has cannulated sheaths that could be used with standard arthroscopes by shortening the hub (Figure 9.11).

The problem of consistently introducing the arthroscope into the hip joint has been resolved if procedure is followed. The new tasks are to perform previously described open procedures requiring arthrotomy with arthroscopy similar to the evolution of arthroscopic surgery in the knee and shoulder.

Since 1983 we have done almost 750 hip arthroscopies using the lateral approach. With the advances in both the lateral and supine techniques, the lateral is still our position of choice as it offers less obstruction in obese patients, allowing soft tissue to drop to the sides, exposing a prominent greater trochanter. As with shoulder arthroscopy, the surgeon's choice will be based on his or her training and comfort.

ANESTHESIA

Most commonly we use general anesthesia. If regional is used, there must be muscle relaxation and paralysis is not necessary. Antibiotic prophylaxis is warranted using one of the cephalosporins.

PATIENT POSITIONING

The patient is placed on a well-padded Jackson or standard operating room table in the lateral decubitus position (Figure 9.12). An axillary roll is positioned, and

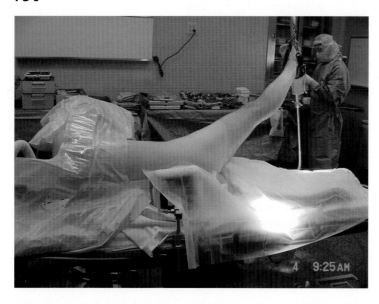

FIGURE 9.1. Patient positioned for total hip replacement in the lateral decubitus position.

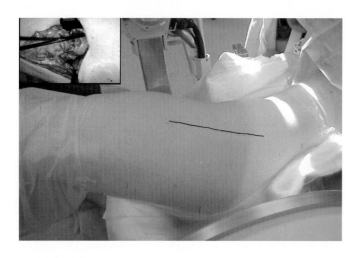

FIGURE 9.2. Patient positioned in the lateral decubitus position; note the Kocher incision for total hip replacement. The inset shows the switching stick over the anterolateral portal in the dissected cadaver.

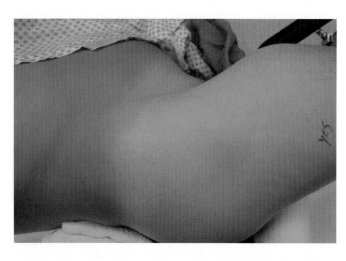

FIGURE 9.3. Patient in lateral decubitus position showing the soft tissue and adipose dropped lateral, exposing the prominent greater trochanter.

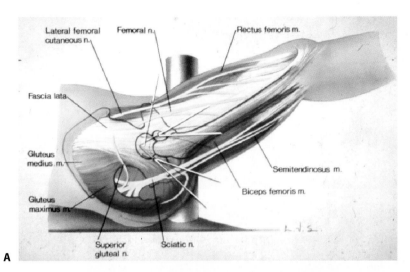

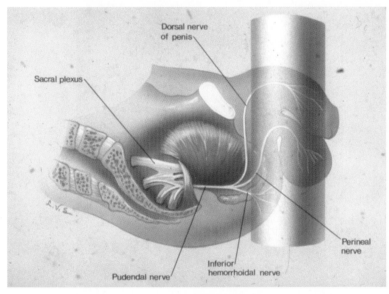

FIGURE 9.4. (A) Diagram of nerves and their relationship to the portals for hip arthroscopy. (B) Diagram showing the course of the pudental nerve and its branches in relationship to the pubis and the peroneal post.

a single posterior hip positioner is used to support the pelvis, which may reduce the risk of pudental neuropraxias by preventing the pelvis from rolling back.

The foot is wrapped with padding, and the foot holder is applied taking care to avoid skin pinching by the device. The leg is held in abduction by the assistant for careful placement of the peroneal post (Figure 9.13). The genitalia are inspected to ensure they are free from compression. Apply the foot holder to the distraction arm and apply only enough traction to support the leg because definitive traction forces should not be applied until the beginning of the operative procedure.

The fluoroscopic C-arm is brought in with the apex under the table and centered at the level of the greater trochanter (Figure 9.14).

Sticky towels or drapes are placed from the iliac crest to 6 inches below the greater trochanter and a sagittal line lateral to the anterior superior iliac spine anterior and the sciatic notch posterior.

The anesthesiologist is at the head of the table, the surgeon stands anterior, and the assistant stands posterior. The scrub technician stands next to the surgeon with the C-arm between them. A Mayo stand is placed above the patient's shoulder for the instruments and arthroscopic cords. We typically drape with split sheets and use a large plastic pouch to catch excess fluids.

TRACTION

For optimal viewing and safe surgery, at least 1.2 cm of distraction is required of the femoroacetabular joint. Two commercial distractors for the lateral approach are available from OSI and Innomed (Savannah, GA), designed by Dr. Glick and Dr. Joseph McCarthy, respectively. The OSI distractor has many advantages in that hip motion is adjustable during surgery and it has a continuous readout tensiometer.

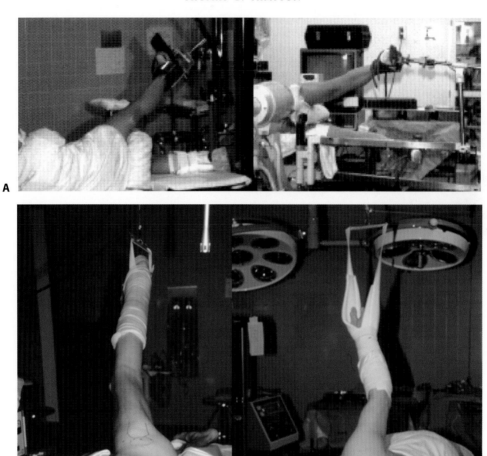

FIGURE 9.5. (A) Traditional fracture tables with the Chick table showing the vertical posterior peroneal post on the left, which may impinge against the sciatic nerve with traction and the leg in extension. (B) The left image shows a patient in abduction traction using a Buck's device and a wall pulley with 45 lb traction. The right view shows patient in the original lateral traction for shoulder arthroscopy using wall pulleys, rope, and weights.

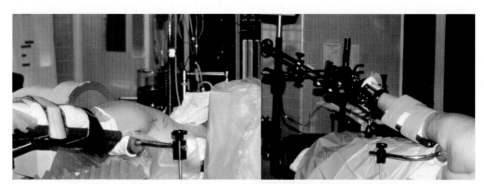

FIGURE 9.6. The Hip Distraktor (Arthronix; no longer available) allows for the use of most operating room tables. A rack supports the leg, preventing valgus forces on the knee, and the foot piece is attached to the traction hand-driven screw, which can be positioned in various degrees of flexion, abduction, and rotation. A tensiometer measures the relative forces applied.

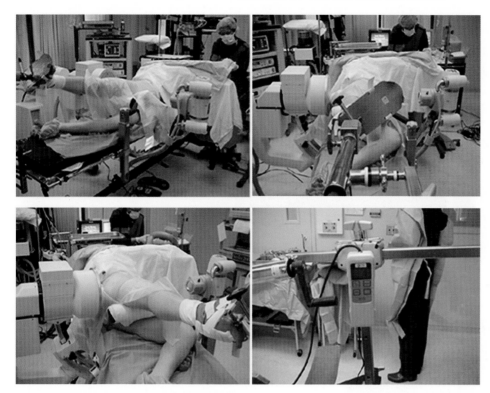

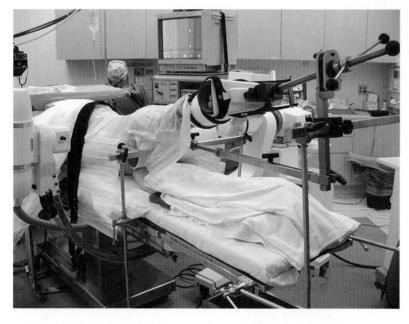

FIGURE 9.7. The OSI Hip distractor on the Jackson table. Note the C-arm is brought beneath the table. The patient's leg can be positioned in varying angles of rotation, flexion, extension, abduction, and adduction. A digital readout tensiometer is used to monitor the traction. The peroneal post has more than 9 cm of padding.

FIGURE 9.8. Patient is lying on a fluoroscopic table in the Innomed hip distractor. Note there is no tensiometer and the leg cannot be flexed or extended once positioned; however, rotation is possible.

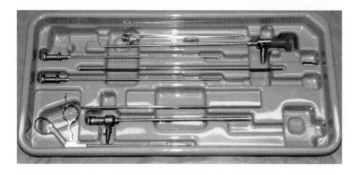

FIGURE 9.9. The Glick Hip Set (Stryker). Note the long arthroscope as well as long instruments and sheaths.

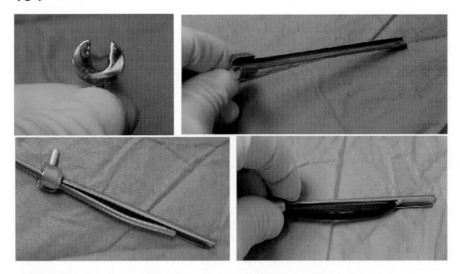

FIGURE 9.10. Slotted cannula allowing introduction of curved instruments into the hip joint.

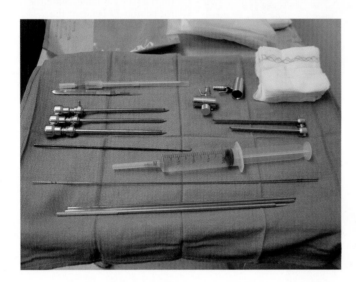

FIGURE 9.11. Dyonics system of sheaths that fit a standard Dyonics arthroscope. Additional instruments are a 14-gauge intracath, no. 11 blade, slotted cannula, switching sticks, and Nitanol wire as well as a syringe with marcaine and epinephrine.

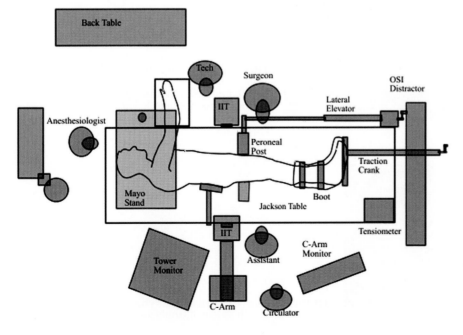

FIGURE 9.12. Operating room layout. Note the patient is in an OSI distractor, and the surgeon and technician are anterior to the patient with the assistant posterior. The C-arm lies between the surgeon and the technician. A Mayo stand lies above the patient for organization of the cords coming from the tower, which is opposite the surgeon. The anesthesiologist is above the head and out of the way.

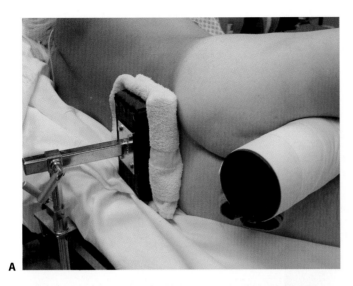

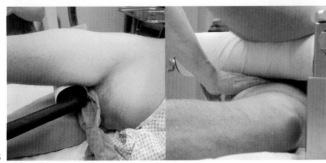

FIGURE 9.13. (A) The patient is lying in a lateral decubitus position with the peroneal post in place. Note the posterior lumbosacral support preventing rollback on the peroneal post. (B) Anterior view of the peroneal post with adequate padding. Note there is adequate space beneath the post, not compressing on the downside leg and offsetting the post toward the operating leg, taking pressure off the pudental nerve.

force, which is entered in the record with the vital signs.

Once the intraarticular portion of the surgery is finished, all the distraction forces are released and the periarticular work can be done without traction concerns.

OPERATING ROOM SETUP

Leg Position

In traction, the hip capsule is maximally relaxed in 15 degrees of flexion, neutral rotation, and 15 degrees of abduction. I use this as a starting position and make adjustments during the procedure. Additionally, the perineal post may be elevated laterally to add an abduction moment for better viewing (Figure 9.15).

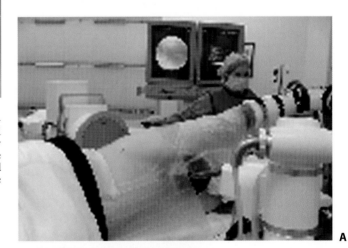

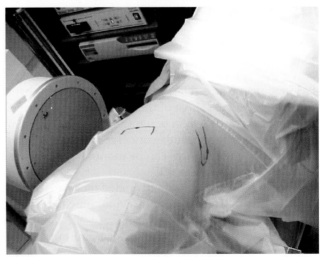

FIGURE 9.14. (A) The C-arm is beneath the patient's table and is brought to the level of the hip joint. The monitor sits across from the surgeon. (B) View of the C-arm from the surgeon's position anterior to the patient. Note it is out of the way of surgery.

Safe traction should be viewed the same as safe tourniquet time and pressure. With the use of evoked potentials, it has been determined that traction forces less than 75 lb for less than 2 hours is safe.[5] I try for traction at less than 50 lb for less than 1 hour to allow for a large margin of safety, and as a result have had no traction-related complications since the technique was implemented.

Realize, however, that "complications may occur from too little or too much traction" (J.M. Glick, personal communication, 2002), and to accomplish the procedure the joint surfaces must be separated to introduce instruments.

The perineal post should have padding of at least 9 cm in diameter and be positioned eccentrically over the pubic symphysis with no compression on the downside thigh. I initiate traction after the case is entirely set up and all the equipment has been turned on and is functioning. We record the traction time and

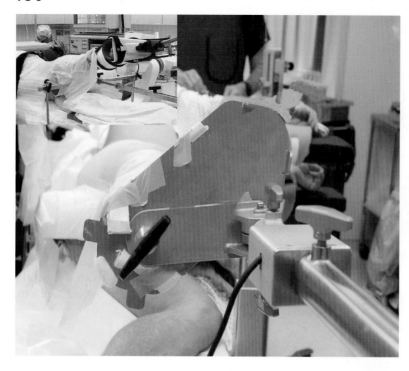

FIGURE 9.15. Leg position is in neutral rotation, taking tension off the hip capsule.

Instruments

The 30-degree arthroscope is best for central viewing. It is easier to get oriented with this angle, and it is the best for getting started. On thin patients standard arthroscopic equipment may be used if the sheath has a short hub. The advantages of the hip kits are that they contain the proper sheath lengths and cannulated systems. The 70-degree arthroscope is best for peripheral viewing and is used to look around the femoral head and to create additional portals. The option for longer arthroscopes should be available for larger patients and for cases in which there is excessive swelling of the thigh.

Both straight and curved graspers are necessary as well as straight and curved shavers (Figure 9.16). To insert curved instruments, a slotted cannula or a flexible plastic sheath is used.

One of the radiothermal probes is used for coagulation, cutting, and ablation of tissues such as capsule or labrum. Because most of these are bendable devices, they can reach the lesion when the metal instruments cannot. The Oratec wands conceived by Marc Philippon and designed for hips can be manually flexed with a trigger handle (Figure 9.17).

Angled neurocurrettes and angled picks are used to treat arthritic defects and remove attached and loose bodies located in difficult areas such as the medial acetabular notch and anteromedial acetabulum.

The Pump

It is generally acceptable to use a pump system because the exact pressure and flow can be controlled and monitored. I recommend using an outflow-dependent pump such as the Stryker Pump, which was designed to work with less fluid demand and that reduces the chance of extravasation into the soft tissues. The pump pressure is set the same as the shoulder or slightly above diastolic pressure.

The Tower

The arthroscopic tower with the monitor and instrument boxes should be placed posterior and slightly cephalad adjacent to the C-arm for optimal viewing of all the settings by the surgeon (Figure 9.18). Think of the surgeon as the pilot of an aircraft. The pilot would not have control of the plane if he or she depended

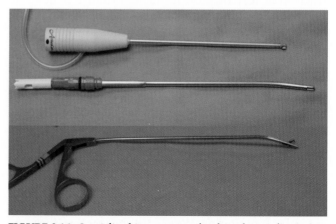

FIGURE 9.16. Specialized instruments that have longer dimensions and curves to reach around the femoral head or into the acetabulum.

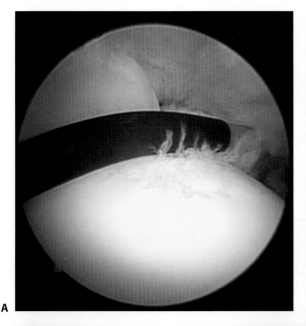

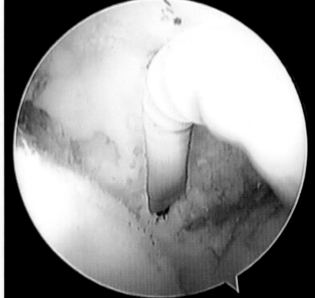

A   B

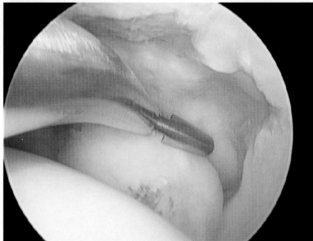

FIGURE 9.17. (A) Arthroscopic view of a curved radiothermal instrument around the femoral head. (B) Arthroscopic view of a flexible chisel operating on the acetabular articular cartilage. (C) Arthroscopic view of a curved grasper removing a loose body from the notch.

C

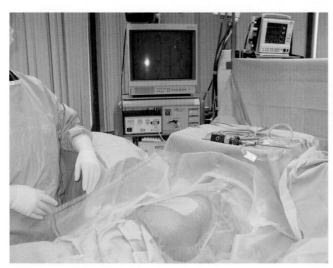

FIGURE 9.18. Surgeon's view of the arthroscopic tower opposite his position. Note the Mayo stand organizing the instruments coming from cephalad within easy reach for the surgeon.

on the flight attendant for engine speed or altimeter readings.

The cords from the tower are brought onto the Mayo stand (Figure 9.19) and organized for the surgeon to easily reach for the shaver and wands. It is more efficient and safe for the Mayo stand to act as neutral ground, whereby only one person accesses it to avoid accidental glove punctures or lacerations.

THE PROCEDURE

The portals for the lateral approach are identical to the supine approach. After everything is set up, the patient is prepped and draped, and all the instruments, camera, and shaver sets are plugged in, and the foot controls are positioned with everything functioning correctly, before initiating traction. For slight and flex-

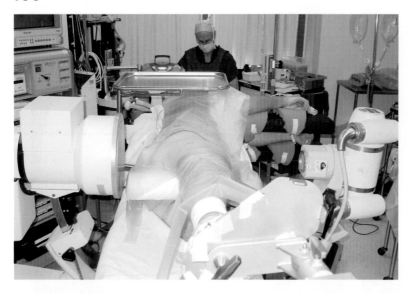

FIGURE 9.19. Patient setup before draping. Note the position of the C-arm. The Mayo stand sits above the patient's shoulder for organization of instruments and easy access to operative field.

ible patients, start with 25 to 50 lb force, and with large stiff patients, use 50 to 75 lb.

Using the C-arm fluoroscope, start with the anterolateral portal (Figure 9.20), observing the 14-gauge 5.25-inch intracath pass between the head of the fe-

mur and acetabulum, closer to the femur to avoid puncturing the labrum. Listen for a hiss as the joint suction seal is broken and observe the traction forces reduce on the tensiometer readout (Figure 9.21). Obtain the desired distraction (usually greater than 1.2

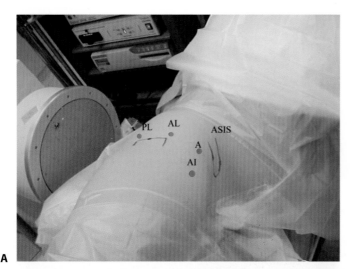

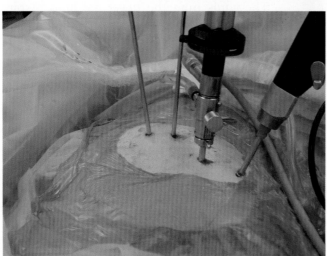

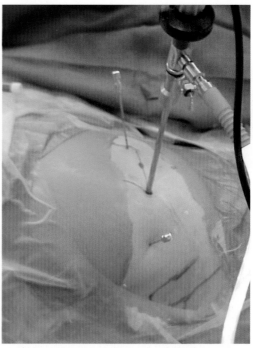

FIGURE 9.20. (A) Patient in a lateral decubitus position with the right hip marked. Note the trochanter and the anterosuperior iliac spine with the portals marked out. A, anterior; AI, anteroinferior; AL, anterolateral; ASIS, anterosuperior iliac spine; PL, posterolateral. (B) Right hip with the arthroscope in the anterolateral portal; the needle is in the posterolateral portal and the anterior portal. (C) Accessory portals include the anteroinferior lateral and anteroinferior medial portal in addition to the anterolateral and posterolateral portals. The arthroscope is in the anteroinferior lateral and the shaver is in the anteroinferior medial portal.

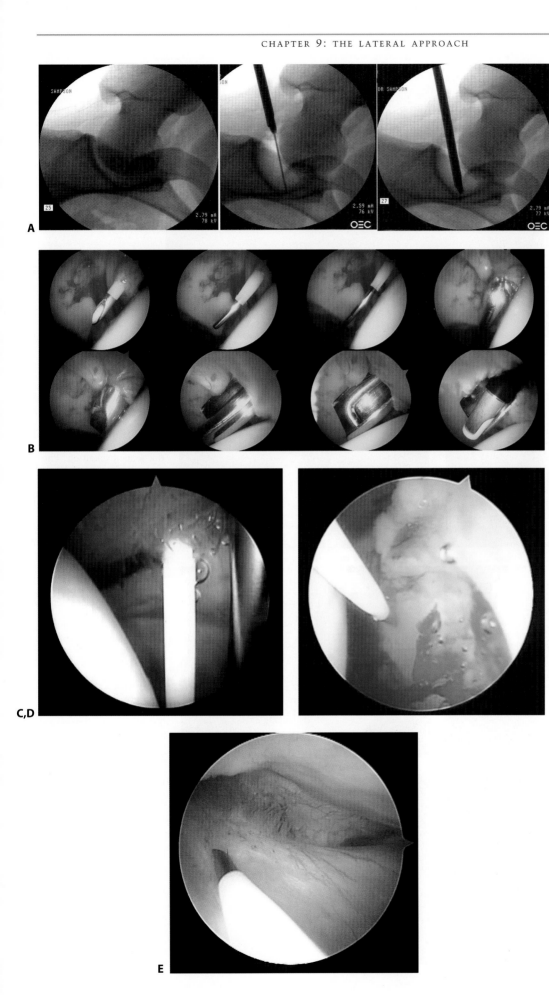

FIGURE 9.21. (A) Fluoroscopic images from the C-arm showing the progression of traction, release of the suction seal, and introduction of the Nitanol wire, and finally the introduction of the arthroscope. (B) Arthroscopic view of a left hip. The sequence shows the introduction of the 14-gauge intracath, following which the Nitanol wire has been introduced. The arthroscopic cannulated sheath with its trochar is introduced into the joint, and then a slotted cannula is introduced over a switching stick. Finally, introduction of a curved instrument is seen in the last image. (C) The introduction of a 14-gauge intracath and a switching stick that has been previously introduced. (D) Arthroscopic view of a Nitanol wire introduced through an intracath into the notch. (E) Arthroscopic view of the inferior pouch with the Nitanol wire being introduced through the intracath. Note the reflection of the iliopsoas and the femoral head seated in the socket with the transverse ligament in the distance.

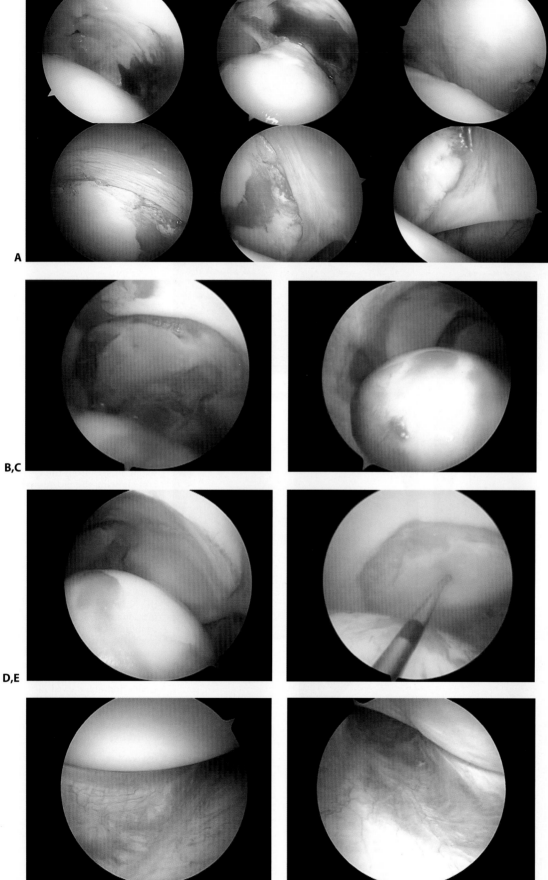

FIGURE 9.22. (A) Arthroscopic view of initial sweep of the 30-degree arthroscope. This image begins with the foveal view, noting the atrophic fat pad. The femoral head is better viewed with the scope backed up. The scope is then rotated posteriorly, showing the labral structures and articular cartilage, and then brought laterally, showing the lateral portion of the labrum at the labral cartilaginous junction. The scope is then rotated anteriorly, showing the labral cartilaginous junction and the anterior labrum. Finally, the scope is swept anteriorly and medially, demonstrating the labral structures and the anterior sulcus. (B) Arthroscopic view anterior central with a 70-degree scope. (C) A 70-degree scope showing the posterior view of the femoral head and labrum. (D) A 70-degree arthroscope showing the anterolateral acetabulum and femoral head and anteromedial sulcus. (E) A 30-degree arthroscopic view showing anterior central position with fluid in the joint and the Nitanol wire in the fat pad. (F) Arthroscopic view of the anteromedial sulcus with the femoral head seated in the acetabulum, noting the anterior labrum and capsule with a reflection of the iliopsoas. (G) Arthroscopic view in the anteromedial sulcus looking posteriorly. Note the transverse acetabular ligament, femoral neck, and head junction.

cm). Insert a Nitanol wire through the catheter, and incise the skin with a no. 11 blade. Push the cannulated arthrosopic sheath over the wire and into the joint while advancing it concentrically over the wire to prevent kinking and wire breakage.

If it is difficult to advance into the joint, suspect the wire is going through the labrum. In such instances, it is best to start over and reposition to avoid labral avulsions or tears. In some cases with stiff hips, the anterior capsule is very thick and difficult to penetrate. For this situation, it is best to begin with the posterolateral portal or gently cut the capsule with a long Beaver blade through the arthroscopic sheath before advancing into the joint. Entry into the joint should always be controlled and gentle to avoid scuffing of the cartilage.

Introduce a 30-degree arthroscope and visually sweep the joint under air. Next, create the posterolateral portal with the same technique with the added benefit of viewing the entry of the intracath and Nitanol wire and instruments while observing the cartilage and labrum. I believe this approach is much safer and reduces iatrogenic injury. The anterior portal is reserved for those cases requiring it and in many cases is not used.

VISUAL SWEEP AND ANATOMY

The acetabulum and its structures are viewed first and visually divided into thirds. Initially, the femoral head cannot be entirely viewed with the hip distracted; however, the hidden portions will be observed when looking in the pericapsular area later in the procedure (Figures 9.22 through 9.26).

With the 30-degree scope, start observing the ac-

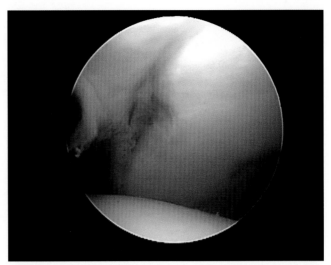

FIGURE 9.24. Arthroscopic view of a normal posterior cleft at the labral cartilaginous junction.

etabular notch and the fat pad. Petechial hemorrhage is normal due to the traction forces pulling negative pressure on the vessels.

Atrophy of the fat pad is abnormal. Look for loose bodies and rice bodies and notch osteophytes or masses. Advance the scope deep to view the ligamentum teres. Look for tears or avulsions. The transverse acetabular ligament is hard to see unless the patient has hyperlaxity.

Rotate the scope posterior and inferior and pick up the posterior labrum at the articular margin, noting the posterior third. Look behind the labrum for loose bodies, then follow the labrum lateral and anterior, noting a normal cleft in the posterior articular margin with a small labral cartilage sulcus. This is not an old avulsion fracture or evidence for subluxation posteri-

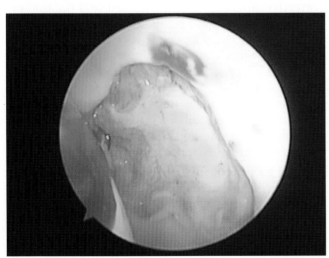

FIGURE 9.23. Arthroscopic view of an atrophic fat pad in the notch of the acetabulum.

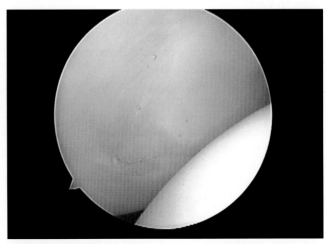

FIGURE 9.25. Arthroscopic view of an articular cartilage blister forming, the beginning of a peel-off lesion at the posterior labral cartilaginous junction.

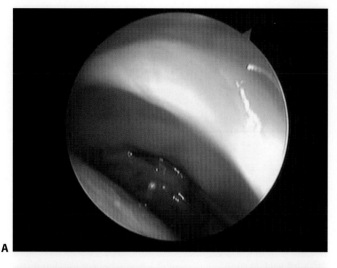

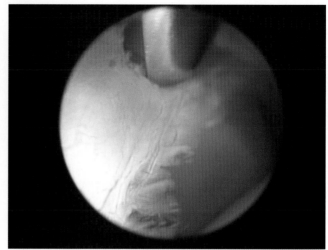

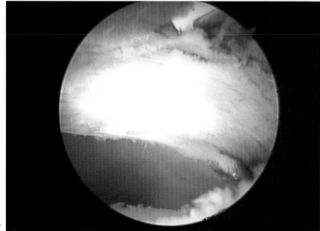

FIGURE 9.26. (A) Arthroscopic view of the superior sulcus above the lateral labrum, below the capsule. (B) Arthroscopic view of a frayed lateral labrum in the superior sulcus beneath the capsule. (C) Arthroscopic view of debridement of a degenerative lateral labrum looking from the superior sulcus.

orly. Note any labral fraying or tears and articular changes.

Look at the mid third and note any labral cartilage separations or fraying and degenerative changes. The surface may be smooth or have a cobblestone appearance in early degeneration.

As the scope is rotated to the anterior third, the labrum may give a backlighting of the joint as the light reflects off the anterior capsule through the labrum. Look for hypertrophy of the labrum in patients with dysplasia. The acetabular cartilage may be soft or may appear blistered or delaminated in dysplastics with anterior groin pain and instability or popping. Look anterior beyond the labrum in the sulcus for synovitis and loose bodies. Move the scope to the superior sulcus of the joint to see the nonarticular side from anterior to posterior. Look for evidence of cysts and spurring and labral tears. During all these maneuvers, a probe or switching stick is used to probe.

Next observe as much of the femoral head with the same method and if necessary rotate the leg while in traction. At this point, I switch to a 70-degree scope to look deeper into the notch and have a better view

of the femoral head fovea with its ligamentum teres attachment.

After viewing from the anterolateral portal, the same procedure is carried out from the posterior portal if one is not satisfied with the initial viewing. The corrective surgery is then performed, and the traction is completely released to allow the hip to be moved in rotation and flexion.

With the hip in slight flexion and neutral rotation, the intracath is inserted through the anterolateral portal, aiming along the femoral neck toward the head–neck junction (Figure 9.27). While observing under fluoroscopy, a small pop is felt as the needle passes through the capsule and the effusion dribbles out of the needle. Pass a Nitanol wire and bounce it off the inferior capsule to confirm it is intraarticular (Figure 9.28). Advance the arthroscopic sheath over the wire and begin viewing the anterior, inferior, and posterior pericapsular space.

First, note the femoral head seated in the labrum as it transforms into the transverse acetabular ligament (Figure 9.29). The zona orbicularis crosses the field, and one may see the vincula-like vessel

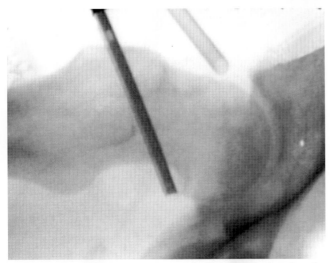

FIGURE 9.27. Fluoroscopic view with the C-arm showing the arthroscope position in the inferior pouch and a cannula near the head–neck junction laterally.

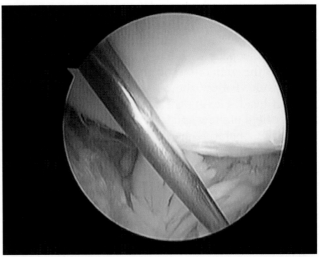

FIGURE 9.28. Arthroscopic view of a Nitanol wire in the inferior pouch. Note the reactive synovitis.

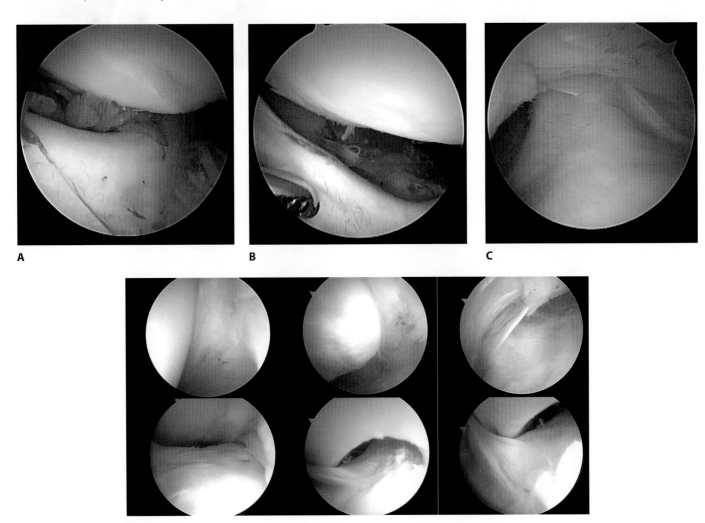

A

B

C

D

FIGURE 9.29. (A) Arthroscopic view of the inferior pouch with lateral distraction of the femoral head. Note the synovitis intraarticular on the inside of the labrum and transverse ligament. (B) Arthroscopic view of the transverse ligament with the hip femoral head distracted laterally. Note the inflamed ligamentum teres. (C) Arthroscopic view of the zona orbicularis. The femoral neck transverses the zona orbicularis. (D) Sequence of a sweep of the inframedial capsule starting with the anteromedial sweeping inferiorly. Note the exposed femoral head and the labrum. Inferiorly there is vincula-like structure representing a branch of the medial femoral circumflex artery to the inferior portion of the femoral head (top row). The bottom row demonstrates the view distal to the zona obicularis on the femoral neck. The zona obicularis is then seen coursing above the femoral neck, and finally a capsular insertion onto the femoral neck.

going into the femoral neck. Push the scope deep and posterior to view the sulcus and look for loose bodies.

As the scope is withdrawn, rotate it inferior to appreciate the reflection of the iliopsoas tendon on the capsule. Follow the reflection proximal over the femoral head. Flexing the hip relaxes the capsule for a larger field of view and improves the mobility of the scope and operative instruments. An anteroinferior portal may be created at the level of the femoral neck midway between the head–neck junction and lesser trochanter for both the arthroscope and operative instruments.

At the completion of the procedure, close the wounds and apply a standard dressing. An intraarticular injection of bupivicaine will make recovery and the trip home more satisfactory.

In the recovery room, have the patient begin actively flexing and extending the hip, as this will give the patient confidence. Crutches are used, with the amount of weight bearing dependent on the diagnosis. Most patients are allowed to fully weight bear unless they have had femoral head–neck ostectomy for femoroacetabular impingement or any femoral neck bone removal.

The dressings are removed in 24 hours, and the patient is allowed to shower. Therapy is started a week later to regain motion and strength.

DISCUSSION

The lateral approach to hip arthroscopy provides a reproducible and safe technique for entering the joint in a patient of any size with any degree of stiffness. Most orthopedic surgeons are familiar with this position from their experience doing hip replacements. Careful attention to the technique may help avoid complications such as arterial injuries or neuropraxias caused by traction. A well-padded peroneal post (>9 cm diameter) and traction of less than 75 lb for less than 2 hours provides *safe traction*. I recommend removing the traction forces as soon as the intraarticular portion of the procedure has been completed. Time will show that most intraarticular and pericapsular procedures will be amenable to arthroscopic treatment.

References

1. Burman M: Arthroscopy of the direct visualization of joints. J Bone Joint Surg [Am] 1931;4:669–695.
2. Eriksson E, Arvidsson L, Arvidsson H: Diagnostic and operative arthroscopy of the hip. Orthopedics 1986;9(2):169–176.
3. Glick JM, et al: Hip arthroscopy by the lateral approach. Arthroscopy 1987;3(1):4–12.
4. Glick JM: Hip arthroscopy. The lateral approach. Clin Sports Med 2001;20(4):733–747.
5. Sampson TG, Fargo LA: Hip arthroscopy by the lateral approach: technique and selected cases. In: Byrd JW (ed). Operative Hip Arthroscopy. New York: Thieme, 1998:105–121.

10

The Supine Approach

J.W. Thomas Byrd

Hip arthroscopy can be performed with equal success whether the patient is positioned supine or laterally. This choice largely depends on the surgeon's preference. However, the supine position has advantages, which are outlined as follows. Positioning is easy and can be accomplished in just a few minutes. The supine position allows the use of a standard fracture table and avoids the necessity of highly specialized, infrequently used distraction devices. The layout of the operating room is user friendly to the surgeon, assistants, and operating room staff. Orientation to the joint is familiar, as orthopedic surgeons are accustomed to this position from their experiences in managing hip fractures. Access to the anterior portions of the joint is also easier, which is important as this is where much of the hip pathology resides.

Another potentially important advantage of the supine position regards the issue of fluid extravasation. As with any joint, some fluid leaks outside the capsule. However, there have been several reports of significant accumulation of fluid within the abdomen or retroperitoneum, resulting in transient vascular compromise of the lower extremities and even cardiac arrest.[1,2] These reports have been limited to the lateral position. This problem may be attributable to the effect of gravity as the abdominal and pelvic cavity creates a sink into which the fluid collects. Although inordinate fluid extravasation is always a potential concern, these severe examples have not been encountered with the patient positioned supine.

DICTUMS ON HIP ARTHROSCOPY

Regardless of the position or technique that is chosen for performing this procedure, several dictums should be thoroughly understood. First, a successful outcome is most clearly dependent on proper patient selection. A technically well-executed procedure fails if performed for the wrong reason. This may include failure of the procedure to meet the patient's expectations. Second, the patient must be properly positioned for the case to go well. Poor positioning ensures a difficult procedure. Third, simply gaining access to the hip joint is not an outstanding technical accomplishment. The paramount issue is accessing the joint in as atraumatic a fashion as possible. Because of the constrained architecture and dense soft tissue envelope of the hip joint, the potential for inadvertent iatrogenic scope trauma is significant and, perhaps to some extent, unavoidable. Thus, every reasonable step should be taken to keep this concern to a minimum. Perform the procedure as carefully as possible and be certain that it is being performed for the right reason.

OPERATING ROOM SETUP

Anesthesia

The procedure is performed as an outpatient procedure under general anesthesia. Epidural is an appropriate alternative, but an adequate motor block is required to ensure muscle relaxation.

Patient Positioning

The patient is positioned supine on the fracture table. An oversized (12 cm outer diameter) formed urethane perineal post is used, positioned laterally against the medial thigh of the operative leg (Figure 10.1). Lateralizing the perineal post adds a slight transverse component to the direction of the traction vector (Figure 10.2). It also distances the post from the area of the pudendal nerve, lessening the risk of compression neuropraxia.

The operative hip is positioned in extension and approximately 25 degrees of abduction. Slight flexion might relax the capsule and facilitate distraction, but this also causes tension on the sciatic nerve, which could increase the risk of traction neuropraxia. Neutral rotation of the extremity during portal placement is important for proper orientation, but freedom of rotation of the footplate during the procedure facilitates visualization of the femoral head.

The contralateral extremity is abducted as necessary to accommodate positioning of the image intensifier between the legs. Before distracting the operative hip, slight traction is applied to the nonoperative leg; this stabilizes the torso on the table and keeps the pelvis from shifting during distraction of the operative hip.

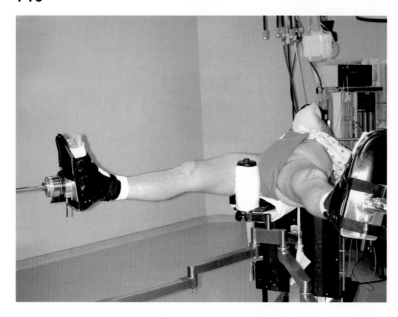

FIGURE 10.1. The patient is positioned on the fracture table so that the perineal post is placed as far laterally as possible toward the operative hip resting against the medial thigh.

Traction is then applied to the operative extremity and distraction of the joint confirmed by fluoroscopic examination. Usually, about 50 lb of traction force is adequate. Sometimes more force is necessary for an especially tight hip, but this should be undertaken with caution.

If adequate distraction is not readily achieved, allowing a few minutes for the capsule to accommodate to the tensile forces often results in relaxation of the capsule and adequate distraction without excessive force. Also, a vacuum phenomenon is apparent fluo-

roscopically. This is created by the negative intracapsular pressure caused by distraction. This seal is released when the joint is distended with fluid at the time of surgery and may further facilitate distraction. However, the effect is variable and should not be depended on to overcome inadequate traction.[3]

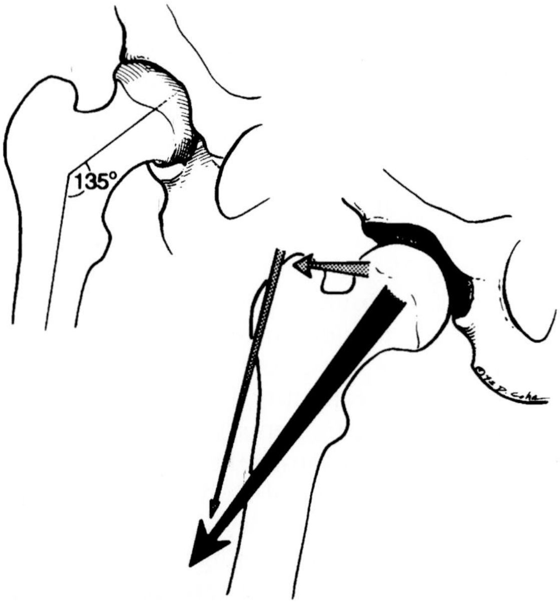

Once the ability to distract the hip joint has been confirmed, the traction is released. The hip is then prepped and draped and traction reapplied when ready to begin arthroscopy (Figure 10.3). The surgeon, assistant, and scrub nurse are positioned on the operative side of the patient. The monitor and arthroscopy cart with an attached sterile Mayo stand containing the video-articulated arthroscopes and power shaver are positioned on the contralateral side (Figure 10.4).

Equipment

Most standard fracture tables can accommodate the few specific needs of hip arthroscopy (Figure 10.5A–D). A tensiometer is a helpful tool that can be incorporated into the footplate and is especially useful for monitoring the intraoperative ability to maintain adequate distraction. A large-sized perineal post with generous padding more safely distributes the pressure on the perineum and facilitates lateralization of the operative hip.

An image intensifier is used for all cases. This is important for ensuring precise portal placement. Simply accessing the joint is often not difficult. More important are care and precision in portal placement to minimize the risk of iatrogenic damage.

Both the 30- and 70-degree video-articulated arthroscopes are routinely used to optimize visualization. Interchanging the two scopes allows excellent visualization despite the limited maneuverability caused by the bony architecture of the joint and its

135°

FIGURE 10.2. The optimal vector for distraction is oblique relative to the axis of the body and more closely coincides with the axis of the femoral neck than the femoral shaft. This oblique vector is partially created by abduction of the hip and partially accentuated by a small transverse component to the vector.

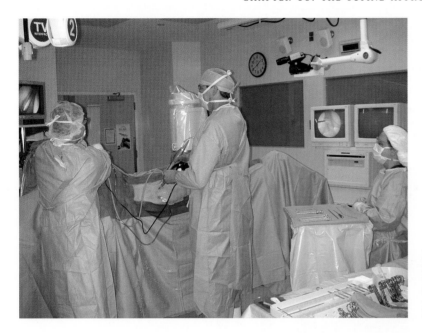

FIGURE 10.3. The surgeon, assistant, and scrub nurse are positioned on the operative side. The arthroscopy cart with monitor is on the nonoperative side. The C-arm, covered with a sterile drape, is positioned between the legs with the fluoroscopic monitor at the foot.

dense soft tissue envelope. The 30-degree scope provides the best view of the central portion of the acetabulum and femoral head and the superior portion of the acetabular fossa, whereas the 70-degree scope is best for visualizing the periphery of the joint, the acetabular labrum, and the inferior portion of the fossa.

A fluid pump provides significant advantages in the hip. A high-flow system can provide optimal flow without having to use excessive pressure. This is important for visualization and safety. Adequate flow is essential for good visualization necessary to perform the procedure effectively and in an expedient manner. Flow cannot be as precisely modulated with a gravity system, creating difficulties both with visualization and extravasation. However, the surgeon must always be cognizant that the pump is functioning properly.

Extra-length cannulas are specifically designed to accommodate the dense soft tissue envelope that surrounds the hip (Figure 10.6). The extra length has been accomplished by shortening the accompanying bridge, which allows these cannulas to be used with a stan-

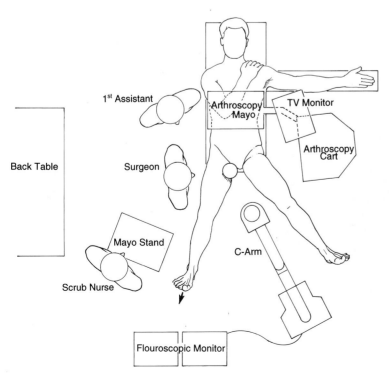

FIGURE 10.4. Schematic of the operating room layout showing the position of the surgeon, assistant, scrub nurse, arthroscopy cart, monitor and Mayo stand, scrub nurse's Mayo, C-arm, and back table.

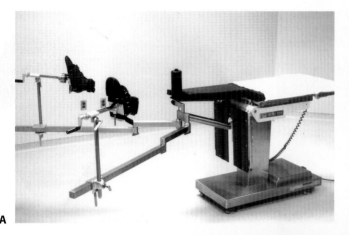

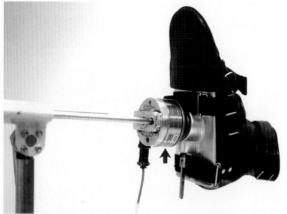

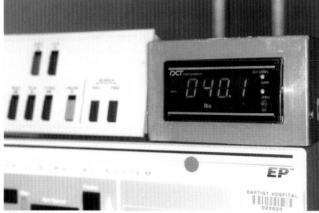

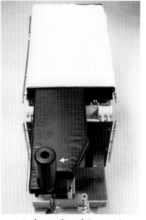

FIGURE 10.5. (A) Modifications to this standard fracture table facilitate safe and effective hip arthroscopy. (B) The tensiometer (arrow) is built into the footplate applied to the operative extremity. (C) The digital display is mounted on the arthroscopy cart, allowing constant intraoperative monitoring of the traction force. (D) The oversized perineal post is lateralized (arrow) toward the operative side on the table. The profile of the underlying pelvic support has been reduced (broken line) on the operative side so that it does not protrude laterally underneath the buttock. This feature can be switched for either a right or left hip.

dard arthroscope. Special cannulated obturators also allow passage of the cannula/obturator assembly over a Nitanol guidewire prepositioned in the joint through 6-inch, 17-gauge spinal needles (Figure 10.7). The

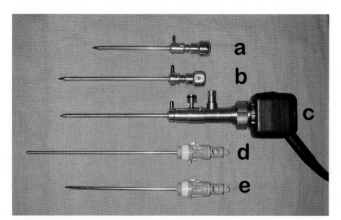

FIGURE 10.6. A standard arthroscopic cannula (a) is compared with the extra-length cannula (b). A modified bridge (c) has been shortened to accommodate the extra-length cannula with a standard length arthroscope. Extra-length blades (d) are also available compared with the standard length blades (e).

scrub nurse's Mayo stand contains the instruments routinely needed for each case (Figure 10.8). The 5.0-mm cannula is used for initial introduction of the arthroscope while the inflow is attached. The diameter allows adequate flow for the fluid management system attached through the bridge. Once all three portals have been established, the inflow can be switched to one of the other cannulas and the 5.0-mm cannula replaced with a 4.5-mm cannula. The use of three 4.5-mm cannulas allows complete interchangeability of the arthroscope, instruments, and inflow. The 5.5-mm cannula is available for larger shaver blades.

Extra-length blades are available. Curved designs are especially helpful for maneuvering within the spherical geometry of the joint. These can be passed through specially designed slotted cannulas (Figure 10.9) that accommodate the curved shaver blades as well as other hand instruments. Specially designed hand instruments must be longer, but also of sturdy construction to minimize the risk of instrument breakage.

Thermal ablation devices demonstrate specific advantages in the hip. The small diameter allows access

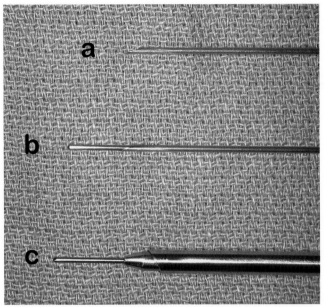

FIGURE 10.7. The cannulated obturator system allows for greater ease and reliably establishing the portals once proper positioning has been achieved with the spinal needle. The 6-inch, 17-gauge spinal needle (a, b) accommodates passage of a Nitanol wire (b, c). Specially treated, the wire is resistant to kinking. The cannulated obturator allows for passage of the obturator/cannula assembly over the guidewire (c).

to recesses within the joint difficult to access with mechanical blades. Also, because of the limits on maneuverability, it can be difficult for the shaver to excise damaged articular cartilage or labrum and create a stable edge. Thermal devices are often much more effective at creating a smooth transition zone, preserving more healthy tissue.

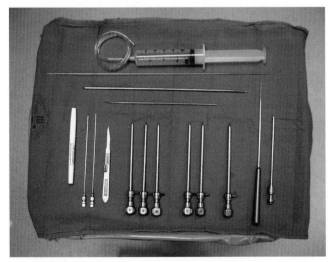

FIGURE 10.8. The scrub nurse's Mayo stand contains basic instruments necessary for initiating the arthroscopic procedure including a marking pen; no. 11 blade scalpel; 6-inch, 17-gauge spinal needles; 60-ml syringe of saline with extension tubing; a Nitanol guidewire; three 4.5-, two 5.0-, and one 5.5-mm cannulas with cannulated and solid obturators; a switching stick; a separate inflow adapter; and modified probe.

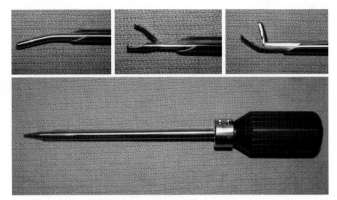

FIGURE 10.9. A slotted cannula with its accompanying cannulated obturator accommodates passage of curved shaver blades and larger hand instruments into the joint.

GENERAL TECHNIQUE

The technique described here has proved to be effective and reproducible.[4–6]

Portals

Three standard portals are used for hip arthroscopy: anterior, anterolateral, and posterolateral (Figures 10.10, 10.11).[7] The site of the anterior portal coincides with the intersection of a sagittal line drawn distally from the anterior superior iliac spine and a transverse line across the superior margin of the greater trochanter. The direction of this portal courses approximately 45 degrees cephalad and 30 degrees toward the midline. The anterolateral and posterolateral portals are positioned directly over the superior aspect of the trochanter at its anterior and posterior borders.

Anterior Portal

The pathway of the anterior portal penetrates the muscle belly of the sartorius and the rectus femoris before entering the anterior capsule (Figure 10.12). At the portal level, the lateral femoral cutaneous nerve has usually divided into three or more branches. Consequently, the portal usually passes within several millimeters of one of these branches. Because of the multiple branches, the nerve is not easily avoided by altering the portal position. Rather, it is protected by using meticulous technique in portal placement. Specifically, the nerve is most vulnerable to a deeply placed skin incision that lacerates one of the branches. Therefore, the initial stab wound should be made carefully through the skin only.

The average minimum distance from the anterior portal to the femoral nerve is 3.2 cm. The relationship of the ascending branch of the lateral circumflex femoral artery is variable but averages 3.6 cm inferior to the anterior portal.

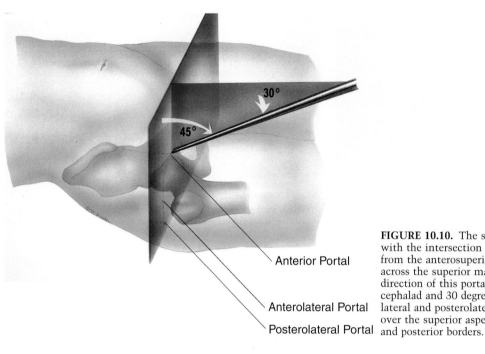

FIGURE 10.10. The site of the anterior portal coincides with the intersection of a sagittal line drawn distally from the anterosuperior iliac spine and a transverse line across the superior margin of the greater trochanter. The direction of this portal courses approximately 45 degrees cephalad and 30 degrees toward the midline. The anterolateral and posterolateral portals are positioned directly over the superior aspect of the trochanter at its anterior and posterior borders.

Anterior Portal

Anterolateral Portal

Posterolateral Portal

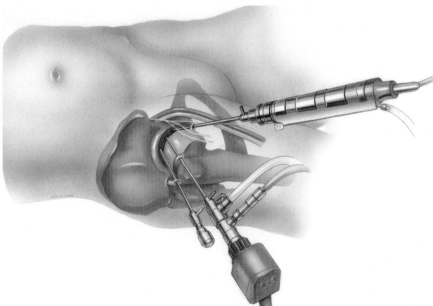

FIGURE 10.11. The relationship of the major neurovascular structures to the three standard portals. The femoral artery and nerve lie well medial to the anterior portal. The sciatic nerve lies posterior to the posterolateral portal. Small branches of the lateral femoral cutaneous nerve lie close to the anterior portal. Injury to these is avoided by using proper technique in portal placement. The anterolateral portal is established first because it lies most centrally in the safe zone for arthroscopy.

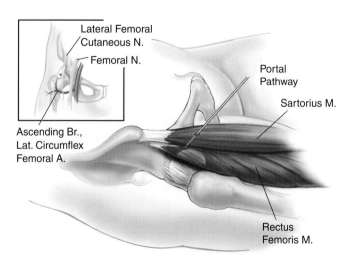

Lateral Femoral Cutaneous N.

Femoral N.

Portal Pathway

Sartorius M.

Ascending Br., Lat. Circumflex Femoral A.

Rectus Femoris M.

FIGURE 10.12. Anterior portal pathway/relationship to lateral femoral cutaneous nerve, femoral nerve, and lateral circumflex femoral artery. (Courtesy of Smith & Nephew Endoscopy, Andover, MA.)

Anterolateral Portal

The anterolateral portal penetrates the gluteus medius before entering the lateral aspect of the capsule at its anterior margin (Figure 10.13). The superior gluteal nerve lies an average of 4.4 cm superior to the portal.

Posterolateral Portal

The posterolateral portal penetrates both the gluteus medius and minimus before entering the lateral capsule at its posterior margin (Figure 10.14). Its course is superior and anterior to the piriformis tendon. The portal lies closest to the sciatic nerve at the level of the capsule, with the distance averaging 2.9 cm. An average distance of 4.4 cm separates the portal from the superior gluteal nerve.

Portal Placement

The anterolateral portal lies most centrally in the *safe zone* for arthroscopy and thus is the portal placed first.[7] Subsequent portal placements are assisted by direct arthroscopic visualization. This initial portal is placed by fluoroscopic inspection in the anteroposterior (AP) plane. However, orientation in the lateral plane is equally important. With the leg in neutral rotation, femoral anteversion leaves the center of the joint just anterior to the center of the greater trochanter. Thus, the entry site for the anterolateral portal at the anterior margin of the greater trochanter corresponds with entry of the joint just anterior to its midportion. This correct entry site of the joint is

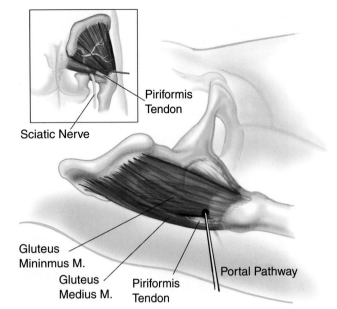

FIGURE 10.14. Posterolateral portal pathway/relationship to the sciatic nerve and superior gluteal nerve. (Courtesy of Smith & Nephew Endoscopy, Andover, MA.)

achieved by keeping the instrumentation parallel to the floor during portal placement (Figure 10.15).

When distracting the hip, a vacuum phenomenon usually is present (Figure 10.16A). Prepositioning for the anterolateral portal is performed with a 6-inch, 17-gauge spinal needle under fluoroscopic control (Figure 10.16B). The joint is then distended with approxi-

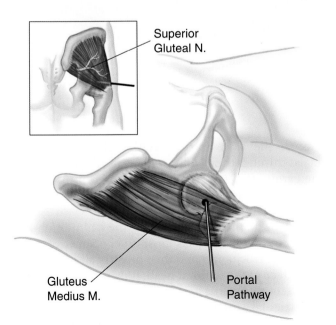

FIGURE 10.13. Anterolateral portal pathway/relationship to superior gluteal nerve. (Courtesy of Smith & Nephew Endoscopy, Andover, MA.)

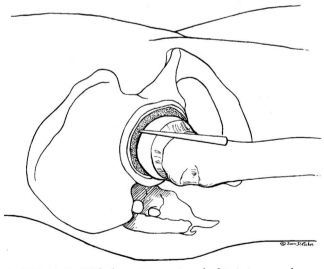

FIGURE 10.15. With the patient supine, the hip is in neutral rotation with the kneecap pointing toward the ceiling. A needle placed at the anterior margin of the greater trochanter (anterolateral position) is maintained in the coronal plane by keeping it parallel to the floor as it enters the joint. Due to femoral neck anteversion, the entry site will be just anterior to the joint's center. If the entry site is too anterior, it becomes crowded with the anterior portal. If it is too posterior, it becomes difficult to properly visualize the entry site for the anterior portal. (From Byrd,[8] with permission of Arthroscopy.)

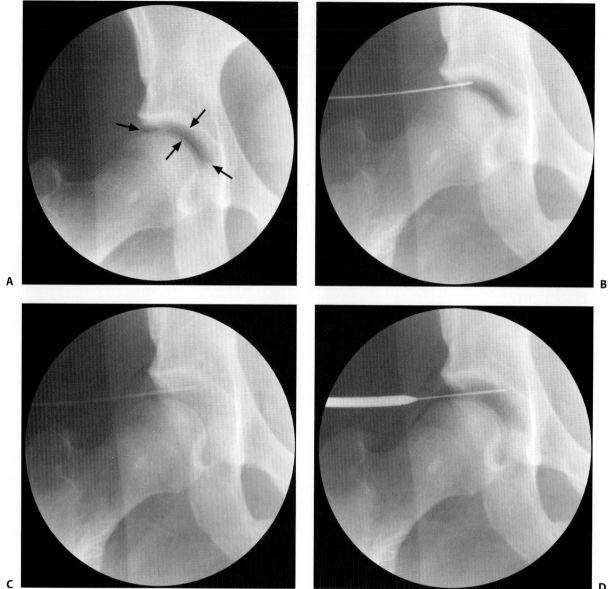

FIGURE 10.16. Anteroposterior (AP) fluoroscopic view of a right hip. (A) A vacuum effect is apparent because of the negative intracapsular pressure created by distraction of the joint (arrows). (B) A spinal needle is used in prepositioning for the anterolateral portal. The needle courses above the superior tip of the trochanter and then passes under the lateral lip of the acetabulum entering the hip joint. (C) Distension of the joint disrupts the vacuum and facilitates adequate distraction. (D) The cannula/obturator assembly is being passed over the Nitanol wire that had been placed through the spinal needle.

mately 40 ml fluid and the intracapsular position of the needle confirmed by backflow of fluid. Distension of the joint enhances distraction (Figure 10.16C).

It is important to note that the needle may inadvertently penetrate the lateral acetabular labrum during initial placement into the joint.[8] This puncture can be felt because pushing the needle through the labrum results in greater resistance than when just penetrating the capsule. If the needle pierces the labrum, once the joint has been distended, it is a simple process to back the needle up and reenter the capsule below the level of the labrum. Failure to recognize this can result in avoidable violation of the labrum by the cannula. A stab wound is made

through the skin at the needle. The guidewire is placed through the needle and the needle is removed. The cannulated obturator with the 5.0-mm arthroscopy cannula is passed over the wire into the joint (Figure 10.16D).

When establishing the portal, the cannula/obturator assembly should pass close to the superior tip of the greater trochanter and then directly above the convex surface of the femoral head. It is important to keep the assembly off the femoral head to avoid inadvertent articular surface scuffing.

Sometimes blood is present within the joint due to the traction force necessary to distract the surfaces. This is difficult to clear until a separate egress has been established. However, venting fluid with the spinal needle from anterior will clear the field of view.

Once the arthroscope has been introduced, the anterior portal is placed next. Positioning is now facilitated by visualization from the arthroscope as well as fluoroscopy. The 70-degree scope works best for directly viewing where the instrumentation penetrates the capsule. Pre-positioning is again performed with the 17-gauge spinal needle, entering the joint directly underneath the free edge of the anterior labrum. As the cannula/obturator assembly is introduced, it is lifted up to stay off the articular surface of the femoral head while passing underneath the acetabular labrum.

If proper attention is given to the topographic anatomy in positioning the anterior portal, the femoral nerve lies well medial to the approach.[7] However, the lateral femoral cutaneous nerve lies quite close to this portal. It is best avoided by using proper technique in portal placement. The nerve is most vulnerable to laceration by a skin incision placed too deeply.

Rarely, access for the anterior portal may be blocked by an overlying osteophyte or simply the architecture of the patient's acetabular bony anatomy. If necessary, arthroscopy can still be effectively performed using just the lateral two portals.

Last, the posterolateral portal is introduced. The fluoroscopic guidelines are similar to the anterolateral portal. Rotating the lens of the arthroscope posteriorly brings the entry site underneath the posterior labrum into view. Placement under arthroscopic control ensures that the instrumentation does not stray posteriorly, potentially placing the sciatic nerve at risk. The hip remains in neutral rotation during placement of the posterolateral portal. External rotation of the hip would move the greater trochanter more posteriorly and, because this is the main topographic landmark, the sciatic nerve might be at greater risk for injury (Figure 10.17).

Portal Placement for Peripheral Joint

After arthroscopy of the interior of the hip is complete, the instruments can be removed and traction released for access to the peripheral compartment. The hip is flexed approximately 45 degrees, which relaxes the anterior capsule (Figure 10.18). From the anterolateral entry site, the spinal needle penetrates the capsule on the anterior neck of the femur under fluoroscopic control (Figure 10.19A,B). Using the guidewire, the cannula/obturator assembly is then placed (Figure 10.19C). The 5-mm cannula is preferred with the inflow attached to the scope.

For instrumentation, an ancillary portal is placed 4 cm distal to the anterolateral portal. Once again prepositioning is performed with the 17-gauge spinal needle, directly observing through the arthroscope where the needle enters the peripheral compartment (see Figure 10.19D). Many loose bodies reside in this area and can be retrieved. This portal also provides superior access to the synovial lining and capsule, which is important for performing a thorough synovectomy and also aids when performing a thermal capsulorrhaphy.

DIAGNOSTIC ARTHROSCOPY

When preparing for hip arthroscopy, the surgeon formulates a tentative treatment plan based on the preliminary diagnosis. However, the definitive treatment strategy will be dictated by the findings observed at arthroscopy. With the current limitations of investigative techniques, the arthroscopic findings may differ significantly from those implied by the preoperative studies. Thus, a systematic and thorough initial inspection of the joint is imperative. Once all aspects of the intraarticular pathology have been identified, the surgeon can then embark on intervention with

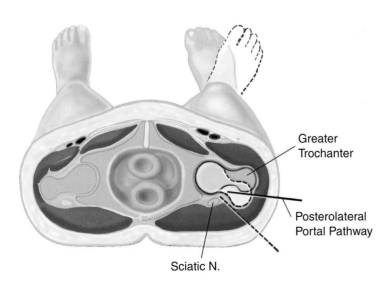

Greater Trochanter

Posterolateral Portal Pathway

Sciatic N.

FIGURE 10.17. Neutral rotation of the operative hip is essential for protection of the sciatic nerve during placement of the posterolateral portal. (Courtesy of Smith & Nephew Endoscopy, Andover, MA.)

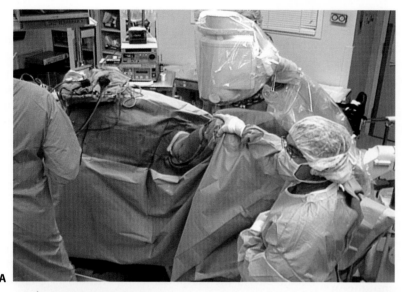

A

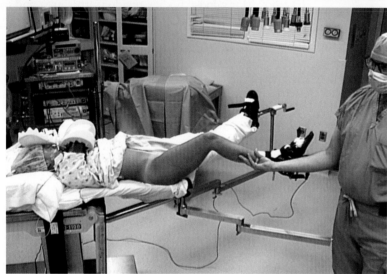

B

FIGURE 10.18. (A) The operative area remains covered in sterile drapes while the traction is then released and the hip flexed 45 degrees. (B) Position of the hip without the overlying drape.

appropriate time management to address all aspects within the joint. The surgeon should avoid spending considerable time on one obvious aspect of the pathology to only then realize that there is other coexistent damage that needs to be addressed.

Using the three-portal technique (anterior, anterolateral, and posterolateral), inspection begins from the anterolateral portal (see Figure 10.11). This is the first portal established because it lies most centrally in the safe zone for arthroscopy. Inspection begins with the 70-degree scope as this provides the best view of the outer margins of the joint and is used for allowing direct arthroscopic visualization of where the other two portals are placed. The anterolateral portal provides the best view of the anterior portion of the joint (Figure 10.20).

Next, the arthroscope is placed in the anterior portal. Viewing laterally, the relationship of the lateral two portals underneath the lateral labrum is seen (Fig-

ure 10.21). The surgeon should be especially cognizant to critique the entry site of the anterolateral portal because this is the one portal that is placed only under fluoroscopic guidance without benefit of arthroscopic visualization of where the portal enters the joint. Viewing medially from the anterior portal, the surgeon can see the most inferior limit of the anterior labrum (Figure 10.22).

The arthroscope is then placed in the posterolateral portal, which provides the best view of the posterior regions of the joint, especially the posterior labrum (Figure 10.23). The posterior labrum is the portion that is least often damaged and has the most consistent morphological appearance. Thus, viewing this area is often used as a reference in assessing variations of the anterior or lateral labrum and accompanying pathology.

Each of the three portals provides a different perspective on the acetabular fossa (Figure 10.24). The 70-

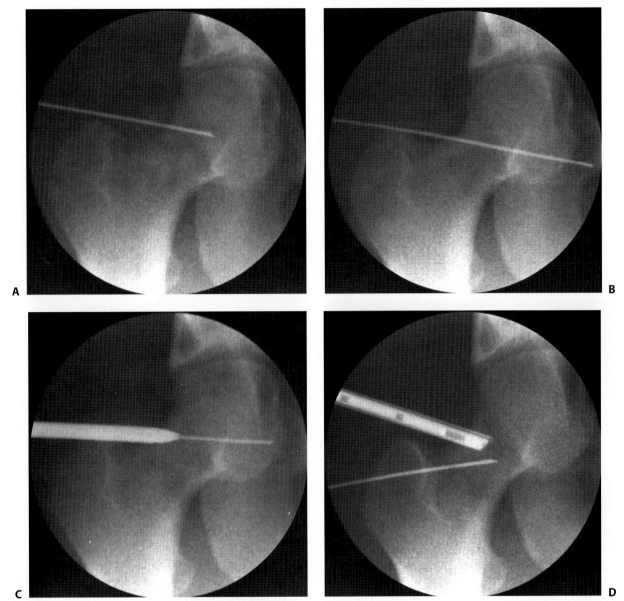

FIGURE 10.19. AP fluoroscopic view of the flexed hip. (A) From the anterolateral entry site, the 17-gauge spinal needle has been repositioned on the anterior neck of the femur. The spinal needle can be felt perforating the capsule before contacting the bone. (B) The guidewire is placed through the spinal needle. It should pass freely to the medial capsule as illustrated. (C) The cannula/obturator assembly is being placed over the guidewire. (D) The position of the 30-degree arthroscope is shown while a spinal needle is being placed for an ancillary portal.

degree scope provides a direct view of the ligamentum teres, which resides in the inferior portion of the fossa. The transverse acetabular ligament can also be partially viewed coursing underneath the ligamentum teres. After the inspection with the 70-degree scope is completed, the 30-degree scope is then used, reversing the sequence of steps between the three portals. The 30-degree scope provides a better view of the central portion of the femoral head and acetabulum and the superior portion of the acetabular fossa.

Once the traction has been released and the hip flexed, the arthroscope is repositioned from the anterolateral portal on the anterior neck of the femur, providing an excellent perspective of the peripheral compartment (Figures 10.25, 10.26). This position brings into view structures that cannot be seen from inside the joint and also provides a different peripheral perspective on some of the intraarticular structures. The medial synovial fold is consistently visualized adjacent to the anteromedial neck of the femur.

Normal Variants

The lateral and the anterior portions of the labrum are the most variable. Sometimes this portion of the labrum is thin, poorly developed, and hypoplastic, and at other times it may appear enlarged. In the presence of acetabular dysplasia, the lateral labrum is especially

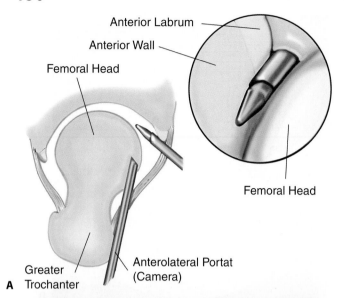

A commonly encountered observation in adults is a stellate-appearing articular lesion immediately above the acetabular fossa, referred to as the *stellate crease* (Figure 10.29). When seen, it is unlikely to be of clinical significance as a contributing cause of pain and is of uncertain long-term prognostic significance regarding susceptibility to future degenerative disease. Occasionally, this must be distinguished from traumatic articular lesions that can occur in this same area, especially from a lateral blow to the hip impacting the femoral head against the superomedial acetabulum.

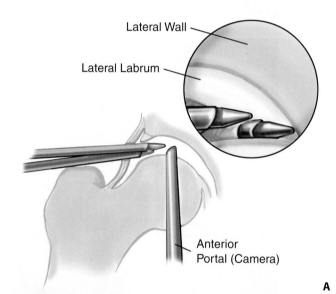

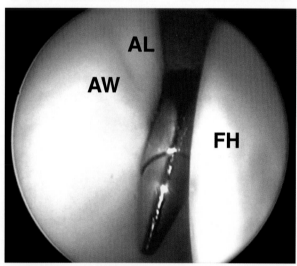

FIGURE 10.20. (A) Arthroscopic view of a right hip from the anterolateral portal. (Courtesy of Smith & Nephew Endoscopy, Andover, MA.) (B) Demonstrated are the anterior acetabular wall (AW) and the anterior labrum (AL). The anterior cannula is seen entering underneath the labrum, and the femoral head (FH) is on the right.

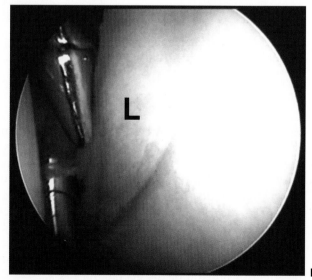

FIGURE 10.21. (A) Arthroscopic view from the anterior portal. (Courtesy of Smith & Nephew Endoscopy, Andover, MA.) (B) Demonstrated are the lateral aspect of the labrum (L) and its relationship to the lateral two portals.

hypertrophic, having a more stabilizing and weight-bearing role substituting for the absent lateral portion of the bony acetabulum. A labral cleft is sometimes present (Figure 10.27); this is a normal finding and should not be misinterpreted as a traumatic detachment. The distinguishing features are absence of tissue that appears damaged and absence of any attempted healing response that would be expected in the presence of trauma.

Remnants of the triradiate cartilage may be evident in adulthood as a physeal scar, void of overlying articular cartilage, extending in a linear fashion along the medial aspect of the acetabulum anterior and/or posterior to the fossa (Figure 10.28). This should not be misinterpreted as an old fracture line.

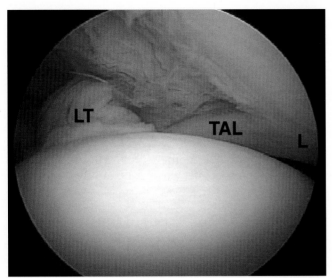

FIGURE 10.22. View inferomedially from the anterior portal demonstrates where the inferior aspect of the anterior labrum (L) becomes contiguous with the transverse acetabular ligament (TAL) below the ligamentum teres (LT).

OPERATIVE ARTHROSCOPY

Loose Bodies

Loose bodies can be extracted, and arthroscopy offers an excellent alternative to arthrotomy, previously indicated for this condition.[9–11] The three standard portals offer access to most parts of the joint where symptomatic loose bodies reside. Removal of free-floating pieces can be a challenge. If there is soft tissue attachment, debridement should leave a small tag of tissue attached that tethers the loose body, making it easier to grasp. Manipulating the position of the inflow cannula often flushes pieces up toward the instrumentation. Many can be debrided with shavers or flushed through large-diameter cannulas. Larger ones can be morselized and removed piecemeal; however, some may be too large for removal through a cannula. Sturdy graspers with various angles are available. Once a portal tract has been developed with a cannula, then, with a little attention to detail, the cannula system can be removed and the larger grasper can be passed along the remaining tract to the joint in a freehand fashion. Make sure to enlarge the capsular incision with an arthroscopic knife and the skin incision so that, as the fragment is retrieved, it will not be lost in the tissues at either the capsule or subcutaneous level. Also note that many loose bodies can reside undetected in the peripheral compartment. Thus, inspecting this area is often important as part of a thorough assessment.

One issue regards timing of arthroscopy following acute trauma. Fluid extravasation can occur due to loss of the capsular integrity or through an acetabular fracture. Waiting several weeks may result in sufficient soft tissue healing to create a fluid seal; however, this must be weighed against the consequences of secondary damage incurred from the entrapped fragments. A high-flow fluid management system can allow adequate flow for visualization without requiring high pressure, which could accentuate extravasation. However, it is always imperative to be cognizant of the rate of fluid ingress. It is also important that the

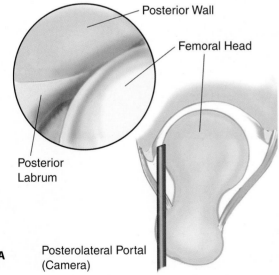

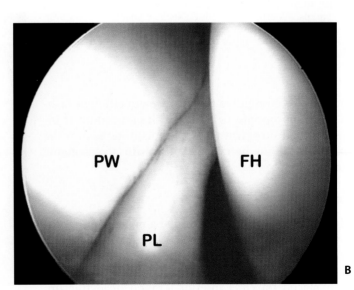

FIGURE 10.23. (A) Arthroscopic view from the posterolateral portal. (Courtesy of Smith & Nephew Endoscopy, Andover, MA.) (B) Demonstrated are the posterior acetabular wall (PW), posterior labrum (PL), and the femoral head (FH). [JWT Byrd, Operative Techniques in Sports Medicine 10:184, 2002, with permission.]

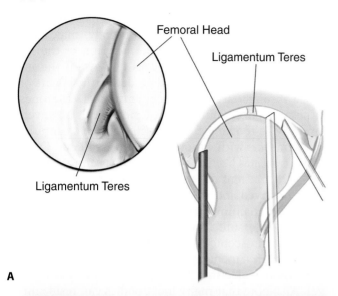

A

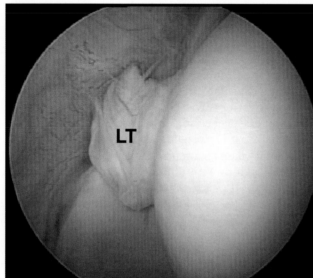

B

FIGURE 10.24. (A) The acetabular fossa can be inspected from all three portals. (Courtesy of Smith & Nephew Endoscopy, Andover, MA.) (B) The ligamentum teres (LT), with its accompanying vessels, has a serpentine course from its acetabular to its femoral attachment.

procedure be completed in a timely and efficient fashion. It is appropriate to abandon the procedure if inappropriate fluid extravasation is encountered or if the procedure cannot be completed within a reasonable amount of time.

CASE 1

A 16-year-old obese girl sustained a posterior dislocation of her right hip (Figure 10.30A). A closed reduction was performed. Postreduction radiography demonstrated a nonconcentric reduction as well as a nondisplaced Pipkin I inferior femoral head fracture (Figure 10.30B). A CT scan demonstrated at least two entrapped intraarticular fragments (Figure 10.30C). Arthroscopy revealed numerous fragments, which were

excised (Figure 10.30D–F). The postoperative radiograph demonstrates removal of the intraarticular fragments with a concentric reduction, while the inferior femoral head fracture remains nondisplaced (Figure 10.30G).

Labral Tears

Traumatic labral tears may respond remarkably well to arthroscopic debridement.[12–16] However, at arthroscopy, be especially cognizant of any underlying

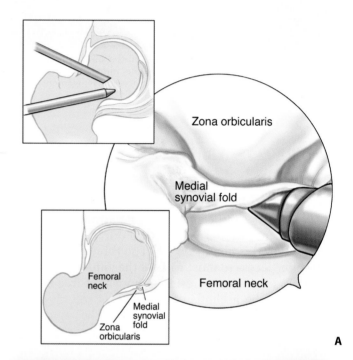

A

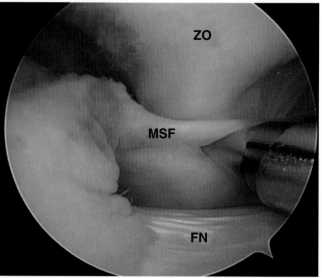

B

FIGURE 10.25. (A) Peripheral compartment viewing medially. (B) Demonstrated are the femoral neck (FN), medial synovial fold (MSF), and the zona orbicularis (ZO).

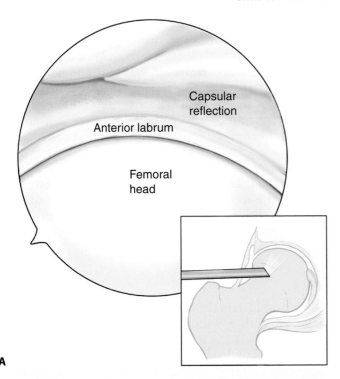

A

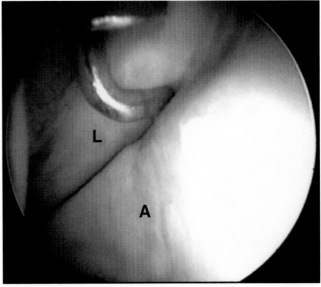

FIGURE 10.27. The cleft identified by the probe sometimes separates the margin of the acetabular articular surface (A) from the labrum (L). This is a normal variant without evidence of trauma or attempted healing response.

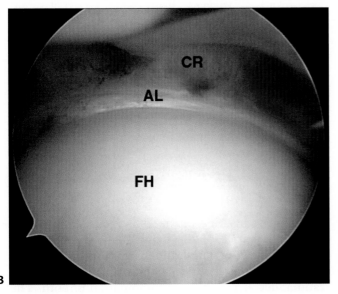

B

FIGURE 10.26. (A) Peripheral compartment viewing superiorly. (B) Demonstrated is the anterior portion of the joint including the articular surface of the femoral head (FH), anterior labrum (AL), and the capsular reflection (CR).

degeneration that may have predisposed to the acute tear. Also, there will often be some accompanying articular damage. The extent of this may be a significant influencing factor on the eventual response to debridement.

Labral tears can be adequately accessed through the three standard portals. Similar to a meniscus in the knee, the task is to remove unstable and diseased labrum, creating a stable transition to retained healthy tissue. The most difficult aspect is usually creating the stable transition zone. Thermal devices have been quite useful at ablating unstable tissue adjacent to the healthy portion of the labrum. Caution is necessary because of the concerns regarding depth of heat penetration, but with judicious use, these devices have been exceptionally useful for precise labral debridement despite the constraints created by the architecture of the joint.

The natural evolution in arthroscopic management of labral pathology is from debridement to repair. Cur-

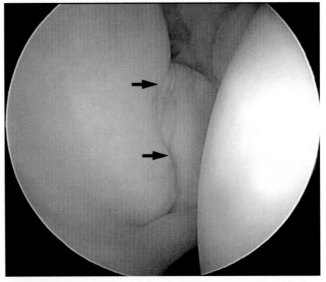

FIGURE 10.28. The physeal scar (arrows) is an area devoid of articular surface that may extend posteriorly from the acetabular fossa (as shown here) or anteriorly, demarcating the area of the old triradiate physis.

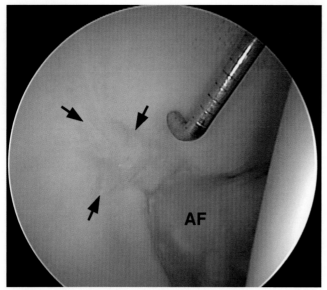

FIGURE 10.29. The stellate crease is frequently found directly superior to the acetabular fossa (AF) characterized by a stellate pattern of chondromalacia (arrows). This appears to be a normally occurring process, even in young adults, without clear prognostic significance.

rent methods of acetabular labral repair are in their infancy. A few such repairs have been attempted with mixed results. Reliable techniques remain to be developed but are probably not far off. In addition to technical advancements, there is much that remains regarding our understanding of labral morphology and pathophysiology. Considerable variation exists in the normal appearance of the labrum including a labral cleft at the articular labral junction, which can be quite large.[12] It is important to distinguish this from a traumatic detachment, which can also occur. Additionally, many labral tears, even in the presence of a significant history of injury, seem to occur due to some underlying predisposition or degeneration. Under these circumstances, even with reliable techniques, repair of a degenerated or morphologically vulnerable labrum would be unlikely to be successful.

Case 2

A 20-year-old Division I collegiate hockey player was referred with a 2-year history of progressively worsening sharp stabbing mechanical right hip pain. Magnetic resonance imaging (MRI) revealed evidence of labral pathology (Figure 10.31A). Arthroscopy revealed the extent of damage, which was debrided with marked symptomatic improvement (Figure 10.31B,C).

Chondroplasty (Microfracture)

Chondroplasty can be effectively performed for lesions of both the acetabular and femoral surfaces. Curved shaver blades are helpful for negotiating the con-

straints created by the convex surface of the femoral head. Due to limitations of maneuverability, thermal devices have again been especially helpful in ablating unstable fragments. However, cautious and judicious use around articular surface is even more important because of potential injury to surviving chondrocytes.

Microfracture of select grade IV articular lesions has been beneficial.[17] As with other joints, microfracture is best indicated for focal lesions with healthy surrounding articular surface. The lesion most amenable to this process is encountered in the lateral aspect of the acetabulum. Microfacture is followed by 8 to 10 weeks of protected weight bearing to neutralize the forces across the hip joint while emphasizing range of motion.

Case 3

A 47-year-old female professional fitness instructor presented with a 9-month history of right hip pain following a twisting injury. Radiography revealed evidence of isolated superolateral joint space narrowing suggestive of early osteoarthritis due to an inverted labrum (Figure 10.32A). Arthroscopy revealed an inverted labrum with associated grade IV articular loss of the superior acetabulum (Figure 10.32B). Debridement and microfracture were performed (Figure 10.32C,D). Postoperatively, she was kept on a strict protected weight-bearing status for 10 weeks, emphasizing range of motion to stimulate a fibrocartilaginous healing response. She demonstrated a successful outcome with significant symptomatic improvement at 8-year follow-up.

Rupture of Ligamentum Teres

Injury to the ligamentum teres is increasingly recognized as a source of hip pain. The disrupted fibers catch within the joint and can be quite symptomatic.[18,19] This disruption may be the result of trauma, degeneration, or a combination of both. The tear may be partial or complete, with the goal of treatment being to debride the entrapping, disrupted fibers.

The acetabular attachment of the ligamentum teres is situated posteriorly at the inferior margin of the acetabular fossa and attaches on the femoral head at the fovea capitis. The disrupted portion of the ligament is avascular, but the fat pad and synovium contained in the superior portion of the fossa can be quite vascular. Debridement is facilitated by a complement of curved shaver blades and a thermal device. The disrupted portion of the ligament is unstable and delivered by suction into the shaver. A thermal device can also ablate tissue while maintaining hemostasis within the vascular pulvinar.

Access to this inferomedial portion of the joint is best accomplished from the anterior portal. External

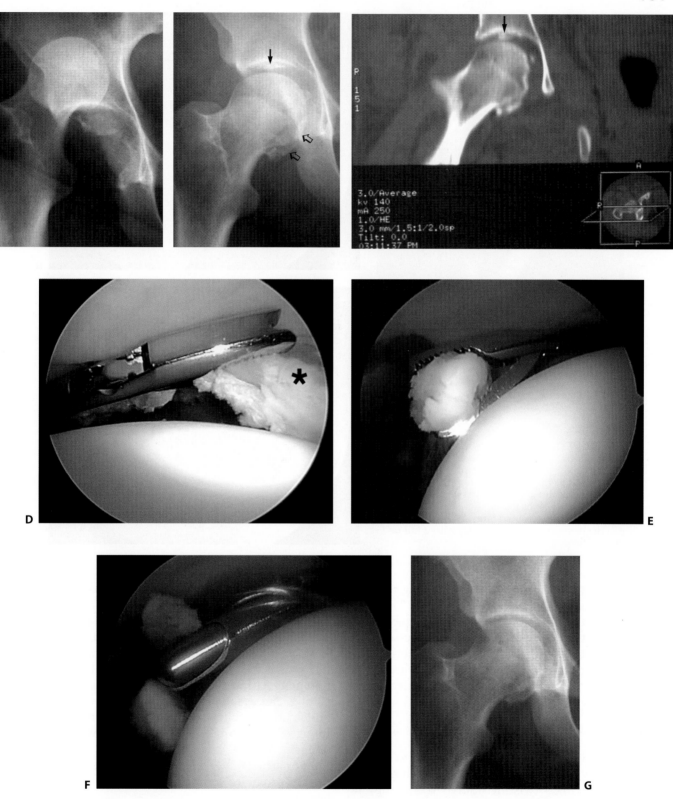

FIGURE 10.30. A 16-year-old obese girl sustained an injury to her right hip. (A) AP radiograph demonstrates a posterior fracture dislocation. (B) Postreduction radiograph reveals a nonconcentric reduction with bone fragment entrapped within the weight-bearing portion of the joint (arrow) and minimally displaced fracture of the femoral head (open arrows). (C) Coronal computed tomography (CT) reconstruction further illustrates the largest entrapped fragment (arrow) within the joint. (D) Arthroscopic view from the anterolateral portal demonstrates the largest fragment (asterisk), which has been grasped with an instrument brought in from the posterolateral portal. (E) Now viewing from the posterolateral portal, fragments are identified within the acetabular fossa. One is retrieved with a grasper. (F) Smaller fragments are debrided with a full-radius resector. (G) Postoperative radiograph demonstrates a concentric reduction, and the inferior femoral head fragment remains in place.

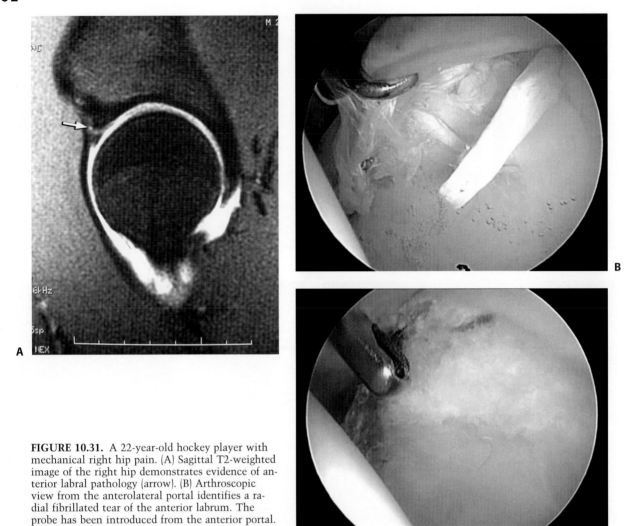

FIGURE 10.31. A 22-year-old hockey player with mechanical right hip pain. (A) Sagittal T2-weighted image of the right hip demonstrates evidence of anterior labral pathology (arrow). (B) Arthroscopic view from the anterolateral portal identifies a radial fibrillated tear of the anterior labrum. The probe has been introduced from the anterior portal. (C) The damaged tissue is debrided with a full-radius resector.

rotation of the hip also helps in delivering the ligament to the shaver brought in anteriorly. The most posterior portion of the fossa and the acetabular attachment of the ligament may be best accessed from the posterolateral portal. Indiscriminate debridement of the ligamentum teres should be avoided because of its potential contribution to the vascularity of the femoral head.

Case 4

A 16-year-old female cheerleader was referred with a 2-year history of intermittent pain and catching of her left hip following a twisting injury. Arthroscopy revealed a rupture of the ligamentum teres (Figure 10.33A); this was debrided with prompt symptomatic improvement (Figure 10.33B,C).

Synovial Disease

Various types of primary synovial disease have been encountered in the hip.[20] More often, secondary synovial proliferation may occur in response to other intraarticular pathology. A focal pattern of synovitis may occur emanating from the pulvinar within the acetabular fossa and is limited to this area. These lesions may be dense and fibrotic or exhibit proliferative villous characteristics. Presumably because of entrapment within the joint, these lesions can be quite painful and respond remarkably well to simple debridement. More diffuse synovial patterns involve the lining of the capsule. A complete synovectomy cannot be performed, but a generous partial synovectomy can be carried out. This procedure necessitates access to the peripheral compartment after the traction has been released.

Case 5

A 22-year-old woman was referred with a 3-year history of poorly defined left hip pain with no antecedent history of trauma. Radiographs revealed evidence of periarticular subchondral cyst formation suggestive of pigmented villonodular synovitis (Figure 10.34A),

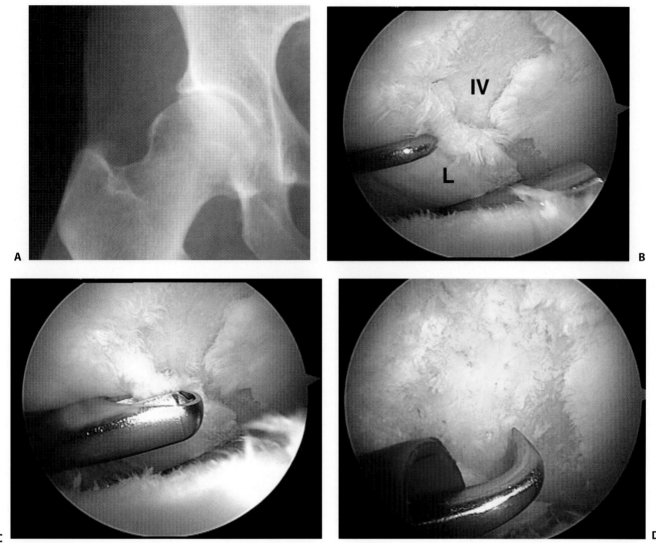

FIGURE 10.32. A 47-year-old woman with 9-month history of right hip pain. (A) Radiographs reveal evidence of superolateral joint space narrowing, which has been described as indicative of early osteoarthritis due to an inverted labrum. (B) The hip is viewed from the anterior portal. The probe marks the torn edge of the labrum (L) adjacent to an area of grade IV articular loss (IV) from the acetabulum. (C) The torn edge of the labrum has been debrided, and chondroplasty is being performed. (D) This grade IV lesion demonstrated healthy surrounding articular surface and thus was a candidate for microfracture performed with an arthroscopic awl.

which was further supported by MRI findings (Figure 10.34B). Arthroscopy revealed the characteristic lesion of pigmented villonodular synovitis arising from the acetabular fossa, which was debrided (Figure 10.34C–F). More extensive disease emanated from the synovial lining of the capsule, which was most fully assessed by arthroscopy of the peripheral joint (Figure 10.34G).

Impinging Fragments

Impinging bone fragments may respond well to arthroscopic excision.[20] These fragments are usually the result of trauma. Degenerative osteophytes rarely benefit from arthroscopic excision as the symptoms are usually more associated with the extent of joint deterioration and not simply the radiographically evident osteophytes that secondarily form. Posttraumatic fragments can impinge on the joint causing pain and blocking motion. These fragments are often extracapsular and require a capsulotomy, extending the dissection outside the joint for excision of the bone fragments. This necessitates thorough knowledge and careful orientation of the extraarticular anatomy and excellent visualization at all times during the procedure. In general, the dissection should stay directly on the bone fragments and avoid straying into the surrounding soft tissues. Various techniques aid in maintaining optimal visualization. A high-flow pump is especially helpful, maintaining a high flow rate without excessive pressure, which would worsen extravasation. Hypotensive anesthesia, placing epinephrine in the arthroscopic fluid, and electrocautery or other thermal

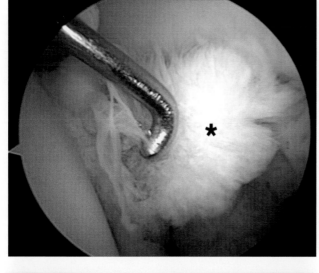

A

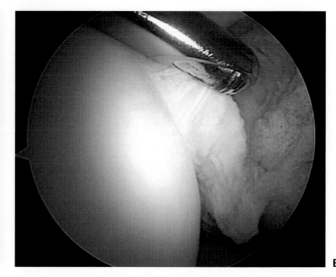

B

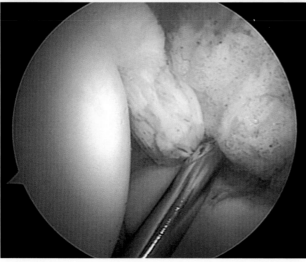

C

FIGURE 10.33. A 16-year-old cheerleader with left hip pain following a twisting injury. Arthroscopic view from the anterolateral portal. (A) Disruption of the ligamentum teres (asterisk) is identified. (B) Debridement is begun with a synovial resector introduced from the anterior portal. (C) The acetabular attachment of the ligamentum teres and the posterior aspect of the fossa is addressed with a shaver from the posterolateral portal.

device for hemostasis all aid in visualization for effectively performing the excision.

CASE 6

An 18-year-old high school football player was treated conservatively for an avulsion fracture of the anterior inferior iliac spine of the left hip. The avulsed fragment ossified (Figure 10.35A,B), creating a painful block to flexion and internal rotation. Dissecting through the capsule anteriorly, the ossified fragment was excised arthroscopically (Figure 10.35C–F), eliminating the fragment (Figure 10.35G) and regaining full painfree range of motion.

Instability

Hip instability can occur but is much less common than seen in the shoulder because the hip joint has a more constrained ball-and-socket bony architecture. Recurrent posterior instability is usually associated

with trauma.[21,22] Atraumatic instability can occur due to an incompetent capsule, usually seen in hyperlaxity states such as Ehlers–Danlos syndrome. Our observation has been that most atraumatic instability is anteriorly directed. In fact, when viewing the peripheral compartment, the femoral head can often be observed to sublux anteriorly during external rotation, even in asymptomatic individuals. In symptomatic cases, thermal capsulorrhaphy can be performed, addressing the capsule in a fashion similar to that described for the shoulder. Postoperative compliance with a limited range-of-motion protocol is imperative to achieving the optimal capsular response to the thermal treatment.

CASE 7

A 17-year-old girl was referred for progressively worsening symptoms of right hip instability. Her medical history was remarkable for Ehlers–Danlos syndrome with severe ligamentous laxity of multiple joints. She

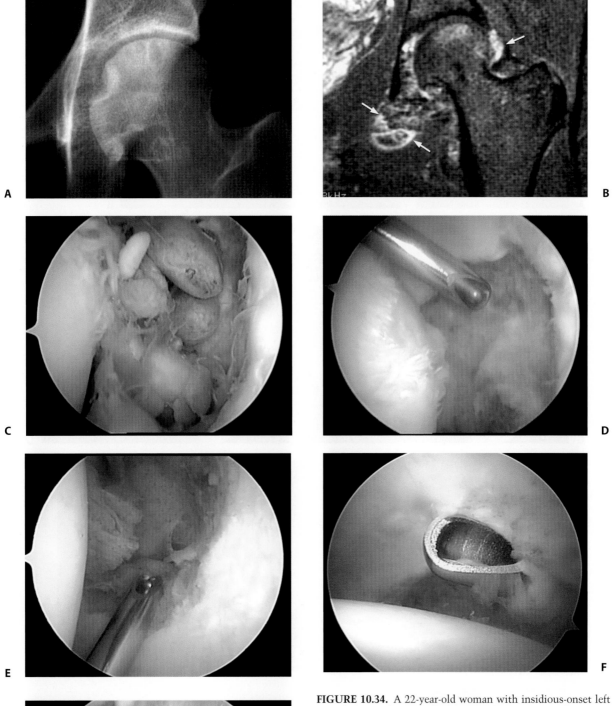

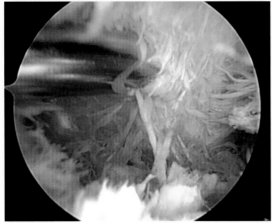

FIGURE 10.34. A 22-year-old woman with insidious-onset left hip pain. (A) AP radiograph demonstrates joint space preservation with multiple subchondral cysts of the femoral head suggestive of pigmented villonodular synovitis. (B) Coronal T2-weighted image of the hip demonstrates evidence of proliferative synovial disease (arrows). (C) The hip is viewed from the anterolateral portal. Synovial disease characteristic of pigmented villonodular synovitis is identified in the acetabular fossa. (D) Debridement of the fossa is begun with the shaver from the anterior portal. (E) Debridement of the fossa is then completed from the posterolateral portal. (F) Synovial disease of the posterior capsule extending underneath the posterior labrum is best debrided from the posterolateral portal because this portion of the capsule is not well accessed from the peripheral compartment. (G) With the traction released and the hip flexed, the arthroscope is then repositioned from the anterolateral portal into the peripheral compartment. Extensive synovial disease is present, which is debrided with a shaver introduced from an ancillary portal. This view especially illustrates the *seaweed* appearance ascribed to pigmented villonodular synovitis.

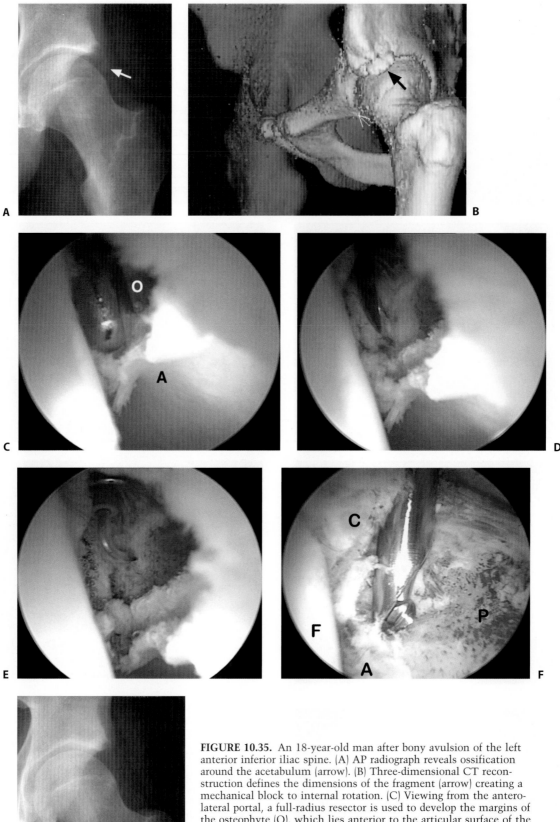

FIGURE 10.35. An 18-year-old man after bony avulsion of the left anterior inferior iliac spine. (A) AP radiograph reveals ossification around the acetabulum (arrow). (B) Three-dimensional CT reconstruction defines the dimensions of the fragment (arrow) creating a mechanical block to internal rotation. (C) Viewing from the antero-lateral portal, a full-radius resector is used to develop the margins of the osteophyte (O), which lies anterior to the articular surface of the acetabulum (A). (D) An arthroscopic knife is used to incise the capsule, which is partially contained within the fragment. (E) Hemostasis, important for optimal visualization, is maintained with judicious use of the arthroscopic cautery. (F) The anterior capsule (C) has been fully released, and a burr is used to excise the fragment, exposing the anterior column of the pelvis (P). The anterior margin of the acetabulum (A) is at the bottom of the picture, and a portion of the femoral head (F) is in view on the left. (G) The postoperative radiograph reveals the extent of bony resection.

had undergone previous successful capsulorrhaphy of her right shoulder. She had sustained a relatively atraumatic dislocation episode of her right hip 5 years previously that was reduced in an emergency room. Subsequently, she had experienced multiple subluxation/dislocation episodes that she had learned to reduce on her own or with the assistance of a family member. She had developed protective behavior to avoid these episodes but, even with precautions, would intermittently experience symptoms of her hip going out, causing her to fall. On examination, her greatest sense of instability and apprehension was created when translating the femoral head anteriorly with forced abduction and external rotation. Radiography revealed normal joint geometry, and an MRI was unremarkable. Because of persistent symptoms

despite adequate precautionary measures, arthroscopy was recommended. A chronic disruption of the ligamentum teres was identified (Figure 10.36A). The disrupted fibers were debrided and thermal capsulorrhaphy was performed (Figure 10.36B–D). Postoperatively, range of motion was restricted for 8 weeks in a hip spica brace. She responded well with elimination of her pain and episodes of subluxation.

Status Post Total Hip Arthroscopy

Arthroscopy can be performed in the presence of a hip prosthesis. However, the indications are limited.[23–26] With a capacious capsule, it may be easy to distract the joint and insert the instruments with the technique as used for a native joint. Normally, distraction should

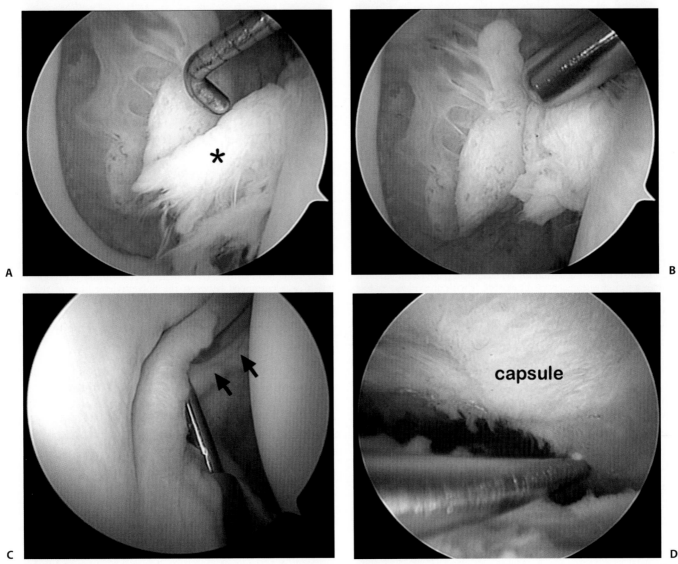

FIGURE 10.36. A 17-year-old girl with a history of recurrent atraumatic right hip instability. (A) Viewing from the anterolateral portal, a chronic disruption of the ligamentum teres is identified (asterisk). (B) The disrupted fibers are debrided. (C) Viewing posteriorly, thermal shrinkage is begun with the laser introduced from the posterolateral portal. Note the band created (arrows) indicating a brisk capsular response. (D) Now viewing the peripheral compartment with the traction released and hip flexed, the anterior capsular laxity is most completely addressed with the laser introduced through an ancillary peripheral portal.

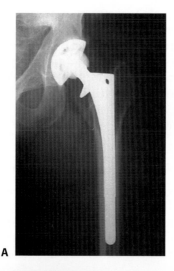

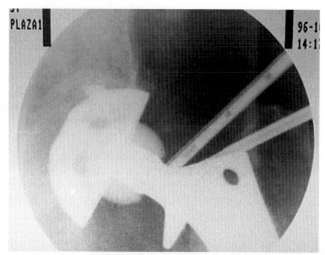

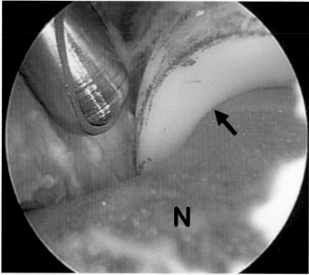

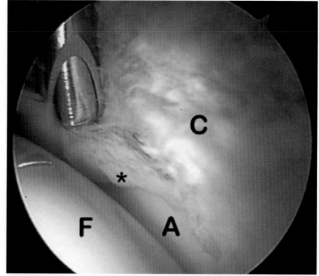

FIGURE 10.37. A 38-year-old man with unexplained left hip pain, 21 months following a total hip replacement. (A) AP radiograph reveals a well-positioned press-fit prosthesis with no evidence of loosening. (B) Fluoroscopic view demonstrates the position of the arthroscope and shaver along the base of the neck, thus avoiding the articular surface of the prosthesis. (C) Debridement of the fibrous tissue exposes the neck of the prosthesis (N) and its junction with the ceramic head (arrow). (D) A dense portion of fibrous tissue (asterisk) was entrapped between the polyethylene liner of the acetabulum (A) and the femoral head component (F). Peripheral to this is the reformed capsule (C).

not require much force. For some cases, it is less potentially damaging to the components to introduce the portals initially along the neck of the prosthesis. If fibrotic tissue is present, this can be debrided, developing a space for visualization of the components.

Case 8

A 38-year-old man was referred for evaluation of his left hip. He had undergone a previous press-fit total hip arthroplasty with an uneventful postoperative course (Figure 10.37A). He developed acute pain when he stepped awkwardly off a step, jarring his left leg. He subsequently presented with an 18-month history of pain with any weight-bearing activities, and an extensive workup was negative for evidence of fracture, loosening, or infection. An arthroscopic evaluation

was performed, identifying dense adhesions partially entrapped within the joint (Figure 10.37B–D). Postoperatively, the patient experienced resolution of the pain that had been plaguing him for the previous year and a half.

References

1. Sampson TG: Complications of hip arthroscopy. Clin Sports Med 2001;20:831–836.
2. Bartlett CS, DiFelice GS, Buly RL, et al: Cardiac arrest as a result of intraabdominal extravasation of fluid during arthroscopic removal of a loose body from the hip joint of a patient with an acetabular fracture. J Orthop Trauma 1998;12:294–299.
3. Byrd JWT, Chern KY: Traction vs. distension for distraction of the hip joint during arthroscopy. Arthroscopy 1997;13:346–349.
4. Byrd JWT: Hip arthroscopy utilizing the supine position. Arthroscopy 1994;10:275–280.

5. Byrd JWT: Hip arthroscopy: the supine position. Instr Course Lect 52:721–730; 2002.

6. Byrd JWT, Jones KS: Prospective analysis of hip arthroscopy with five year follow up. Presented at AAOS 69th annual meeting, Dallas, TX, February 14, 2002.

7. Byrd JWT, Pappas JN, Pedley MJ: Hip arthroscopy: an anatomic study of portal placement and relationship to the extra-articular structures, Arthroscopy 1995;11:418–423.

8. Byrd JWT: Avoiding the labrum in hip arthroscopy. Arthroscopy 2000;16:770–773.

9. Byrd JWT: Hip arthroscopy for post-traumatic loose fragments in the young active adult: three case reports. Clin Sport Med 1996;6:129–134.

10. McCarthy JC, Bono JV, Wardell S: Is there a treatment for synovial chondromatosis of the hip joint. Arthroscopy 1997;13:409–410.

11. Medlock V, Rathjen KE, Montgomery JB: Hip arthroscopy for late sequelae of Perthes disease. Arthroscopy 1999;15:552–553.

12. Byrd JWT: Labral lesions: an elusive source of hip pain: case reports and review of the literature. Arthroscopy 1996;12:603–612.

13. Lage LA, Patel JV, Villar RN: The acetabular labral tear: an arthroscopic classification. Arthroscopy 1996;12:269–272.

14. Farjo LA, Glick JM, Sampson TG: Hip arthroscopy for acetabular labrum tears. Arthroscopy 1999;15:132–137.

15. Santori N, Villar RN: Acetabular labral tears: result of arthroscopic partial limbectomy. Arthroscopy 2000;16:11–15.

16. Byrd JWT, Jones KS: Prospective analysis of hip arthroscopy with two year follow up. Arthroscopy 2000;16:578–587.

17. Byrd JWT, Jones KS: Inverted acetabular labrum and secondary osteoarthritis: radiographic diagnosis and arthroscopic treatment. Arthroscopy 2000;16:417.

18. Gray AJR, Villar RN: The ligamentum teres of the hip: an arthroscopic classification of its pathology. Arthroscopy 1997;13:575–578.

19. Byrd JWT, Jones KS: Traumatic rupture of the ligamentum teres as a source of hip pain. Arthroscopy 20(4):385–391; 2004.

20. Byrd JWT: Hip arthroscopy: patient assessment and indications. Instr Course Lect 2003;52:711–719.

21. Seldes RM, Tan V, Hunt J, Katz M, Winiarsky R, Fitzgerald RH Jr: Anatomy, histologic features, and vascularity of the adult acetabular labrum. Clin Orthop 2001;382:232–240.

22. McCarthy JC, Noble PC, Schuck MR, Wright J, Lee J: The watershed labral lesion: its relationship to early arthritis of the hip. J Arthroplasty 2001;16(8 suppl 1):81–87.

23. Hyman JL, Salvati EA, Laurencin CT, et al: The arthroscopic drainage, irrigation, and debridement of late, acute total hip arthroplasty infections: average 6-year follow-up. J Arthroplasty 1999;14:903–910.

24. Nordt W, Giangarra CE, Levy IM, Habermann ET: Arthroscopic removal of entrapped debris following dislocation of a total hip arthroplasty. Arthroscopy 1987;3:196–198.

25. Vakili F, Salvati EA, Warren RF: Entrapped foreign body within the acetabular cup in total hip replacement. Clin Orthop 1980;150:159–162.

26. Shifrin LZ, Reis ND: Arthroscopy of a dislocated hip replacement: a case report. Clin Orthop 1980;146:213–214.

11

Hip Arthroscopy Without Traction

Michael Dienst

For the past two decades, different centers in Europe,[1–19] the United States,[20–37] and Japan[38–40] have been contributing to the development of standardized techniques and specification of indications for arthroscopy of the hip joint (HA), with most authors advocating the use of traction.[6,22,25,41] The technique of hip arthroscopy without traction, however, has been disregarded. Only a few investigators have presented their experiences using this procedure.[9,11,13,34,35,42–44]

More recent reports have proposed different advantages of the nontraction technique. Klapper et al. also emphasized the low complication rate of this procedure.[34] Although traction is required for inspection of the direct weight-bearing cartilage, the acetabular fossa and the ligamentum teres, arthroscopy without traction is ideally situated for evaluation of the hip joint periphery.[13,43]

Based on the classification of the arthroscopic compartments of the hip joint, the following review presents detailed steps on performing this technique. A systematic mapping of that part of the joint that can be inspected without traction is included. Indications and contraindications are then specified and illustrated with selected case examples.

ARTHROSCOPIC COMPARTMENTS OF THE HIP JOINT

Placement of portals and maneuverability of the arthroscope and instruments within the hip joint are more difficult than in other joints. This difficulty is related to various anatomic features: a thick soft tissue mantle, close proximity of two major neurovascular bundles, a strong articular capsule, a relatively small intraarticular volume, permanent contact of the articular surfaces, and the sealing of the deep, central part of the joint by the acetabular labrum. Thus, if no traction is applied to the hip, only a small film of synovial fluid separates the articular surface of the femoral head from the lunate cartilage and acetabular labrum (*artificial space*).

The anatomy of the acetabular labrum must be considered when accessing the hip joint. The labrum seals the joint space between the lunate cartilage and the femoral head. Even under complete muscle relaxation during anesthesia, the labrum maintains a vacuum force of about 120 to 200 N, which keeps the femoral head within the socket.[45–47] To overcome the vacuum force and passive resistance of the soft tissues, traction is needed to separate the head from the socket, to elevate the labrum from the head, and to allow the arthroscope and other instruments access to the narrow artificial space between the weight-bearing cartilage of the femoral head and acetabulum. However, if traction is applied, the joint capsule with the iliofemoral, ischiofemoral, and pubofemoral ligaments is tensioned and the joint space peripheral to the acetabular labrum decreases. Thus, to maintain the space of the peripheral hip joint cavity for better visibility and maneuverability during arthroscopy, traction should be avoided.

In consequence, Dorfmann and Boyer[11,13] divided the hip arthroscopically into two compartments separated by the labrum (Figure 11.1). The first is the *central compartment*, comprising the lunate cartilage, the acetabular fossa, the ligamentum teres, and the loaded articular surface of the femoral head. This part of the joint can be visualized almost exclusively with traction. The second is the *peripheral compartment*, consisting of the unloaded cartilage of the femoral head, the femoral neck with the medial, anterior, and lateral synovial folds (Weitbrecht's ligaments), and the articular capsule with its intrinsic ligaments including the zona orbicularis. This area can be seen without traction and is described subsequently here.[43]

OPERATIVE TECHNIQUE

Operating Room Setup

The placement of personnel and equipment for HA without traction does not differ from the general HA setup (Figure 11.2). Surgeon, assistant, and scrub nurse

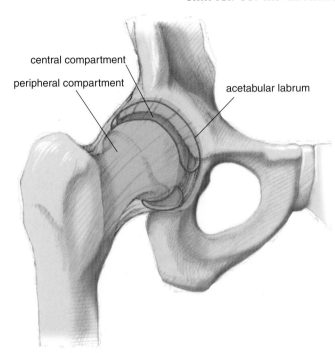

FIGURE 11.1. Arthroscopic compartments of the hip joint according to Dorfmann and Boyer.[11,13] (Reprinted with permission from Dienst et al.[44])

Positioning, Distension, and Portals

Hip arthroscopy with and without traction can be performed in the lateral[20,22] or supine position.[25,39,43] Some authors claim that there are advantages to the lateral position, including better access to the posterolateral area[48,49] and better application of traction in line with the femoral neck.[50] However, for HA without traction, I favor the supine position.[13,35,43,51] From my experience, the decision whether to use the supine or lateral position for the traction technique appears to be more a matter of individual training and habit of use. However, the almost exclusive use of the anterolateral portal (as indicated below) during HA without traction makes the supine position preferable for this part of HA.

Cadaver experiments and in vivo experience[52] have shown that free draping and a good range of movement are important to relax parts of the capsule and increase the intraarticular volume of the area that is inspected (Figure 11.3A,B).[53] This consideration is important for safe movement of the scope to avoid damage to the cartilage of the femoral head and synovial folds and unwanted sliding of the scope out of the joint. The distending effect of irrigation fluid pressure is of minor importance because the pressure should not be increased over 70 mm Hg to reduce the risk of development of a severe soft tissue edema. Klapper et al.[34] do not use a pump and prefer to control distension of the capsule and irrigation pressure by adjusting the sus-

with instrument table are on the ipsilateral side. The image intensifier is placed on the opposite side. The arthroscopy unit with video monitor and image intensifier with monitor are placed toward the foot.

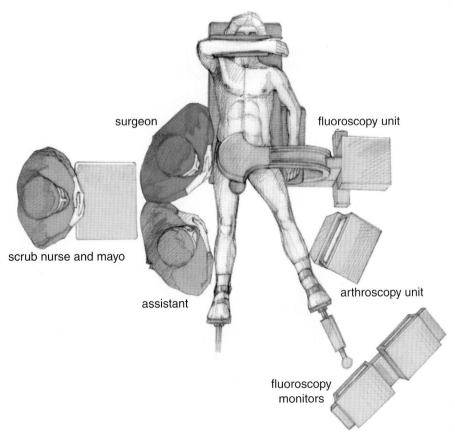

FIGURE 11.2. Operating room setup. (Reprinted with permission from Dienst et al.[44])

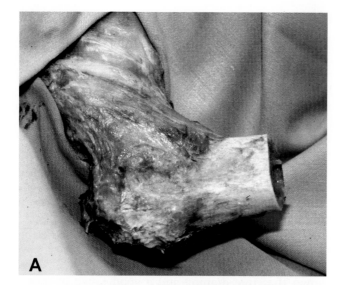

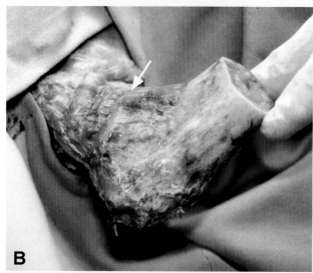

FIGURE 11.3. Anterior hip joint capsule in extension (A) and flexion (B). Flexion leads to a relaxation of the strong anterior iliofemoral ligament (arrow) and to a significant increase of the intraarticular joint space of the anterior and medial head and neck area (cadaveric hip joint).

pension height of the water bags and the three-way stopcock on the inflow site of the arthroscope.

In general, I combine HA without traction and HA with traction. As indicated below, the combination of both techniques is important to allow a complete diagnostic arthroscopic examination of the hip. From my experience, the traction part should be done before the nontraction scoping because positioning for traction is more demanding. In particular, exact placement of the counterpost is crucial to avoid complications. This placement can be done only under nonsterile conditions.

Technique

For HA without traction, the patient is placed supine on a standard traction table or a standard operating

table with an additional traction frame or robotic limb-positioning device. The bony landmarks and the femoral neurovascular bundle are palpated and the longitudinal axis of the femoral neck is determined with the image intensifier. Landmarks and axis of the femoral neck are marked on the skin for orientation during joint access and the surgical procedure. The portal zones are divided into anterior, anterolateral, lateral, and posterolateral (Figure 11.4). From Dorfmann and Boyer's[13] and our experience,[43,44] a comprehensive overview can be obtained from the an-

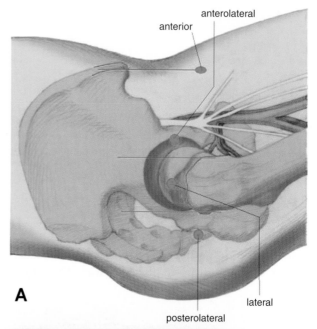

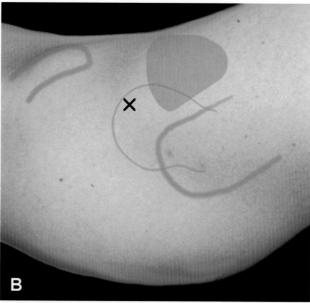

FIGURE 11.4. (A, B) Portals to the hip joint. For HA without traction, only portals within the anterior and the anterolateral zone are used (B). The standard portal is the anterolateral portal between the anterosuperior iliac spine and greater trochanter (X); additional portals for outflow and further instruments can be placed more distally and medially (gray area). (A reprinted with permission from Dienst et al.[44])

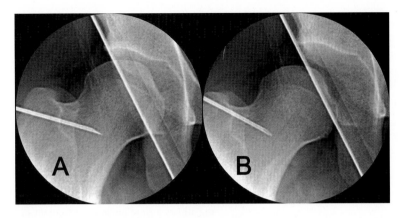

FIGURE 11.5. Intraoperative fluoroscopy for confirmation of entry to the joint and correct portal placement. (A) Puncture of the anterior recess at the transition between the femoral neck and head with a cardiac needle and (B) distension of the joint with 40 ml saline in combination with 10 to 20 kg traction. Correct intraarticular position is demonstrated by displacement of the femoral head. (Reprinted with permission from Dienst et al.[44])

terolateral portal only. Because the soft tissue mantle is relatively thin and the position of the portal is near the lateral cortex of the femoral neck, maneuverability of the arthroscope is sufficient for moving the arthroscope into the medial recess, gliding over the anterior surface of the femoral head to the lateral recess, and frequently passing the lateral cortex of the femoral neck for inspection of the posterior recess.[43]

First access to the hip joint periphery can be achieved with or without traction. I prefer a slight force to apply tension to the anterior capsule and to confirm entry to the joint by displacement of the femoral head by distension. The hip is flexed to about 20 degrees, the knee is extended, and 10 to 20 kg traction is applied only for the initial access to the joint. A long needle (diameter: approximately 1–2 mm) is introduced via the anterolateral portal and directed to the transition between the anterior aspect of the femoral head and neck. Here, the capsule is elevated from the neck, which allows easier access of the needle into the joint. Entry to the joint is then confirmed by distension of the joint with up to 40 ml saline, which leads to a visible lateral and caudal displacement of the femoral head under fluoroscopy as the hip is under traction (Figure 11.5A,B). The standard reflux test, return of fluid through the needle, is more inconsistent because of occlusion of the needle by hypertrophic synovium.

A guidewire is then inserted through the needle. The blunt guidewire can be advanced medially until

it bounces against the medial capsule. The capsular penetration is then dilated (dilating trochars, cannulated trochar) and the arthroscope is introduced in the peripheral compartment under fluoroscopy (Figure 11.6A–C). Traction is then released and the counterpost removed.

The knee is flexed to about 45 degrees and held by either a specially designed long bar at the end of the table or an assistant; the degree of flexion, rotation, and abduction of the hip joint are controlled (Figure 11.7). A second portal is placed under arthroscopic control in the anterior and the anterolateral zone (see Figure 11.4B). Irrigation is used to clear the view via the scope sheath and outflow via the additional portal. Standard and extra-long 25- and 70-degree lenses are used for the diagnostic round.

DIAGNOSTIC ROUND AND ANATOMY OF THE PERIPHERAL HIP JOINT CAVITY

Similar to the knee joint, the key to an accurate and complete diagnosis of lesions within the hip joint is a systematic approach to viewing. A methodical sequence of examination should be developed, progressing from one part of the joint cavity to another and systematically carrying out this sequence in every hip.

For arthroscopic examination, the peripheral compartment of the hip can be divided routinely into the

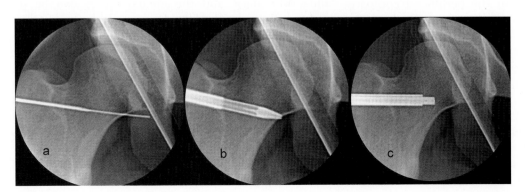

FIGURE 11.6. Introduction of the arthroscope to the hip joint periphery: guidewire (a), dilating trochars (b), starting position of the arthroscope (c). (Reprinted with permission from Dienst et al.[44])

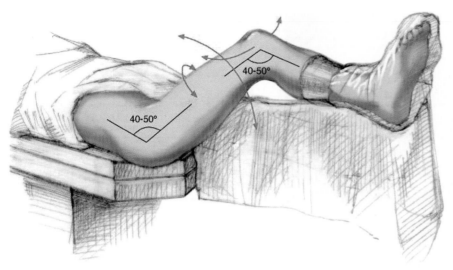

FIGURE 11.7. Positioning for HA without traction. The patient is placed supine. Removal of the counterpost and free draping allows a good range of movement of the hip. Held by the traction bar, flexion, rotation, and abduction can be controlled. (Reprinted with permission from Dienst et al.[44])

following areas: anterior neck area, medial neck area, medial head area, anterior head area, lateral head area, lateral neck area, and posterior area. From my experience, the peripheral compartment can be best viewed during a diagnostic round trip starting from the anterior surface of the femoral neck (Figure 11.8). Under slow rotation and sliding of the arthroscope over the femoral neck and head, the arthroscope is brought into the different areas of the peripheral compartment of the hip.

Anterior Neck Area

Entering the peripheral compartment from the anterolateral portal the scope is lying on the anterior surface of the femoral neck. The first view (see Figure 11.8A) allows inspection of the anterior and medial neck area with the anterior and medial synovial folds, the anteromedial surface of the femoral neck, the anteromedial part of the zona orbicularis, and the ligamentum iliofemorale (Y-shaped ligament of Bigelow). With the 25-degree lens of the arthroscope directed medially, a medial synovial fold (*iliopectineal fold*)[13] can be found consistently. It is usually not adhering to the femoral neck and passes proximally from the medial border of the femoral head distally to the lesser trochanter. This structure is a helpful landmark, especially if visibility within the peripheral compartment is limited by synovial disease.[13] The anterior synovial fold is adherent to the neck and only recognizable by its single fibers covering the bone of the neck. It can be partially torn by entering the joint with the sharp trochar, which should be avoided by using blunt instruments. Anatomic dissections showed that 80% to 90% of the synovial folds contain small branches of the circumflex femoral arteries.[54] In each fold, one to three small arteries with a mean cross-sectional area of 0.13 mm^2 for the anterior fold and 0.18 mm^2 for the medial fold were found. Larger ves-

sels were found in the lateral fold. Even if the major blood supply to the femoral head comes from the posterior branches, tearing of the folds should be avoided to decrease intraarticular bleeding. Dorfmann reported that he has seen local inflammation and hypertrophy of the medial synovial fold, which may be the sequelae of a chronic impingement of the fold between head, neck, and zona orbicularis.[52] Resection of the fold leads to improvement.

By rotating the arthroscopic lens cranially, the anterior margin of the femoral head, the anterior recess with the anterior capsule, and the zona orbicularis (see Figure 11.8B) can be inspected. Caudally, a complete view to the inferior reflection of the articular capsule at the intertrochanteric crest can be achieved with the 70-degree lens (see Figure 11.8C). Here, the articular cavity should be scanned for loose bodies. Biopsies of the synovium can be taken easily without a risk to labrum and cartilage via portals that are placed in the anterior or the anterolateral zone.

Medial Neck Area

Moving the scope medially over the medial synovial fold, the medial neck area can be examined. By rotating the 25-degree lens, the medial margin of the femoral head, the medial wall of the capsule with the zona orbicularis and the medial recess can be inspected. Rotating the lens downward, the zona orbicularis vanishes posterior to the femoral neck. By external rotation of the hip joint, a larger area of the posteromedial surface of the neck and head can be inspected. Changes in hip position, a short period of high-flow irrigation, and use of a suction forceps via the additional working portal or manual ballotement from posterior may be necessary to bring loose bodies from posterior into the medial or anterior recess. The 70-degree lens is replaced by the 25-degree lens and directed upward to the medial head area.

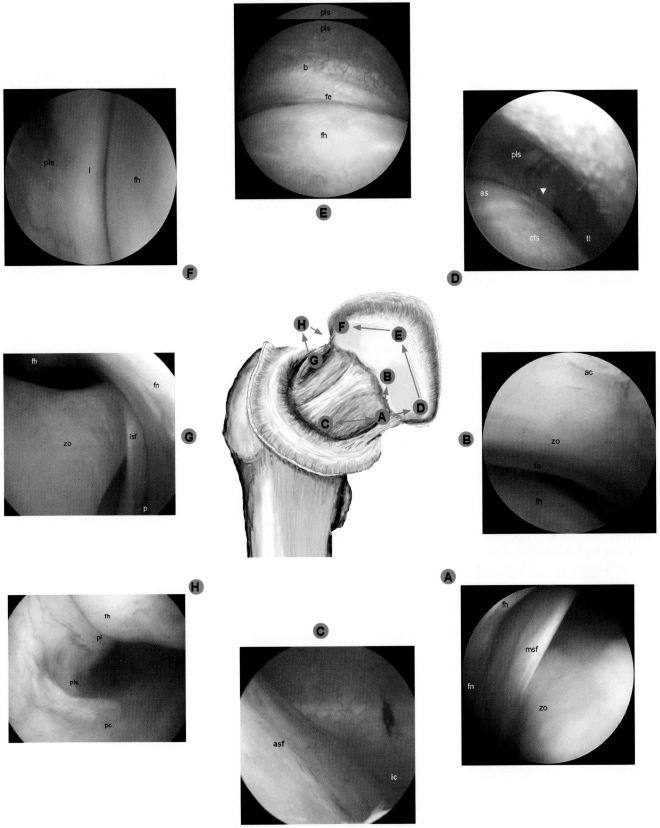

FIGURE 11.8. Diagnostic round and arthroscopic anatomy of the peripheral compartment of a right hip. (A) Anteromedial neck area: medial synovial fold (msf), femoral head (fh), femoral neck (fn), anteromedial capsule with the zona orbicularis (zo). (B) Upward view to the junction between the anterior neck and head area: anterior cartilage surface of the femoral head (fh), anterior part of the zona orbicularis (zo), anterior capsule (ac), free edge (fe) of the zona orbicularis. (C) Anterior neck area: downward view with the anterior synovial fold (asf) and reflection of the capsule at the intertrochanteric crest (ic). (D) Medial head area: articular surface (as) and cartilage-free surface (cfs) of the medial femoral head, anterior horn of the labrum (arrowhead), perilabral sulcus (pls), transverse ligament (tl). (E) Anterior head area: cartilage of the femoral head (fh), free edge of the labrum (fe), base of the labrum (b), perilabral sulcus (pls). (F) Lateral head area: cartilage of the femoral head (fh), lateral portion of the labrum (l), perilabral sulcus (pls). (G) Lateral neck area: lateral margin of the femoral neck (fn) and head (fh); lateral synovial fold (lsf) building a small subplical pouch (p), zona orbicularis (zo). (H) Posterior area: posterior surface of the femoral head (fh), posterior labrum (pl), perilabral sulcus (pls), thin posterior capsule (pc). (Reprinted with permission from Dienst et al.[43])

Medial Head Area

If the patient is not obese, the standard scope can be moved medially into the medial head area. Otherwise, longer scopes must be used. At the medial corner of the joint, inspection of the anterior horn of the labrum and the anteromedial part of the transverse ligament is possible (see Figure 11.8D). The labrum is close to the chondral surface of the femoral head. A small gap or synovium can be seen between the femoral head and the transverse ligament, which connects the base of both horns and both edges of the lunate cartilage.

Anterior Head Area

By gentle rotation, sliding tangentially over the cartilage of the femoral head and withdrawing the arthroscope, the labrum and anterior cartilage of the femoral head can be inspected from the medial to the anterior and lateral head area (see Figure 11.8E). The more the hip is flexed, the more the labrum is lifted from the head, which allows a partial inspection of the central compartment. In particular, the labrum has to be probed for labral cysts and tears, which are most frequently found in this location. A shaver or electrothermic instruments can be slid underneath the labrum and debridement of the labrum can be performed. Cysts can be decompressed.

Lateral Head Area

Moving the arthroscope laterally to the lateral head area can be hindered by a tight zona orbicularis. Flexion of the hip up to 45 degrees, with 20 to 40 degrees of abduction and slight external rotation of the hip, may ease passing of the arthroscope, thus allowing inspection of the lateral part of the labrum and cartilage of the head (see Figure 11.8F). Alternatively, the scope can be withdrawn distally to the neck for inspection of the lateral neck area first. Then the scope is moved forward to the lateral head area.

Lateral Neck Area

From an anterolateral portal, sweeping directly along the lateral side of the femoral head down into the posterior area is hindered by the zona orbicularis. Consequently, the scope is withdrawn distally to the circular fibers of the capsule and the lateral neck area is inspected first (see Figure 11.8G). Here, the zona orbicularis can be seen running posteriorly around the neck. A lateral synovial fold can be seen quite consistently. This fold runs from the greater trochanter upward along the lateral side of the neck to the lateral margin of the head. It is often posteriorly adherent to the neck and forms a small pouch. Thus, the lateral fold is not as prominent as the medial one. Anatomic dissections have revealed that the lateral fold

contains small arteries of larger diameter (mean, 0.28 mm^2) than the anterior and medial fold.[54] As recommended for the other folds, tearing of the folds should be avoided.

Posterior Area

Access to the posterior area can be achieved by moving the scope straight posteriorly between the zona orbicularis and the lateral synovial fold. After insertion of the 70-degree lens, the posterolateral and lateral part of the labrum, head, and neck and the posterior synovium can be inspected (see Figure 11.8H). The lateral and the posterior areas are more difficult to inspect compared with the anterior and medial areas. Hypertrophy of the synovium and tight joints (e.g., osteoarthritic hip joints with capsular fibrosis) can significantly decrease orientation and mobility for passing the arthroscope to the lateral and posterior areas. In addition, the posterior area is the smallest because the posterior wall and labrum cover most of the head in extension and the attachment of the joint capsule is 2 to 3 cm proximal to the intertrochanteric crest, thus more proximal than on the anterior surface.[53] If the arthroscope cannot be brought in this part of the joint without traction, placement of a posterolateral portal appears to be dangerous without traction. The greater trochanter blocks the view of the posterolateral parts of the femoral neck. Thus, if a portal was placed without traction, the starting point on the skin would be too far posteromedial, bringing the sciatic nerve at risk for direct injury. In these circumstances, we therefore recommend inspecting the posterior area during the traction part of the procedure. Under traction, the trochanter is pulled distally, and the arthroscope introduced via the lateral or anterolateral portal can slide over the posterolateral labrum to the posterior perilabral sulcus. Here, at least partial inspection of the posterior area of the peripheral compartment can be performed.

By slowly withdrawing the scope to the anterior surface of the neck, the diagnostic round trip of the peripheral part of the hip is finished.

INDICATIONS AND CONTRAINDICATIONS

The indications for HA without traction do not differ from those described for the traction technique. The traction and nontraction techniques should be combined to allow a complete diagnostic inspection of the hip joint. Performing HA solely as a nondistraction method should be limited to children and situations in adults in which distraction is not sufficient to introduce instruments into the central compartment of the hip.

The author does not have experience with HA of children and adolescents. Personal communications with other hip arthroscopists,[55,56] who have performed HA in children with septic arthritis and Perthes disease, reveal that a traction table is not necessary in patients younger than 12 to 14 years. Soft tissues, including the hip joint capsule and pericapsular ligaments, are so lax at this age that HA can be performed solely as a combination of nontraction and manual traction.

A minimum distraction of the central compartment of the hip of about 8 to 10 mm should be confirmed under fluoroscopy before placement of the first portal. In patients with osteoarthritis of the hip joint, shortening and fibrosis of the joint capsule and pericapsular tendons may lead to less distraction of the hip. Under those circumstances, introducing cannulas between head and socket must not be tried. Otherwise, labral and cartilage damage are likely. However, proceeding with the nontraction technique for an exclusive scope of the hip joint periphery may be considered. Certain pathology, as indicated below, can be found and addressed here.

Unclear Hip Pain

With respect to the limited sensitivity and specificity of preoperative radiologic methods for intraarticular hip joint lesions, indicating hip arthroscopy for patients with unclear hip pain is not uncommon.[17,23,25,36,48,57–59] However, preoperative evaluation should exclude spinal, abdominal-inguinal, neurologic, and rheumatologic diagnoses before the patient is considered for a hip scope. In addition, radiologic imaging of intraarticular loose bodies and labral and cartilage lesions has improved since the advent of computed tomography (CT) and magnetic resonance (MR) arthrograms (MRA) (personal communication, J.W. Thomas Byrd, Nashville, TN).[52,60,61] Intraarticular application of radiopaque material and air (double-contrast CT) or gadolinium (MRA) enhances the contrast between intraarticular structures.

Relief of pain with a local anesthetic is another strong indicator that the hip is the source of pain. If the etiology remains unclear, a complete diagnostic inspection of the hip joint is mandatory. Especially in this situation, it is important to combine the traction with the nontraction technique. As described in case example 1, loose bodies can be easily missed if only the central compartment is scanned. Synovial diseases such as a chondromatosis or an inflammatory synovitis typically manifest first in the hip joint periphery. Here, access to the synovium for biopsy and synovectomy is easy and is less harmful.

Loose Bodies

Radiologic evidence of loose bodies may be the classical indication for hip arthroscopy.[2,22,23,34,38,50,59,62–64] Loose bodies prefer to accumulate in the peripheral recesses. This realization is important in assessing preoperative radiographs or CT or MR imaging and also for operative planning.[13,43] The medial neck area, the perilabral recesses, and the recess underneath the transverse ligament especially need to be scanned. The technique of removal depends on the size and consistency of the loose bodies. Small loose bodies may be easily washed or sucked out via an additional portal cannula. In contrast to the limitation of the cannula diameter to 5 or 6 mm during arthroscopy with traction of the central compartment (narrow gap between labrum and femoral head), the nontraction technique allows the use of larger cannulas. This is helpful especially for synovial chondromatosis, where chopping up of the chondromas can be time consuming. Larger loose bodies must be chopped up with a shaver or more aggressive instruments if they have a bony core (see case 2). Inspection and removal of loose bodies in the posterior area of the peripheral compartment of the hip is more demanding. As indicated earlier, it may be difficult to pass the lateral femoral neck and bring the 70-degree scope into the posterior area, particularly if visibility is decreased by synovitis or the joint is tight. Sometimes, rotation of the hip, manual ballotement, or intraarticular suction can bring loose bodies from the posterior area into the visible anterior or medial areas.[35] To confirm a complete loose body removal, especially in synovial chondromatosis, an intraoperative arthrogram can be helpful before joint evacuation.

Synovial Diseases

If the hip joint is under distraction, the synovium (pulvinar) of the acetabular fossa can be seen. However, only small parts of the synovial lining of the medial, anterior, and lateral capsule are visible. From our and other authors' experience, this part of the synovium can best be seen without traction.[13,43] As indicated, chondromas tend to accumulate in the medial neck area, the perilabral recesses, and the recess underneath the transverse ligament. Here, cannulas can be easily placed via another anterolateral or anterior portal for synovial biopsies (reactive or specific synovitis, PVNS), synovectomies, and removal of chondromas. In addition, other pathologic conditions such as cysts of the labrum, anterior capsule, and communications with the iliopectineal bursa have to be ruled out. Particularly in patients with rheumatoid arthritis, an iliopectineal cyst has to be considered as a source of a painful hip. Depending on the size of the cyst, arthroscopic decompression may be performed. However, in case of larger cysts with fibrotic walls and related compression syndromes or recurrence, open excision may be the treatment of choice.

Septic Arthritis

Arthroscopic treatment of a septic arthritis of the hip joint should include a debridement of detritus and necrotic tissue, a lavage with at least 3 to 4 L irrigation fluid, placement of a drain into the femoral neck area, and antibiotic treatment for at least 7 days.[65–68] The author does not have experience with this disease or complication, but recommends combining the traction with the nontraction technique. During traction, the labrum and the zona orbicularis hinder flow of the irrigation fluid to and back from the peripheral recesses. Direct access to the peripheral areas without traction ease direct inspection, washing, and debridement of necrotic tissues and detritus. In addition, placement of a drain can easily be performed.

Labral Lesions

Klapper and Silver[35] and Dorfmann and Boyer[13] used the nontraction technique for arthroscopic treatment of labral lesions. From the author's experience, a good indication for the nontraction technique is a labral cyst, which is better accessed from the peripheral side. A typical location of a labral cyst is the anterior labrum close to the iliopsoas tendon. Here, the differential diagnosis should include an iliopectineal, capsular cyst. From the author's experience, tears of the labrum are more difficult to address with the nontraction technique. An instrument can be passed underneath the labrum for partial resection or trimming only if the labrum can be elevated from the femoral head by flexion. However, traction is usually preferred because labral lesions are commonly found at the articular side of the labrum. In addition, under traction the labrum does not adhere to the femoral head and allows better access for mechanical or electrothermal instruments.

Chondral Lesions

A review of the literature reveals that considerable numbers of HA are performed for traumatic and nontraumatic (osteoarthritis, osteochondritis dissecans) chondral lesions. In osteoarthritis-associated lesions such as loose bodies, labral lesions and synovitis can be frequently found preoperatively and intraoperatively.[51]

CONTRAINDICATIONS

Hip arthroscopy in a recent acetabular fracture has been reported with a risk of leakage of irrigation fluid into the retroperitoneal space and abdomen.[69–71] In patients with advanced osteoarthritis of the hip, the benefit of an arthroscopic debridement is small. In addition, access to the hip joint periphery may be hindered by femoral head osteophytes, thickening and fibrosis of the capsule, and hypertrophy of the synovium.

COMPLICATIONS

The possibility of complications during HA without traction is minor. Because no traction is used, the perineum and pudendal nerve are not at risk. Instruments do not have to pass between labrum and cartilage of the femoral head, and thus tearing the labrum and scuffing the load-bearing cartilage of the femoral head is unlikely. The zone of portal placement is safe if only anterolateral portals are used. Byrd et al.[21] showed that the superior gluteal nerve is the only structure with significance relative to the anterolateral portal and has been shown to be at least 3.2 cm from the portal. If the portal is placed further medially and proximally, the lateral femorocutaneous nerve is more at risk. To avoid direct cutting of one of the branches of the superficial nerve, skin incisions must be made superficially. Dilators and portal sheath should be introduced stepwise using blunt instruments. Forceful lever movements in the presence of portal sheaths should be avoided. Skin sutures must be placed superficially.[44] If paresthesias of the lateral femorocutaneous nerve occur, those are usually transient and regress within a few days. After perforation of the articular capsule, scuffing of the articular cartilage of the anterior part of the femoral head and the anterior synovial fold covering the anterior femoral neck is possible.[43] As for HA with traction, unnecessary perforations of the articular capsule must be avoided. Leakage of fluid into the periarticular soft tissues cause an increasing narrowing of the joint cavity. The shaft, particularly that of the 70-degree arthroscope, should remain inside the joint and not come too close to the capsule because the optic of the 70-degree arthroscope exceeds the shaft more than that of the 30-degree arthroscope. This carries the danger of direct fluid leaking from the sheath into the periarticular soft tissues. For this reason, we recommend that shafts and portal sheaths be used that are not fenestrated. In particular, after sliding out of the joint, the irrigation pressure should be kept as low as possible.[44]

CASE EXAMPLES

Case 1: Synovial Chondromatosis of the Peripheral Compartment

HISTORY AND PREOPERATIVE FINDINGS

A 57-year-old female patient was referred with a 4-year history of progressive right hip pain. A diagnostic HA was performed 2 years ago without any significant pathologic intraarticular findings. However, analysis of the operative report revealed that only the central compartment of the hip joint was scoped under traction. The patient complained of a pain radiating in her right groin and anterior proximal thigh that

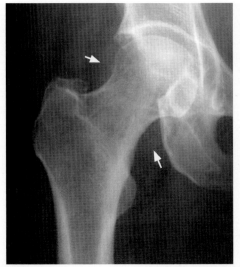

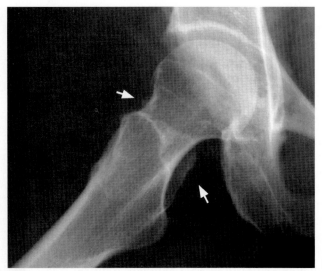

FIGURE 11.9. Case 1. Anteroposterior (A) and lateral (B) radiographs of the right hip indicating osseous spots (arrows) around the femoral neck.

was worse during activity and movements of the hip. She reported infrequent catching and locking episodes. On physical examination, the groin was moderately tender to palpation, trochanter irritation sign was negative, and labral impingement and apprehension significantly positive. Her range of motion was decreased for flexion and internal rotation. Radiographic examination revealed small calcifications projecting around the femoral neck (Figure 11.9A,B). Subsequently, a MRI of the right hip was taken showing multiple calcified loose bodies in the peripheral compartment with a significant effusion and signal increase of the synovium (Figure 11.10A,B). No loose bodies were seen within the central compartment including the

acetabular fossa. The preoperative diagnosis of synovial chondromatosis was established.

HIP ARTHROSCOPY

Arthroscopy was performed to confirm the diagnosis and remove the chondromas. First, the central compartment was scoped under traction. As preoperatively seen on MRI, the joint space between the femoral head and lunate cartilage and the acetabular fossa was free of chondromas. The synovium of the pulvinar was unremarkable. Because no pathologic lesions were found, the central compartment was evacuated. An anterolateral portal to the peripheral compartment was es-

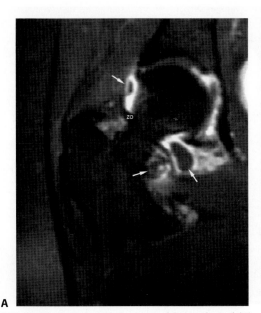

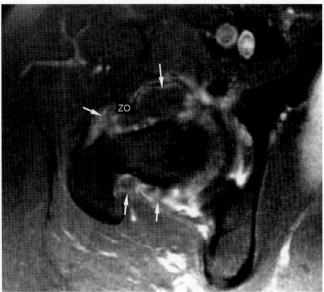

FIGURE 11.10. Case 1. MRI in coronal (A) and axial (B) orientation of the right hip showing multiple chondromas around the femoral neck (arrows). No evidence of chondromas in the acetabular fossa. zo, zona orbicularis.

tablished, and traction was released. The preoperative diagnosis was immediately confirmed: The complete peripheral compartment was packed with chondromas so that visibility was significantly reduced (Figure 11.11). A second anterolateral portal was established in line with the longitudinal axis of the femoral neck. A large flexible cannula was introduced. However, because most of the chondromas were larger than 0.8 cm in diameter with a bony core, a strong forceps had to be introduced to chop up the chondromas before they could be removed and washed out (Figure 11.12). Removal of the chondromas took about 90 minutes. It was not possible to sweep with the arthroscope into the posterior area behind the femoral neck. However, as there were no sessile and attached chondromas, posterior chondromas could be mobilized and sucked into the medial and anterior areas. Complete removal was confirmed with an arthrogram under fluoroscopy. The synovium appeared thickened and inflamed (Figure 11.13).

RESULT

At 1-year follow-up, the patient had maintained good range of motion and pain relief. However, radiographs and an arthrogram revealed recurrence of a few chondromas within the peripheral compartment. As the patient was not complaining of pain or locking, arthroscopy was postponed and follow-up recommended in case of recurrence of symptoms.

DISCUSSION

This case example illustrates how important it is to include the inspection of the peripheral compartment

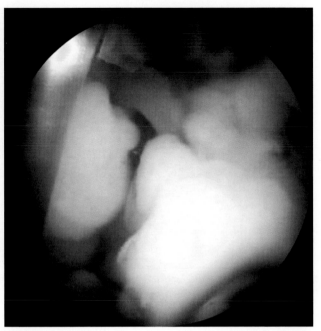

FIGURE 11.12. Case 1. Removal and chopping-up of the chondromas with a forceps.

during HA. The first HA of the central compartment 2 years earlier did not show any evidence of loose bodies as did the second one. However, inspection of the hip joint periphery without traction was characteristic for synovial chondromatosis. From the author's experience, the accumulation of chondromas and loose bodies within the peripheral recesses is a typical finding. Most of the synovium as the source of chondromas is found peripheral to the labrum (with exception of the pulvinar). If the joint is not distracted, as it is

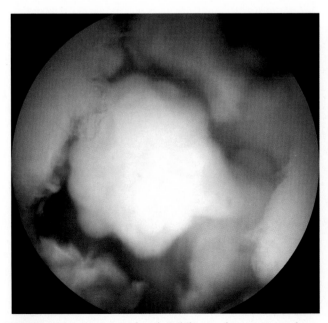

FIGURE 11.11. Case 1. Reduced visibility in the anterior and medial neck area because of multiple chondromas.

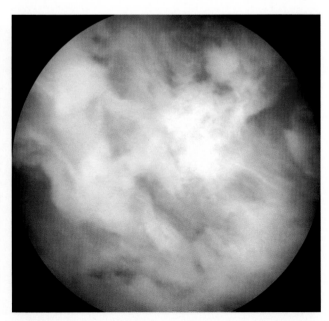

FIGURE 11.13. Case 1. Synovium status post removal of the chondromas, with evidence of chronic inflammation and fibrosis.

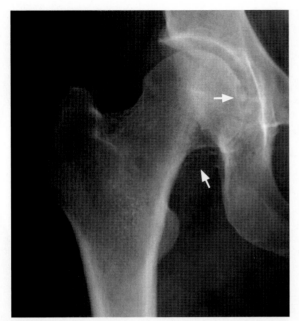

FIGURE 11.14. Case 2. Anteroposterior radiograph of the right hip indicating small radiodense spots medial to the transition of the femoral neck and head and in the acetabular fossa (arrows).

Case 2: Synovial Chondromatosis of Both Compartments

HISTORY AND PREOPERATIVE FINDINGS

A 56-year-old female patient was referred with a 2-year history of right hip pain. She reported frequent catching and locking episodes with giving-way episodes. When those occurred, she also complained of a sharp pain radiating into the anterior distal thigh. Otherwise she was asymptomatic. Radiographs revealed the characteristic findings of synovial chondromatosis with small radiodense spots around the femoral neck and within the fossa acetabuli (Figure 11.14). The diagnosis was confirmed with a MR arthrogram showing chondromas within the peripheral and central compartment (Figure 11.15A,B). Hip arthroscopy for removal of the chondromas was indicated.

HIP ARTHROSCOPY

The patient was placed supine on a fracture table for HA with traction. An anterolateral portal was established under fluoroscopy, and an additional posterolateral portal was placed under arthroscopic control (Figure 11.16). After the diagnosis of synovial chondromatosis was confirmed, four soft chondromas were found within the acetabular fossa and subsequently removed using a forceps and shaver (Figure 11.17). By sliding the 70-degree arthroscope distally to the posterior labrum, no chondromas were seen in the posterior area of the hip joint. The central compartment was then evacuated. An anterolateral portal to the peripheral compartment was established. Chondromas were immediately found in the medial neck and head area underneath the transverse ligament (Figure 11.18) and anterior neck area (Figure 11.19). For extraction of the chondro-

under nonoperative conditions, the labrum and transverse ligament seal the central compartment, keeping the chondromas in the joint periphery.

The recurrence of chondromas is a known problem that always leads to the question whether a synovectomy should have been performed. However, studies have shown that recurrence does not significantly differ if synovectomy was done or not.[71] In addition, open or arthroscopic synovectomy of the hip joint can only be partial, at least with the current techniques. We therefore remove chondromas only.

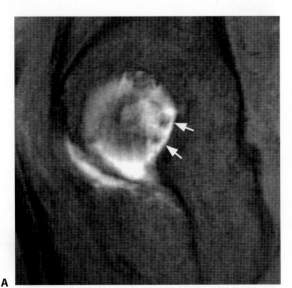

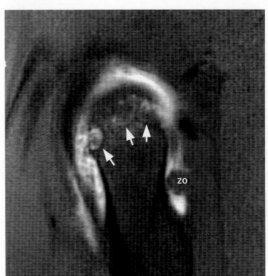

FIGURE 11.15. Case 2. MR arthrogram in sagittal orientation of the acetabular fossa (A) and medial third of the proximal femur (B) showing chondromas within the acetabular fossa and peripheral compartment (arrows). zo, zona orbicularis.

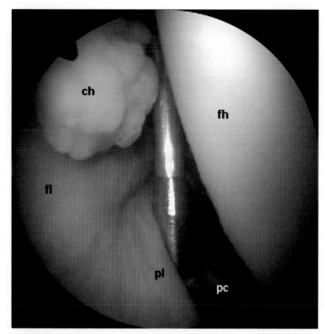

FIGURE 11.16. Case 2. Placement of the posterolateral portal to the central compartment of the hip with traction. Identification of a chondroma (ch). Lunate cartilage (fl), posterior labrum (pl), posterior capsule (pc), femoral head (fh).

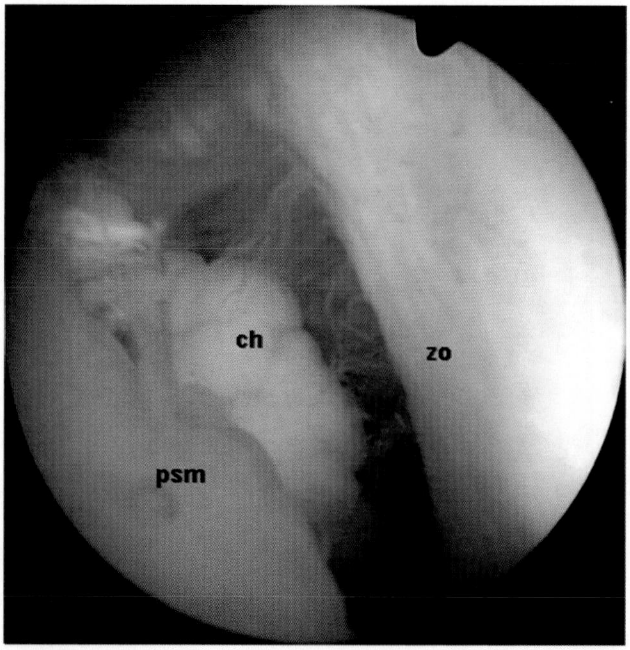

FIGURE 11.18. Case 2. Peripheral compartment with medial neck and head area. Chondroma (ch) between the medial synovial fold (psm) and zona orbicularis (zo).

mas, an additional portal was placed within the anterolateral area in line with the femoral neck. Ten mostly soft chondromas with a small osseous core were removed using a forceps (Figure 11.20) and shaver (Figure 11.21). Arthroscopic scanning of the peripheral compartment revealed a complete removal (Figures 11.22, 11.23).

RESULT

At 3 months and 1 year postoperatively, the referring physician reported a complete relief of the catching and locking symptoms. The patient continued to be painfree.

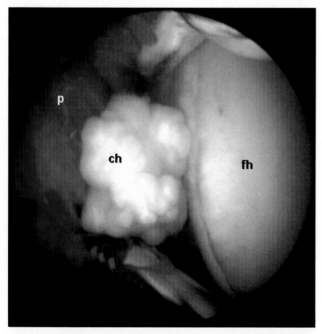

FIGURE 11.17. Case 2. Removal of a chondroma (ch) with a shaver introduced via the posterolateral portal. Pulvinar (p), femoral head (fh).

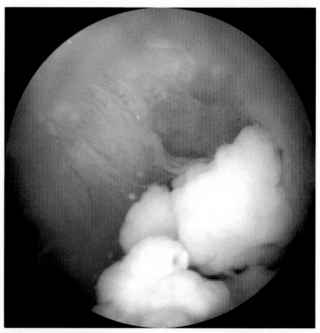

FIGURE 11.19. Case 2. Peripheral compartment with inferior anterior neck area. Chondromas (ch) at the inferior capsular reflection at the intertrochanteric crest (ic).

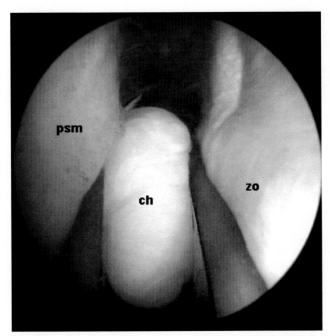

FIGURE 11.20. Case 2. Removal of a chondroma (ch) with a forceps. Medial synovial fold (psm), zona orbicularis (zo).

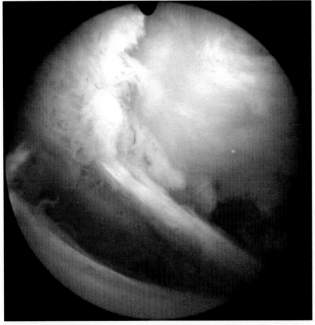

FIGURE 11.22. Case 2. Status post removal. Medial neck area with medial synovial fold (psm), femoral neck (fn), and medial capsule (mc).

DISCUSSION

Contrary to case 1, synovial chondromatosis was present in both compartments. Chondromas were found in the characteristic locations, the acetabular fossa, and the recesses of the anterior neck and medial neck and head areas. The use of the posterolateral portal is ideal for removal of loose bodies within the peripheral compartment, at least in the supine position. Follow-ing gravity, chondromas and loose bodies tend to accumulate in the posterior space between femoral head and lunate cartilage and acetabular fossa, respectively. Here, the posterolateral portal offers an ideal access for instruments and a drainpipe for small chondromas. Because chondromas tend to accumulate in the anterior and medial areas of the peripheral compartment, an anterolateral portal in line with the femoral neck

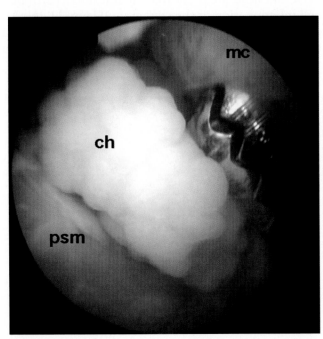

FIGURE 11.21. Case 2. Removal of a chondroma (ch) with a shaver. Medial synovial fold (psm), medial capsule (mc).

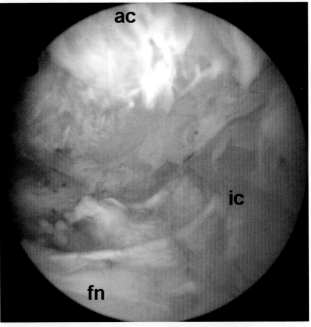

FIGURE 11.23. Case 2. Status post removal. Inferior anterior neck area with femoral neck (fn), capsular reflection at the intertrochanteric crest (ic), and anterior capsule (ac).

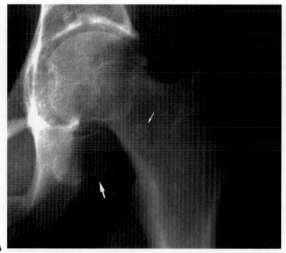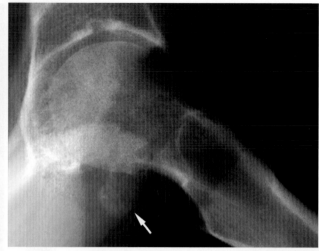

FIGURE 11.24. Case 3. Anteroposterior (A) and lateral (B) radiographs of the left hip showing a big osseous body (large arrow) and a smaller body (small arrow) medial and posterior to the transition of the femoral neck and head.

appears most suitable. An instrument can be introduced reaching even up to the transverse ligament.

Case 3: Loose Body in the Peripheral Compartment

HISTORY AND PREOPERATIVE FINDINGS

A 35-year-old male patient was referred with a history of left hip pain for more than 5 years. He reported a persistent moderate aching in the groin that was aggravated with hip rotation and flexion. For example, when getting in or out of a car, he frequently complained of catching symptoms and giving-way episodes. On radiographs, a large ossified body about 3.5 by 2 by 2 cm medial to the transition of the femoral neck and head was found (Figure 11.24A,B). A smaller one was seen in projection on the femoral neck. A MR arthrogram was suspicious for osteochondromas

within the peripheral compartment of the hip (Figure 11.25A,B). Even if arthroscopic removal appeared difficult with respect to the size and bony consistency of the large round body, we decided to start the procedure with an arthroscopic approach. Because radiographs and MRA only showed cartilage degeneration, without evidence of loose bodies within the central compartment of the hip, we preoperatively planned to perform HA without traction of the peripheral compartment only.

HIP ARTHROSCOPY

A standard anterolateral portal to the peripheral compartment was established. The anterior and medial neck and head areas showed significant hypertrophy and inflammation of the synovium (Figure 11.26). An additional anterolateral portal in line with the femoral neck was placed and an electrocautery unit used to

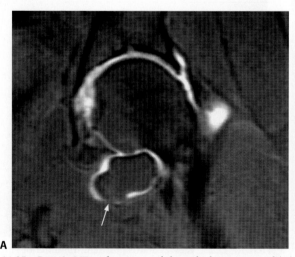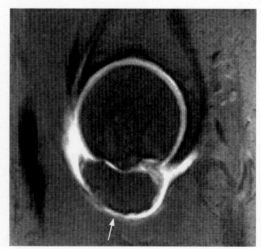

FIGURE 11.25. Case 3. MR arthrograms of the right hip in coronal (A) and sagittal (B) orientation showing a large osseous body (arrows) medial to the transition of the femoral neck and head.

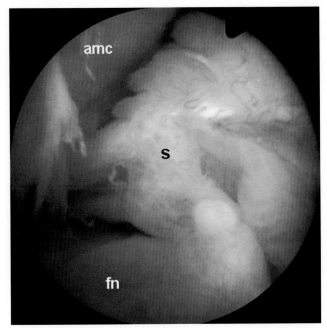

FIGURE 11.26. Case 3. Synovitis (s) in the medial neck area between the femoral neck (fn) and anteromedial capsule (amc).

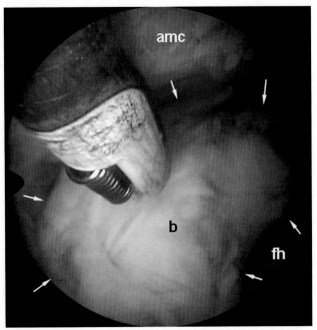

FIGURE 11.28. Case 3. Identification of margins of the large body (b, arrows). Anteromedial capsule (amc), femoral head (fh).

remove the inflamed synovium. After synovectomy within the anterior and medial neck and head area (Figure 11.27), the osseous body could be inspected and probed (Figures 11.28, 11.29). It was molded by the medial wall of the femoral neck and femoral head, bulging out the medial and anteromedial capsule. The body filled the complete medial neck and head area and reached up to the transverse ligament and the me-

dial and the anteromedial labrum. Subsequently, two more smaller loose bodies with a bony core were found and removed. Attempts to remove the large loose body with large threaded K-wires and pins failed because the body could not be mobilized. Thus, a large rongeur was taken from the spine set and piecemeal work was started (Figure 11.30). After 1 hour, the bony loose body was chopped up and removed. There was evi-

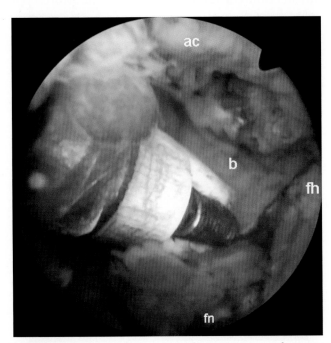

FIGURE 11.27. Case 3. Electrothermal synovectomy with progressive identification of the osseous body (b). Femoral neck (fn), head (fh), anterior capsule (ac).

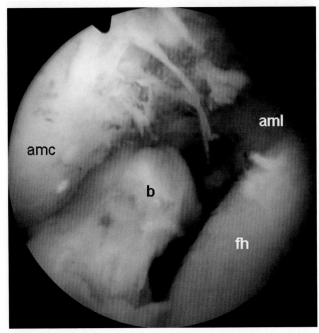

FIGURE 11.29. Case 3. Anterior proximal end of the large body (b). Femoral head (fh), anteromedial capsule (amc), anteromedial labrum (aml).

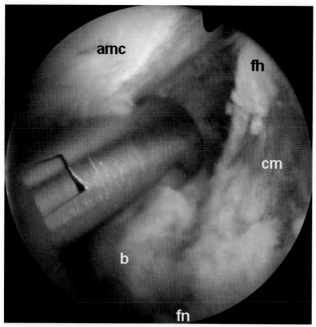

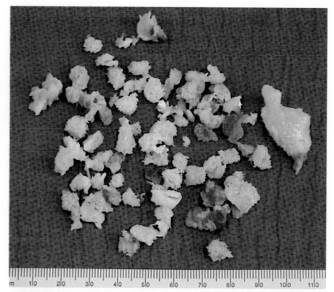

FIGURE 11.32. Case 3. Chopped-up osseous body after removal.

FIGURE 11.30. Case 3: Removal of the osseous body (b) with a rongeur. Notice the kissing chondromalacic lesion (cm) of the femoral head (fh). Femoral neck (fn), anteromedial capsule (amc).

RESULTS

Postoperative radiographs revealed complete loose body removal (Figure 11.33). The patient immediately described a significant improvement of the sharp catching pain and absence of giving-way episodes. This improvement was maintained at the 2-year follow-up.

DISCUSSION

From the author's experience, the location of a large osseous loose body makes an open removal also difficult and time consuming. In addition, the arthroscopic

dence of a full-thickness erosion of the anteromedial cartilage of the femoral head. Arthroscopy and an intraoperative arthrogram revealed a complete removal (Figure 11.31). After surgery, the small pieces of the chopped-up specimen were photographed (Figure 11.32).

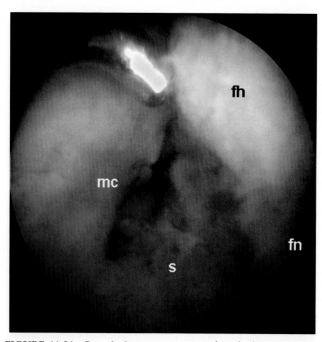

FIGURE 11.31. Case 3. Status post removal with the empty medial neck area, synovitis on the bottom (s), medial capsule (mc), femoral neck (fn), and head (fh).

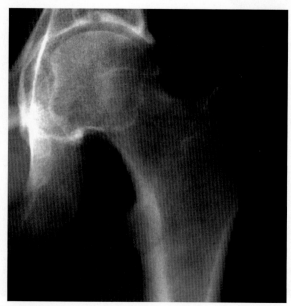

FIGURE 11.33. Case 3. Postoperative anteroposterior radiograph indicating a complete removal.

procedure was minimally invasive and allowed direct full weight bearing and range of movement postoperatively. Contrary to the author's general recommendation to combine HA of the central with the peripheral compartment, in this case only the hip joint periphery was scoped without traction. Our decision was based on the preoperative radiologic findings and expectation that the removal would be time consuming.

CONCLUSIONS

A comprehensive inspection of the hip joint requires the combination of hip arthroscopy with traction and hip arthroscopy without traction. Although traction is necessary for access to the central compartment for evaluation of the direct weight-bearing cartilage, acetabular fossa, and ligamentum teres, the periphery of the joint can best be seen without traction.

Acknowledgments.   The author thanks Dieter Kohn, MD, for his consistent support and advice for development of the technique; Guenther Schneider, MD, for his cooperation for improvement of imaging procedures; and Nicole Koenig, MS, for her help in the preparation of the case examples.

References

1. Keene GS, Villar RN: Arthroscopic anatomy of the hip: a in vivo study. Arthroscopy 1994;10:392–399.
2. Gondolph-Zink B: Aktueller Stand der diagnostischen und operativen Hüftarthroskopie. Orthopäde 1992;21:249–256.
3. Gondolph-Zink G, Noack W, Puhl W: Neue Möglichkeiten zur Erkennung und operativen Therapie der Hüftsynovialitis. Z Rheumatol 1987;46:120–123.
4. Hempfling H, Schäfer H: Arthroscopy and arthrography. A combined procedure. Surg Endosc 1989;3:203–211.
5. Gondolph-Zink B: Die Hüftarthroskopie. Aktuel Probl Chir Orthop 1991;40:35–43.
6. Eriksson E, Arvidsson I, Arvidsson H: Diagnostic and operative arthroscopy of the hip. Orthopedics 1986;9:169–176.
7. Villar RN: Hip Arthroscopy. Oxford: Butterworth Heinemann, 1992.
8. Gondolph-Zink G, Puhl W: Einsatzmöglichkeiten der operativen Hüftarthroskopie. Arthroskopie 1990;3:71–77.
9. Dorfmann H, Boyer T, Henry P, DeBie B: A simple approach to hip arthroscopy. Arthroscopy 1988;4:141–142.
10. Gondolph-Zink B, Puhl W, Noack W: Semiarthroscopic synovectomy of the hip. Int Orthop 1988; 2:31–35.
11. Dorfmann H, Boyer T: Hip arthroscopy utilizing the supine position. Arthroscopy 1996;12:264–267.
12. Hempfling H: Das Hüftgelenk. In: Hempfling H (ed). Farbatlas der Arthroskopie grosser Gelenke, 2nd ed. Stuttgart: Fischer, 1995:511–571.
13. Dorfmann H, Boyer T Arthroscopy of the hip: 12 years of experience. Arthroscopy 1999;15:67–72.
14. Hempfling H Arthroskopie selten betroffener Gelenke. Derzeitiger Stand. Orthopäde 1998;27:251–265.
15. Conn KS, Villar RN Die Labrumläsion aus der Sicht eines arthroskopischen Hüftchirurgen. Orthopäde 1998;27:699–703.
16. Eriksson E, Pitman MI. Arthroscopy and arthroscopic surgery of joints other than the knee. In: Sharihaee H (ed). O'Connor's Textbook of Arthroscopic Surgery. Philadelphia: Lippincott, 1984:311–322.
17. Baber YF, Robinson AHN, Villar RN: Is diagnostic arthroscopy of the hip worthwhile? A prospective review of 328 adults investigated for hip pain. J Bone Joint Surg 1999;81B:600–603.
18. Griffin DR, Villar RN: Complications of arthroscopy of the hip. J Bone Joint Surg 1999;81B:604–606.
19. Santori N, Villar RN: Acetabular labral tears: result of arthroscopic partial limbectomy. Arthroscopy 2000;16:11–15.
20. Hawkins RB: Arthroscopy of the hip. Clin Orthop 1989;249:44–47.
21. Byrd JWT, Pappas JN, Pedley MJ: Hip arthroscopy: an anatomic study of portal placement and relationship to the extraarticular structures. Arthroscopy 1995;11:418–423.
22. Glick JM, Sampson TG, Behr JT, Schmidt E: Hip arthroscopy by the lateral approach. Arthroscopy 1987;3:4–12.
23. McCarthy JC, Busconi B: The role of hip arthroscopy in the diagnosis and treatment of hip disease. Can J Surg 1995;38(suppl):S13–S17.
24. McCarthy JC, Busconi B: The role of hip arthroscopy in the diagnosis and treatment of hip disease. Arthroplasty Rounds 1995;18:753–756.
25. Byrd JWT: Hip arthroscopy utilizing the supine position. Arthroscopy 1994;10:275–280.
26. Byrd JWT, Chern KY: Traction versus distension for distraction of the joint during hip arthroscopy. Arthroscopy 1997;13:346–349.
27. Sampson TG, Glick JM: Indications and surgical treatment of hip pathology. In: McGinty JB, Caspari RB, Jackson RW, Poehling GG (eds). Operative Arthroscopy, 2nd ed. Philadelphia: Lippincott-Raven, 1996:1067–1078.
28. Glick JM, Sampson TG: Hip arthroscopy by the lateral approach. In: McGinty JB, Caspari RB, Jackson RW, Poehling GG (eds). Operative Arthroscopy, 2nd ed. Philadelphia: Lippincott-Raven, 1996:1079–1088.
29. Byrd JWT: Hip arthroscopy: the supine position. In: McGinty JB, Caspari RB, Jackson RW, Poehling GG (eds). Operative Arthroscopy, 2nd ed. Philadelphia: Lippincott-Raven, 1996:1091–1099.
30. Parisien JS: Hip arthroscopy: supine position. In: Parisien JS (ed). Techniques in Therapeutic Arthroscopy. New York: Raven, 1993:23.1–23.9.
31. Glick JM: Complications of hip arthroscopy by the lateral approach. In: Sherman OH, Minkoff J (eds). Arthroscopic Surgery. Baltimore: Williams & Wilkins, 1990:193–201.
32. Byrd JWT: Indications and contraindications. In: Byrd JWT (ed). Operative Hip Arthroscopy. New York: Thieme, 1998:7–24.
33. Sampson TG, Farjo LA: Hip arthroscopy by the lateral approach: technique and selected cases. In: Byrd JWT (ed). Operative Hip Arthroscopy. New York: Thieme, 1998:105–122.
34. Klapper R, Dorfmann H, Boyer T: Hip arthroscopy without traction. In: Byrd JWT (ed). Operative Hip Arthroscopy. New York: Thieme, 1998:139–152.
35. Klapper RC, Silver DM: Hip arthroscopy without traction. Contemp Orthop 1989;18:687–693.
36. Byrd JWT: Labral lesions: an elusive source of hip pain. Case reports and literature review. Arthroscopy 1996;12:603–612.
37. McCarthy JC, Mason JB, Wardell SR: Hip arthroscopy for acetabular dysplasia: a pipe dream? Orthopedics 1998;14:977–979.
38. Ide T, Akamatsu N, Nakajima I: Arthroscopic surgery of the hip joint. Arthroscopy 1991;7:204–211.
39. Suzuki S, Awaya G, Okada Y, Maekawa M, Ikeda T, Tada H: Arthroscopic diagnosis of ruptured acetabular labrum. Acta Orthop Scand 1986;57:513–515.
40. Suzuki S, Kasahara Y, Seto Y, Futami T, Furukawa K, Nishino Y: Arthroscopy in 19 children with Perthes' disease. Pathologic changes of the synovium and the joint surface. Acta Orthop Scand 1994;65:581–584.

41. Villar RN: Hip arthroscopy. J Bone Joint Surg 1995;77B:517–518.
42. Dienst M, Kohn D: Hüftarthroskopie: Minimal-invasive Diagnostik und Therapie des erkrankten oder verletzten Hüftgelenks. Unfallchirurg 2001;104:2–18.
43. Dienst M, Goedde S, Seil R, Hammer D, Kohn D: Hip arthroscopy without traction: in vivo anatomy of the peripheral hip joint cavity. Arthroscopy 2001;17:924–931.
44. Dienst M, Goedde S, Seil R, Kohn D: Diagnostic arthroscopy of the hip joint. Orthop Traumatol 2002;10:1–14.
45. Wingstrand H, Wingstrand A, Krantz P: Intracapsular and atmospheric pressure in the dynamics and stability of the hip. A biomechanical study. Acta Orthop Scand 1990;61:231–235.
46. Weber W, Weber E: Über die Mechanik der menschlichen Gehwerkzeuge nebst der Beschreibung eines Versuches über das Herausfallen des Schenkelkopfes aus der Pfanne im luftverdünnten Raum. Ann Phys Chem 1837;40:1–13.
47. Dienst M, Seil R, Gödde S, et al: Effects of traction, distension and joint position on distraction of the hip joint: an experimental study in cadavers. Arthroscopy 2002;18:865–71.
48. Funke E, Munzinger U: Zur Indikation und Technik der Hüftarthroskopie: Möglichkeiten und Grenzen. Schweiz Rundsch Med Prax 1994;83:154–157.
49. Funke EL, Munzinger U: Complications in hip arthroscopy. Arthroscopy 1996;12:156–159.
50. Norman-Taylor FH, Villar RN: Arthroscopic surgery of the hip: current status. Knee Surg Sports Traumatol Arthroscopy 1994;2:255–258.
51. Dienst M, Seil R, Gödde S, Georg T, Kohn D: Hüftarthroskopie bei radiologisch beginnender bis mäßiggradiger Koxarthrose. Diagnostische und therapeutische Wertigkeit. Orthopäde 1999;28:812–818.
52. Personal communication with H. Dorfmann and T. Boyer, Paris, France.
53. Dvorak M, Duncan CP, Day B: Arthroscopic anatomy of the hip. Arthroscopy 1990;6:264–273.
54. Dienst M, Goedde S, Brang M, Kohn D: Arthroscopic anatomy of the peripheral compartment of the hip: on the frequency and morphology of Weitbrecht's retinacula in cadaver and in vivo. Presented at the 17th annual meeting of the Arthroscopy Association of North America (AANA) 2000, Miami, FL, April 14, 2000.
55. Hoffmann F: Die arthroskopische Behandlung der hämatogenen bakteriellen Koxitis im Säuglings- und Kindesalter. Arthroskopie 1991;4:98–102.
56. Majewski M: Arthroscopic mobilisation of the hip joint in children and adolescents by distension and bump resection. Presented at the 18th annual meeting of the Association of German-speaking Arthroscopists (AGA), Saarbruecken, 2001.
57. Nishii T, Nakanishi K, Sugano M, Naito H, Tamura S, Ochi T: Acetabular labral tears: contrast-enhanced MR imaging under continuous leg traction. Skeletal Radiol 1996;25:349–356.
58. Ikeda T, Awaya G, Suzuki S, Okada Y, Tada H: Torn acetabular labrum in young patients. Arthroscopic diagnosis and management. J Bone Joint Surg 1988;70B:13–16.
59. Villar RN: Arthroscopy. BMJ 1994;308:51–53.
60. Czerny C, Hofmann S, Neuhold A, et al: Lesions of the acetabular labrum: accuracy of MR imaging and MR arthrography in detection and staging. Radiology 1996;200:225–230.
61. Urban M, Hofmann S, Tschauner C, Czerny C, Neuhold A, Kramer J: MR-Arthrographie bei der Labrumläsion des Hüftgelenks. Technik und Stellenwert. Orthopäde 1998;27:691–698.
62. Goldman A, Minkoff J, Price A, Krinick R: A posterior arthroscopic approach to bullet extraction from the hip. J Trauma 1987;27:1294–1300.
63. Villar RN: Hip arthroscopy. Review. B J Hosp Med 1992;47:763–766.
64. Schindler A, Lechevallier JJC, Rao NS, Bowen JR: Diagnostic and therapeutic arthroscopy of the hip in children and adolescents: evaluation of results. J Pediatr Orthop 1995;15:317–321.
65. Bould M, Edwards D, Villar RN: Arthroscopic diagnosis and treatment of septic arthritis of the hip joint. Case report. Arthroscopy 1993;9:707–708.
66. Blitzer CM: Arthroscopic management of septic arthritis of the hip. Arthroscopy 1993;9:414–416.
67. Chung WK, Slater GL, Bates EH: Treatment of septic arthritis of the hip by arthroscopic lavage. J Pediatr Orthop 1993;13:444–446.
68. Carls J, Kohn D: Arthroskopische Therapie der eitrigen Koxitis. Arthroskopie 1996;9:274–277.
69. Byrd JWT: Complications associated with hip arthroscopy. In: Byrd JWT (ed). Operative Hip Arthroscopy. New York: Thieme, 1998:171–176.
70. Bartlett CS, DiFelice GS, Buyly R, et al: Cardiac arrest as a result of intraabdominal extravasation of fluid during arthroscopic removal of a loose body from the hip joint of a patient with an acetabular fracture. J Orthop Trauma 1998;12:294–300.
71. Maurice H, Crone M, Watt I: Synovial chondromatosis. J Bone Joint Surg 1988;70B:807–811.

12

Arthroscopic Iliopsoas Release for Coxa Saltans Interna (Snapping Hip Syndrome)

Thomas G. Sampson

Coxa saltans interna is a hip syndrome resulting in the iliopsoas tendon snapping pathologically over structures beneath it, causing a loud audible click or clunk, which may be associated with pain. It is thought the most common involved structure it courses over is the iliopectineal eminence (Figure 12.1); however, other intraarticular structures may be large loose bodies and exostoses. The differential diagnosis must rule out labral tears, synovial chondromatosis, and abnormal shapes of the femoral head from an old slipped capital femoral epiphysis or hip dysplasia and acetabular retroversion.

The iliacus and the psoas fuse to become one musculotendinous unit as they pass in a sulcus between the anteroinferior iliac spine and the iliopectineal eminence (Figure 12.2). The tendon courses over the anterior hip capsule as it passes posteriorly in the iliopsoas bursa to insert onto the lesser trochanter (Figure 12.3). The tendon assumes a lateral position on the iliopectineal eminence when the hip is in flexion, abduction, and external rotation. As the hip is moved into extension, adduction, and internal rotation, the tendon moves from lateral to medial; however, the musculotendinous portion remains in the groove.[1]

The symptomatic snapping hip is caused by the back-and-forth movement over the anterior hip capsule and femoral head. The etiology may be a hyperextension injury to the hip capsule or tendon itself. Other causes may be from exostoses on the acetabular rim or femoral head as well as the lesser trochanter.[2] The iliopsoas bursa may also become inflamed or hypertrophic, leading to the condition. Of note, the iliopsoas bursa is the largest bursa in the body, measuring 7 cm long and 4 cm in width.

CLINICAL DIAGNOSIS

The patient presents with a vague history of an injury that may have felt like a groin sprain or of having done the splits. Some report a hyperextension injury of the hip. Associated with the injury, the patient may experience the onset of popping or hip clicking that intensifies over time to a consistent snapping sensation that may be heard by anyone around them. The initial pain from the injury typically never resolves, and the snap hurts.

Normal walking is not painful, but pain may limit sports or dancing that involves hip flexion. With the patient supine, the patient can reproduce the snap as he or she flexes and extends the hip. The examiner can eliminate the snap by applying pressure over the anterior hip capsule, which restricts the tendon's movement. Such a maneuver is diagnostic for coxa saltans interna.

IMAGING

Plain radiographs are usually normal and may be helpful to identify exostoses or a spur on the lesser trochanter as well as dysplasia or impingement. Magnetic resonance imaging (MRI) is best to document any thickening of the iliopsoas tendon or fluid in the bursa. Iliopsoas bursography may demonstrate the outline of the tendon as it snaps over the hip capsule and is a dynamic test.[3] Elimination of the pain by a lidocaine injection in the bursa is a positive diagnostic test.

SURGICAL TREATMENT

The classic open surgical approach is through an 8- to 10-cm groin incision, protecting the neurovascular structures and lengthening the tendon 2 cm.[4,5] We have developed an arthroscopic approach in which the iliopsoas tendon is either partially or completely released from the lesser trochanter.

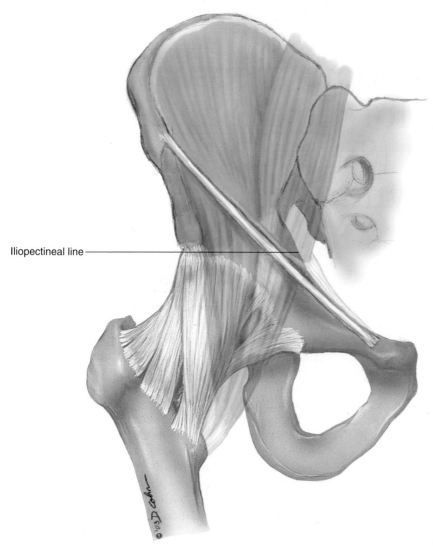

Iliopectineal line

FIGURE 12.1. The iliopsoas courses over the iliopectineal line.

Technique

The patient is positioned for the lateral approach (see Chapter 9).[6,7] After the hip has undergone a diagnostic arthroscopy, the traction is completely released. The foot is maximally externally rotated, thus bringing the lesser trochanter to an anterior position and is viewed orthogonal with the C-arm fluoroscope (Figure 12.4A,B).

Two additional safe portals are needed: the anteroinferior (AI) and far anteroinferior (FAI). Originally, we used the anteroinferior medial (AIM) and AI (Figure 12.5A,B).

Arthroscope Placement

An intracath is directed from the AFI portal to a point just proximal to the lesser trochanter into the iliopsoas bursa. A Nitanol wire is passed through the intracath and the skin is anesthetized with marcaine/ epinephrine. The skin is incised with a no. 11 blade, and the cannulated scope sheath is passed over the wire into the bursa under fluoroscopic control. The inflow is started to distend the bursa.

Instrument Placement

A second AI portal is created in the same manner and a switcher stick is placed. The iliopsoas tendon is palpated while viewing with a 30-degree arthroscope (Figure 12.6A,B). It may be necessary to clear bursa or muscle to view the tendon. A long cannula may aid in passing instruments or to maintain outflow to prevent distension.

The Release

The iliopsoas tendon is sectioned with a radiothermal cutter so as to coagulate bleeders as it is cut. We have

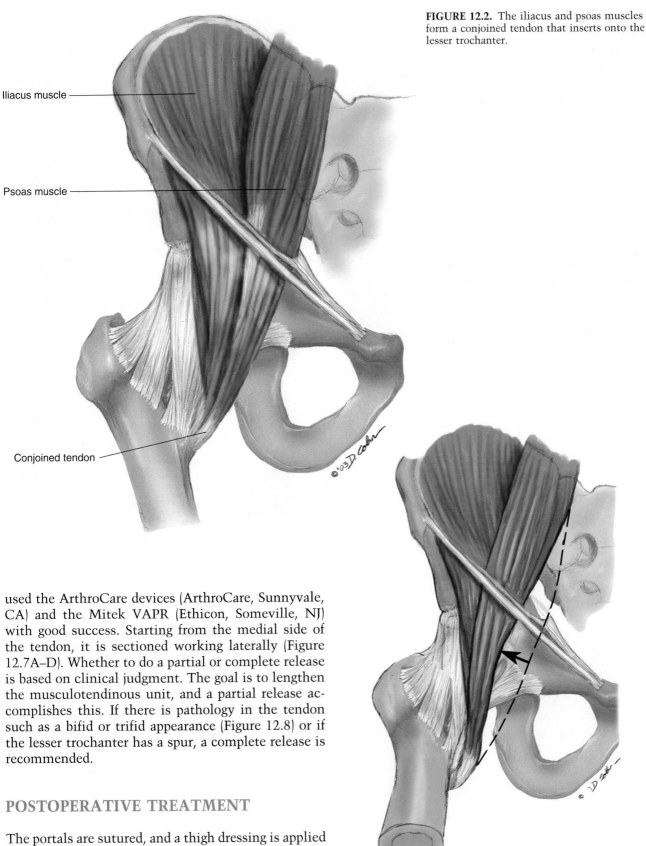

FIGURE 12.2. The iliacus and psoas muscles form a conjoined tendon that inserts onto the lesser trochanter.

Iliacus muscle

Psoas muscle

Conjoined tendon

used the ArthroCare devices (ArthroCare, Sunnyvale, CA) and the Mitek VAPR (Ethicon, Someville, NJ) with good success. Starting from the medial side of the tendon, it is sectioned working laterally (Figure 12.7A–D). Whether to do a partial or complete release is based on clinical judgment. The goal is to lengthen the musculotendinous unit, and a partial release accomplishes this. If there is pathology in the tendon such as a bifid or trifid appearance (Figure 12.8) or if the lesser trochanter has a spur, a complete release is recommended.

POSTOPERATIVE TREATMENT

The portals are sutured, and a thigh dressing is applied with compression. Crutches, with partial weight bearing, are used until the patient has good control of the hip (usually 2 to 3 weeks). Flexion exercises are begun immediately, and strength returns in 3 to 6 weeks after a partial release and 3 to 6 months after a com-

FIGURE 12.3. The iliopsoas lies anterior to the hip capsule and moves lateral with hip flexion, abduction, and external rotation. As the hip is extended, adducted, and internally rotated, the tendon moves in a medial direction.

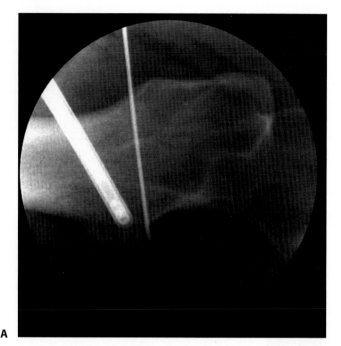

A

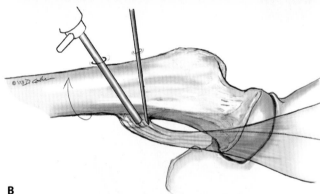

B

FIGURE 12.4. (A) Fluoroscopic view with the C-arm giving an orthogonal view of the lesser trochanter while the hip is externally rotated and instruments are positioned. (B) The arthroscope is placed through the far anteroinferior portal and the cutting instrument through the anteroinferior portal.

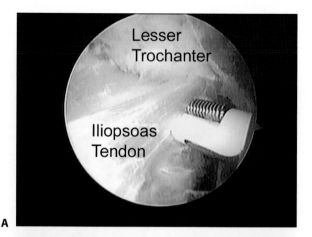

A

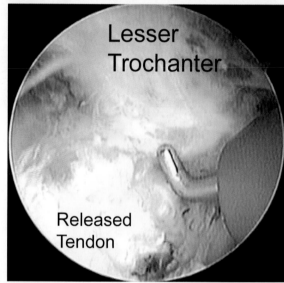

B

FIGURE 12.6. (A) Arthroscopic view of the iliopsoas tendon inserting onto the lesser trochanter. (B) After partial release.

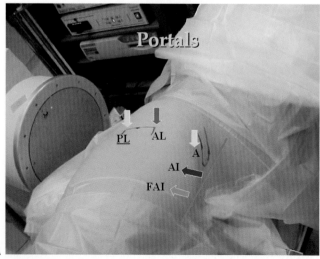

A

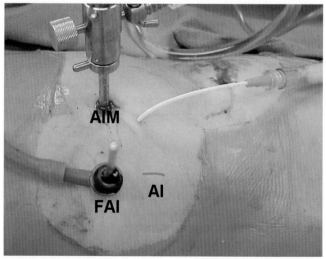

B

FIGURE 12.5. (A) Patient in the lateral decubitus position, the C-arm in place. The portals are posterolateral (PL), anterolateral (AL), anterior (A), anteroinferior (AI), and far anteroinferior (FAI). (B) Technique using the FAI and the anteroinferior medial (AIM) portals (the original method).

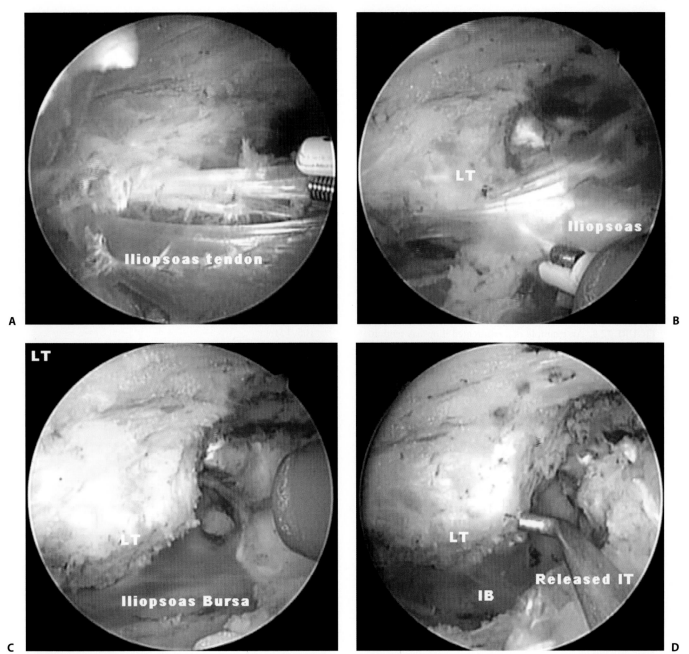

FIGURE 12.7. (A) Sprained iliopsoas tendon inserting onto the lesser trochanter. (B) After partial release with a radiothermal wand. (C) The iliopsoas has been completely released. Note the large bursal space. (D) The probe is on the lesser trochanter (LT). The iliopsoas tendon (IT) is retracted after its release in the iliopsoas bursa (IB).

plete release. Occasionally, a nonpainful mild pop may be present for 3 to 6 months.

RESULTS

Since 1993 we have released 35 iliopsoas tendons for snapping hip syndrome. All were successfully viewed and released using the arthroscopic technique. There were two complications, one with neuropraxia of the lateral femoral cutaneous nerve and one with 4/5 flexor weakness at 6 months. All the rest had full re-

turn of their muscle strength by 3 months. All had resolution of their snap, and 94% had good to excellent results and pain relief.

CONCLUSION

Arthroscopic iliopsoas tendon release has been described. It is a safe and effective way to treat coxa saltans interna and is reproducible. The results are better than the results of open surgery and have fewer complications.

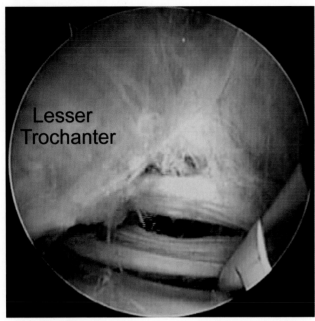

FIGURE 12.8. An example of a trifurcated iliopsoas tendon.

Acknowledgment.   I would like to thank James M. Glick, MD, for his contributions to this chapter.

References

1. Allen WC, Cope R: Coxa saltans: the snapping hip revisited. J Am Acad Orthop Surg 1995;3(5):303–308.
2. Schaberg JE, Harper MC, Allen WC: The snapping hip syndrome. Am J Sports Med 1984;12(5):361–365.
3. Harper MC, Schaberg JE, Allen WC: Primary iliopsoas bursography in the diagnosis of disorders of the hip. Clin Orthop 1987; 221:238–241.
4. Dobbs MB, Gordon JE, Luhmann SJ, et al: Surgical correction of the snapping iliopsoas tendon in adolescents. J Bone Joint Surg [Am] 2002;84(3):420–424.
5. Jacobson T, Allen WC: Surgical correction of the snapping iliopsoas tendon. Am J Sports Med 1990;18(5):470–474.
6. Glick JM, Sampson TG, Gordon RB, et al: Hip arthroscopy by the lateral approach. Arthroscopy 1987;3(1):4–12.
7. Sampson TG, Fargo LA: Hip arthroscopy by the lateral approach: technique and selected cases. In: Byrd JW (ed). Operative Hip Arthroscopy. New York: Thieme, 1988: 105–121.

13

Hip Arthroscopy in Athletes

J.W. Thomas Byrd

Sports-related injuries to the hip joint have received relatively little attention. This trend is changing but, until recently, there have been few publications in peer-reviewed journals and the topic has rarely been presented at scientific meetings. There are three reasons. First, perhaps hip injuries are less common than injuries to other joints. Second, investigative skills for the hip including clinical assessment and imaging studies have been less sophisticated. Third, there have been fewer interventional methods available to treat the hip, including both surgical techniques and conservative modalities, and thus there has been little impetus to delve into this unrecognized area.

The evolution of arthroscopy has been intimately tied to sports medicine. The motivating principle has been a less-invasive technique that facilitates quicker return to unrestricted athletics. It is now recognized that this basic sports medicine principle applies well to all individuals, whether the goal is to accomplish an earlier return to the workplace or simply a return to normal daily activities.

However, hip arthroscopy has followed a distinctly different route. It began as a surgical alternative to only a few recognized forms of hip pathology. These indications included removal of loose bodies that could otherwise only be addressed by an extensive arthrotomy and arthroscopic debridement for degenerative arthritis to postpone the need for hip arthroplasty.[1,2]

Neither of these early indications found much application in an athletic population. However, as the basic methods of hip arthroscopy were developed, it began to be performed for select cases of unexplained hip pain. Arthroscopy revealed that there are numerous intraarticular sources of disabling hip symptoms that were previously unrecognized and are now potentially amenable to arthroscopic intervention[3,4]; these include tearing of the acetabular labrum, traumatic injury to the articular surface, and damage to the ligamentum teres among others.

The indications for hip arthroscopy fall into two broad categories. In one, arthroscopy offers an alternative to traditional open techniques previously employed for recognized forms of hip pathology such as loose bodies or impinging osteophytes. In the other, arthroscopy offers a method of treatment for disorders that previously went unrecognized including labral tears, chondral injuries, and disruption of the ligamentum teres. Most athletic injuries fall into this latter category. In the past, athletes were simply resigned to living within the constraints of their symptoms, often ending their competitive careers, with a diagnosis of a chronic groin injury. Based on the results of arthroscopy among athletes, it is likely that many of these careers could have been resurrected with arthroscopic intervention.[5]

MECHANISM OF INJURY

The mechanism of injury can be as varied as the sports in which athletes participate. In general, hip disorders attributable to a significant episode of trauma tend to respond better to arthroscopy.[6] This is because, other than the damage due to trauma, the athlete usually has an otherwise healthy joint. Individuals who simply develop progressive onset of symptoms in absence of injury tend to experience a less-complete response, because insidious onset of symptoms usually suggests either underlying disease or some predisposition to injury that cannot be fully reversed and may leave the joint vulnerable to further deterioration in the future. Even the presence of an acute injury such as a twisting episode, which is known to cause a tear of the acetabular labrum, may be more likely if the labrum was vulnerable to injury and may represent a less certain response to surgery. This vulnerability can result from abnormal labral morphology or underlying degeneration.

However, these broad generalizations must be tempered in the competitive athlete. Individuals who participate in contact and collision sports simply may not be able to recount which traumatic episode led to the onset of symptoms. Remember that significant intraarticular damage can occur from an episode without the athlete developing incapacitating pain. The athlete may be able to continue to compete and subsequently undergo workup only when symptoms fail to resolve. Injury can occur from any contact or collision sport or sports involving forceful or repetitive twisting of the hip. The aging joint may also be more vulnerable. These parameters do not exclude many sports.

A particular entity has been identified associated with acute chondral damage.[7] It is mostly encountered in physically fit young adult men. The characteristic feature is a lateral impact injury to the area of the trochanter (Figure 13.1). Young adult men are apt to be participating in contact and collision activities where this mechanism is frequent. With good body conditioning, they have little adipose tissue overlying the trochanter, so much of the force of the blow is delivered directly to the bone. This force is then transferred unchecked into the hip joint, resulting in either shearing of the articular surface on the medial aspect of the femoral head at the tidemark, or compression of the articular surface on the superior medial acetabulum, exceeding its structural threshold. The result is a full-thickness articular fragment from the femoral head or articular surface breakdown of the acetabulum, possibly with loose bodies, depending on the magnitude of acetabular chondral, or chondroosseous cell death (Figures 13.2, 13.3). This mechanism is dependent on peak bone density, as otherwise the force would result in fracture rather than delivery of the energy to the surface of the joint. The injury usually results in immediate onset of symptoms, but may not be disabling. It may be assessed as a groin pull, with workup ensuing only when symptoms fail to resolve.

Ice hockey is a sport that seems to present a particularly high prevalence of hip pathology. Hip flexibility is a premium consideration in this sport. The joint is subjected to violent and repetitive torsional maneuvers and also subjected to relatively high-velocity impact loading. Thus, the labrum is susceptible to tearing from the twisting maneuvers, while the articular surface is vulnerable to impact injury. Often, acute epi-

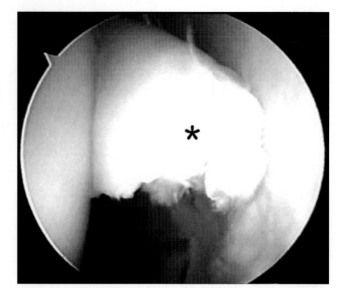

FIGURE 13.2. Arthroscopic view of the left hip of a 20-year-old collegiate basketball player demonstrates an acute grade IV articular injury (asterisk) to the medial aspect of the femoral head.

sodes are simply superimposed on the cumulative effect of years of exposure (Figure 13.4A–C).

Golf is another illustrative sport that seems to have a predilection for precipitating hip symptoms. It is not a contact or collision sport, but the golf swing does incorporate a significant element of twisting on the hip joint. Additionally, it is a sport in which participants can compete with advancing age, even at the professional level. Thus, the greater susceptibility to injury of an aging hip exists, as well as the cumulative effect of repetitive trauma over a prolonged career. Tennis shares many of these same attributes.

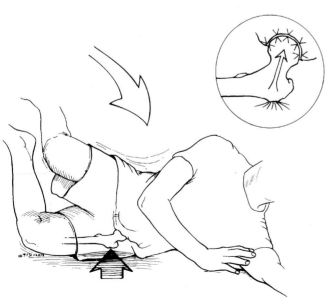

FIGURE 13.1. Fall results in direct blow to the greater trochanter and, in absence of fracture, the force generated is transferred unchecked to the hip joint.

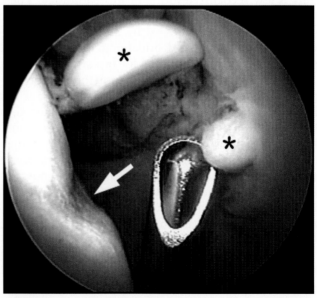

FIGURE 13.3. Arthroscopic view of the left hip of a 19-year-old man who sustained a direct lateral blow to the hip, subsequently developing osteocartilaginous fragments (asterisks) within the superomedial aspect of the acetabulum.

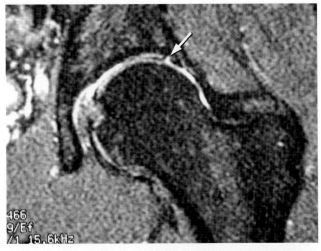

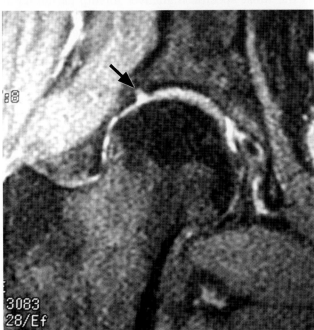

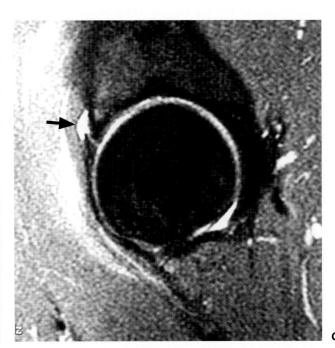

FIGURE 13.4. Three National Hockey League players were referred, each with a 2-week history of hip pain following an injury on the ice. Each case demonstrated magnetic resonance imaging (MRI) evidence of labral pathology (arrows). These cases were treated with 2 weeks of rest followed by a 2-week period of gradually resuming activities. Each of these athletes was able to return to competition and has continued to play for several seasons without needing surgery. (A) Coronal image of a left hip demonstrates a lateral labral tear (arrow). (B) Coronal image of a right hip demonstrates a lateral labral tear (arrow). (C) Sagittal image of a left hip demonstrates an anterior labral tear with associated paralabral cyst (arrow).

In our study of athletes undergoing arthroscopy, injury to the ligamentum teres was the third most common finding (Table 13.1).[5] Historically, rupture of the ligament is associated with hip dislocation. It has been recognized that injury can occur without dislocation, but this has been described only as case reports.[8–11] Disruption appears to be attributable to a twisting injury and is increasingly recognized as a source of intractable hip pain. In our review of 23 cases of traumatic injury to the ligamentum teres, 17 (74%) occurred without accompanying dislocation of the hip.[12]

TABLE 13.1. Diagnoses for Hip Arthroscopy.

Labral pathology (27)	Loose bodies (3)
Chondral damage (23)	Impinging osteophyte (2)
Ligamentum teres damage (11)	Avascular necrosis (1)
Arthritic disorder (7)	Synovitis (1)
Dysplasia (5)	Perthes disease (1)

Source: From Byrd and Jones,[5] with permission of Clinics in Sports Medicine.

PATIENT SELECTION

Successful hip arthroscopy is most clearly dependent on proper patient selection. A well-executed procedure fails when performed for the wrong reasons. Paramount among these is patient expectation. Be certain that the athlete has reasonable goals and knows what can be accomplished with arthroscopy, which is only partially dictated by the nature of the pathology. Remember that there is much we do not fully understand regarding the pathomechanics, pathoanatomy, and natural history of many of these lesions that are now being surgically addressed. However, with the increasing amount of clinical experience, patients can be offered reasonable statistical data on likely outcomes.

Athletes are often set apart by their drive, discipline, and motivation as they push their bodies to their physiologic limits. However, the most uniquely challenging aspect of deciding on surgical intervention in this population is time constraints: How quickly does the surgeon decide to operate and how quickly will the patient recover? This is a year-round issue, whether the athlete is attempting to return for the current season, preparing for the upcoming season, or simply resuming the necessary off-season conditioning regimen. Except for loose bodies, no literature suggests that harm is caused by not recommending early surgical intervention for most of the problems that are now being recognized.[13] Most of these disorders declare themselves over time through failure of response to conservative measures. Unfortunately, for athletes, time is often not an accepted ally.

Extraarticular injuries far outnumber intraarticular problems in the hip region. Thus, it is best to temper the interest in performing an extensive intraarticular workup for every athlete with pain around the hip. However, in our study of athletes who underwent arthroscopy with documented pathology, in 60% of cases the hip was not recognized as the source of symptoms at the time of initial treatment, and the patients were managed for an average of 7 months before the hip was considered as a potential contributing source.[5] The most common preliminary diagnoses were various types of musculotendinous strains (Table 13.2). Thus, it is prudent to at least consider possible intraarticular pathology in the differential diagnosis when managing a strain around the hip joint. Most important is thoughtful follow-up and reassessment when these injuries do not respond as expected.

A careful history and examination usually indicate whether the hip is the source of symptoms. Characteristic features are outlined in Table 13.3. Single-plane activities such as straight-ahead running are often well tolerated, whereas torsional and twisting maneuvers are more problematic in precipitating painful symptoms. Stairs and inclines may be more troublesome, and the same athlete who can run painfree on level surfaces may have more difficulty running hills. Prolonged hip flexion such as sitting can be uncomfortable, and catching symptoms are often experienced when rising from a seated or squatted position.

Hip symptoms are most commonly referred to the anterior groin and may radiate to the medial thigh. However, a characteristic clinical feature is the *C-sign*.[14] A patient describing deep interior hip pain will

TABLE 13.3. Characteristic Exacerbating Features.

Straight plane activity relatively well tolerated
Torsional/twisting activities problematic
Prolonged hip flexion (sitting) uncomfortable
Pain/catching going from flexion to extension (rising from seated position)
Inclines more difficult than level surfaces

use a hand to grip above the greater trochanter, with the thumb lying posteriorly and the fingers cupped within the anterior groin. It may appear that the patient is describing lateral pain such as from the iliotibial band or trochanteric bursa, but characteristically, the patient is reflecting pain within the joint.

On examination, log rolling the leg back and forth is the most specific maneuver for hip pathology because this rotates only the femoral head in relation to the acetabulum and capsule, not stressing any of the surrounding neurovascular or musculotendinous structures. More sensitive examination maneuvers include forced flexion combined with internal rotation or abduction combined with external rotation. Sometimes these produce an accompanying click, but more important is simply whether the maneuvers reproduce the athlete's pain.

For long-standing conditions, athletes may secondarily develop extraarticular symptoms of tendonitis or bursitis or may have coexistent extraarticular pathology. A useful test for distinguishing the intraarticular origin of symptoms is a fluoroscopically guided intraarticular injection of anesthetic. The hallmark is temporary alleviation of symptoms during the anesthetic effect. With the more recent technology of gadolinium arthrography combined with magnetic resonance imaging (MRA), always be certain to include anesthetic with the injection to elicit this useful diagnostic response.

MANAGEMENT STRATEGY

Labral lesions are the most common hip pathology, present in 61% of athletes undergoing arthroscopy.[5] Various studies have demonstrated that articular damage is present in association with more than half of all labral tears.[15–18] Often it is the extent of articular pathology that is the limiting factor as far as success of arthroscopic intervention. MRIs and MRAs are best at identifying labral lesions but poor at demonstrating accompanying articular pathology (Figures 13.5, 13.6, 13.7). Thus, the uncertain presence of articular damage is often the *wild card* in predicting the outcome of arthroscopy and should temper the surgeon's enthusiasm for predicting uniform success in the presence of imaging evidence of labral damage.

In our experience, in cases with documented arthroscopic evidence of joint pathology, MRI has a 42%

TABLE 13.2. Preliminary Diagnoses (Other Than the Hip).

Hip flexor strain (6)	Piriformis syndrome (1)
Lumbar disorder (5)	Sciatica (1)
Unspecified muscle strain (4)	SI disorder (1)
Adductor strain (3)	Stress fracture (1)
Iliopsoas tendonitis (2)	Contusion (1)
Trochanteric bursitis (2)	Malalignment (1)
Hamstring injury (2)	Don't know (1)

Source: From Byrd and Jones,[5] with permission of Clinics in Sports Medicine.

false-negative interpretation, which is reduced to 8% with MRA. However, with MRA, the false-positive interpretation doubles from 10% to 20%, with overinterpretation of labral lesions being the principal source of false-positive results.[19] Lecouvet et al. have also demonstrated MRI evidence of labral pathology among asymptomatic volunteers, and the incidence increases with age.[20] Thus, surgeons must still rely more on their clinical assessment of the athlete rather than simply MRI findings. With the increasing awareness of hip joint injuries in athletes and an increasing number of investigative studies being performed, a significant number of false-positive findings are likely, which could potentially lead the surgeon astray. It is also likely that many athletes participating in contact and collision sports over a long career may demonstrate MRI evidence of hip pathology even in absence of symptoms.

Also, much is not fully understood regarding the natural history of labral lesions. Seldes et al. demon-

strated microvascular proliferation, suggesting a healing capacity of labral tears.[21] It is uncertain whether these will truly heal, but it is clear that some become clinically asymptomatic (see Figure 13.4). For the athlete with protracted mechanical symptoms in association with imaging evidence of hip pathology, the decision is simple; they can choose to live with their symptoms, or select arthroscopy with a reasonable expectation of success. The more difficult challenge is the athlete with more recent injury and MRI evidence of labral pathology. This situation is increasingly encountered as investigative studies are being performed earlier in the course of evaluation.

The following algorithm is proposed for athletes with recent injury, hip joint symptoms, and MRI evidence of labral pathology. The hip should be rested for 2 to 4 weeks to see if symptoms subside. If the pain subsides sufficiently, the athlete can then begin to resume activities and return to competition. If the symptoms are stable, it is unlikely that any further

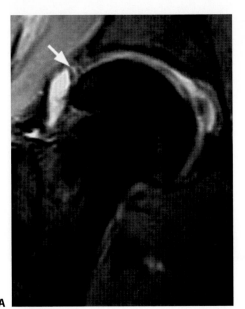

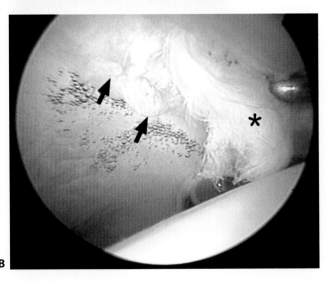

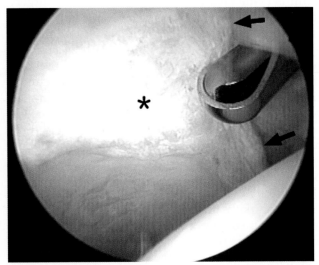

FIGURE 13.5. A 25-year-old top-ranked professional tennis player sustained a twisting injury to his right hip. (A) Coronal MRI demonstrates evidence of labral pathology (arrow). (B) Arthroscopy reveals extensive tearing of the anterior labrum (asterisk) as well as an adjoining area of grade III articular fragmentation (arrows). (C) The labral tear has been resected to a stable rim (arrows), and chondroplasty of the grade III articular damage (asterisk) is being performed.

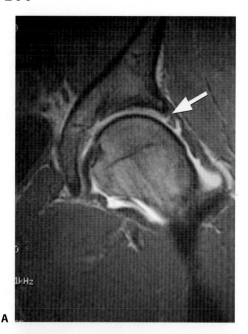

A

FIGURE 13.6. A 25-year-old top-ranked professional tennis player sustained a twisting injury to his left hip. (A) Coronal MRI demonstrates evidence of labral pathology (arrow). (B) Arthroscopy reveals the extent of labral pathology (arrows). (C) However, there was also an area of adjoining grade IV articular delamination (arrows) with exposed subchondral bone (asterisk). Chondroplasty was performed as the lesion was not amenable to microfracture. The athlete recovered successfully, but the length of recuperation was more protracted, with return to competition at 5 months.

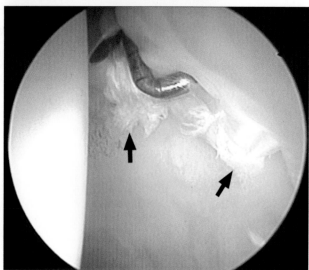

B

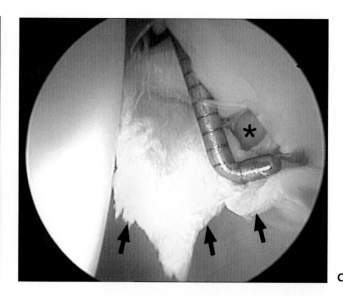

C

harm is being created by not recommending surgery. If baseline symptoms persist, then surgical intervention can be undertaken at a more opportune time.

In general, for in-season injuries, a brief period of rest and a trial of conservative treatment is the most likely course to allow the athlete to return to competition during the current season. Preseason injuries present a greater dilemma. If surgery is still needed after a period of rest, then time is lost that could interfere with the upcoming season. Ultimately, the surgeon must call on his or her experience and that of others to make the best decision for the athlete under the particular circumstances.

It is unlikely that any harm is caused by not recommending surgery but, as with other joints, there are hip *abusers* who can cause further damage by neglecting the joint. Thus, the best perspective to offer

an athlete is that it is unlikely that more harm or damage will occur in the absence of worsening symptoms.

RESULTS

In our study of 42 athletes, the average improvement using a modified Harris hip rating system (100-point maximum) was 35 points (preoperative, 57; postoperative, 92).[5] Ninety-three percent demonstrated at least 10 points of improvement. Also, of those questioned, 76% returned to their sport symptom free and unrestricted or at least at an increased level of performance, while 18% either chose not to return or were unable to return to their primary sport.

After understanding the potential benefits of an arthroscopic procedure, the next issue of paramount

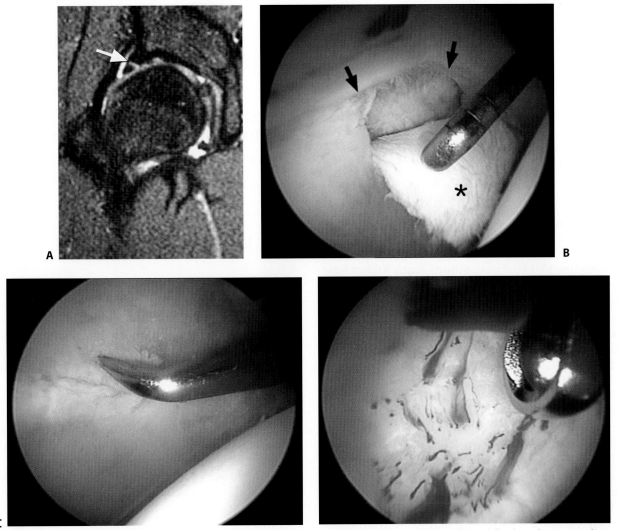

FIGURE 13.7. A 23-year-old elite professional tennis player sustained an injury to his right hip. (A) Coronal MRI demonstrates evidence of labral pathology (arrow). (B) Arthroscopy reveals the labral tear (arrows), but also an area of adjoining grade IV articular loss (asterisk). (C) Microfracture of the exposed subchondral bone is performed. (D) Occluding the inflow of fluid confirms vascular access through the areas of perforation. The athlete was maintained on a protected weight-bearing status emphasizing range of motion for 10 weeks, with return to competition at 3.5 months.

importance among athletes is how quickly they will recover. According to the same study, the greatest improvement (67%) was noted after the first month. Maximal improvement was achieved by 3 months, and these results were maintained among those athletes with 5-year follow-up (Figure 13.8).

Among athletes, the best results have been seen for impinging osteophytes, loose bodies, and rupture of the ligamentum teres (Figure 13.9). Impinging osteophytes are uncommon, but when recognized, the structural problem can be corrected, thus often resulting in pronounced symptomatic improvement. Loose bodies have traditionally been recognized as the clearest indication for arthroscopy. Predictable results have been further confirmed in the athletic population. Rupture of the ligamentum teres is an entity that has infrequently been reported in the literature. A propensity for this injury has been identified among

athletes, being the third leading diagnosis, and it responds remarkably well to arthroscopic debridement. More average results have been reported for labral tearing and chondral injury. The results are poor in the presence of clinical evidence of arthritis, but those patients undergoing microfracture fared better than with simple chondroplasty.

The nature of the onset of symptoms seems at least partially to influence the results. Those with a specific history of a significant traumatic event fared the best (Figure 13.10), whereas those with insidious onset did the worst. Those of acute onset fared only slightly better than insidious, which suggests that, even in the presence of a modest explainable injury, some type of predisposition should be suspected and the results of arthroscopy may be less certain.

Among the reported group of athletes, one-third competed at the collegiate, elite, or professional

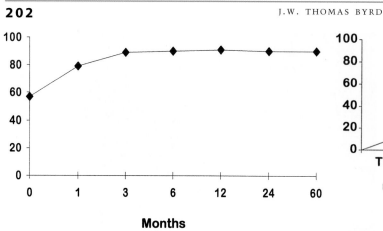

FIGURE 13.8. Average modified Harris hip scores among athletes at various intervals of follow-up.

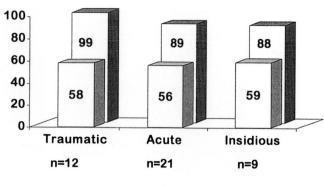

FIGURE 13.10. Results based on the onset of symptoms. (From Byrd and Jones,[5] with permission of Clin Sports Med.)

level (Figure 13.11). These groups had a higher baseline preoperative score than the recreational and high school athletes. This finding suggests that these athletes are functioning near the physiologic limits of the body and at a level at which small deficits may significantly influence the athlete's performance.

CONCLUSIONS

The indications for hip arthroscopy have been well established. The results among athletes appear to be favorable and, in fact, are somewhat better than those reported among a general population.

Intraarticular disorders in athletes may go unrecognized for a protracted period of time, most commonly being diagnosed as a strain. With an increasing awareness of these intraarticular problems and the intensity of services often available to athletes, joint injuries are now being diagnosed earlier. However, this emphasis for earlier diagnosis must be tempered. It is still likely that extraarticular in-

juries vastly outnumber injuries within the joint, and thus one should avoid the temptation for an extensive intraarticular workup for every simple muscle strain. Also, it is unknown whether early diagnosis necessitates early intervention. There is much that is not understood regarding the natural history of some of these intraarticular disorders. Thus, while it is difficult to say that a labral lesion identified by MRI will heal, it is uncertain how many of these may become clinically quiescent and asymptomatic or whether some of the signal changes evident on imaging may be caused by remote trauma that had previously become silent.

Nonetheless, arthroscopy has defined various sources of intraarticular hip pathology. In many cases, operative arthroscopy may result in significant symptomatic improvement. For some, arthroscopy offers a distinct advantage over traditional open techniques, but for many, arthroscopy now offers a method of treatment where none existed before.

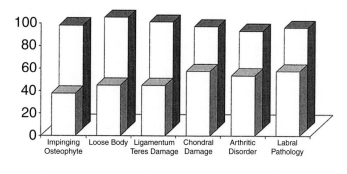

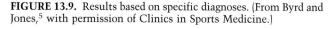

FIGURE 13.9. Results based on specific diagnoses. (From Byrd and Jones,[5] with permission of Clinics in Sports Medicine.)

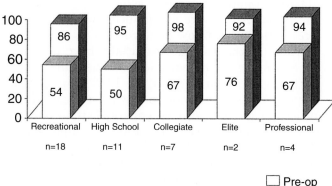

FIGURE 13.11. Results based on level of sport. (From Byrd and Jones,[5] with permission of Clinics in Sports Medicine.)

References

1. Byrd JWT: Hip arthroscopy for post-traumatic loose fragments in the young active adult: three case reports. Clin Sports Med 1996;6:129–134.

2. Villar RN: Arthroscopic debridement of the hip: a minimally invasive approach to osteoarthritis. J Bone Joint Surg 1991;73B:170–171.

3. Byrd JWT: Indications and contraindications. In: Byrd JWT (ed). Operative Hip Arthroscopy. New York: Thieme, 1998:7–24.

4. Sampson TG, Glick JM: Indications and surgical treatment of hip pathology. In: McGinty J, Caspari R, Jackson R, Poehling G (eds). Operative Arthroscopy, 2nd ed. New York: Raven Press, 1995:1067–1078.

5. Byrd JWT, Jones KS: Hip arthroscopy in athletes. Clin Sports Med 2001;20:749–762.

6. Byrd JWT, Jones KS: Prospective analysis of hip arthroscopy: two year follow-up. Arthroscopy 2000;16:578–587.

7. Byrd JWT: Lateral impact injury: a source of occult hip pathology. Clin Sports Med 2001;20:801–816.

8. Delcamp DD, Klarren HE, VanMeerdervoort HFP: Traumatic avulsion of the ligamentum teres without dislocation of the hip. J Bone Joint Surg 1988;70A:933–935.

9. Barrett IR, Goldberg JA: Avulsion fracture of the ligamentum teres in a child. A case report. J Bone Joint Surg 1989;71A:438–439.

10. Ebrahim NA, Salvolaine ER, Fenton PJ, Jackson WT: Calcified ligamentum teres mimicking entrapped intraarticular bony fragments in a patient with acetabular fracture. J Orthop Trauma 1991;5:376–378.

11. Kashiwagi N, Suzuki S, Seto Y: Arthroscopic treatment for traumatic hip dislocation with avulsion fracture of the ligamentum teres. Arthroscopy 2001;17:67–69.

12. Byrd JWT, Jones KS: Traumatic rupture of the ligamentum teres as a source of hip pain. Arthroscopy 2003 (in press).

13. Epstein H: Posterior fracture-dislocations of the hip: comparison of open and closed methods of treatment in certain types. J Bone Joint Surg 1961;43A:1079–1098.

14. Byrd JWT: Investigation of the symptomatic hip: physical examination. In: Byrd JWT (ed). Operative Hip Arthroscopy. New York: Thieme, 1998:25–41.

15. Byrd JWT, Jones KS: Prospective analysis of hip arthroscopy with five year follow up. Presented at AAOS 66th annual meeting, Dallas, TX, February 14, 2002.

16. McCarthy JC, Noble PC, Schuck MR, Wright J, Lee J: The watershed labral lesion: its relationship to early arthritis of the hip. J Arthroplasty 2001;16(8 suppl 1):81–87.

17. Farjo LA, Glick JM, Sampson TG: Hip arthroscopy for acetabular labrum tears. Arthroscopy 1999;15:132–137.

18. Santori N, Villar RN: Acetabular labral tears: result of arthroscopic partial limbectomy. Arthroscopy 2000;16:11–15.

19. Byrd JWT, Jones KS: Diagnostic accuracy of clinical assessment, MRI, gadolinium MRI, and intraarticular injection in hip arthroscopy patients. Am J Sports Med, 2004:4.

20. Lecouvet FE, VandeBerg BC, Malghen J, et al: MR imaging of the acetabular labrum: variations in 200 asymptomatic hips. AJR Am J Roentgenol 1996;167:1025–1028.

21. Seldes RM, Tan V, Hunt J, Katz M, Winiarsky R, Fitzgerald RH Jr: Anatomy, histologic features, and vascularity of the adult acetabular labrum. Clin Orthop 2001;382:232–240.

14

Hip Arthroscopy in Adolescence and Childhood

Keith R. Berend and Thomas Parker Vail

The appropriate application of hip arthroscopy to pediatric conditions requires a broad understanding of children's hip problems. In the end, the success of a hip arthroscopy in treating a pediatric hip condition depends as much on an accurate anatomic diagnosis as it does on technique. A dense constellation of intraarticular and extraarticular anatomic structures exists in close proximity to the hip joint. As such, multiple intraarticular and extraarticular pathologic conditions ranging from developmental to traumatic to infectious can be responsible for hip pain in the young active patient. Indeed, many of these conditions are specific to children and skeletally immature young adults. Traumatic etiologies include apophyseal injury, labral tears, chondral injury with or without loose body formation, and even hip dislocation.[1–4] Legg–Calvé–Perthes disease (LCP), slipped capital femoral epiphysis (SCFE), osteomyelitis, pyarthrosis, psoas compartment abscess, transient synovitis, femoral neck stress fractures, tumors, juvenile rheumatoid arthritis (JRA), and developmental dysplasia (DDH) account for the majority of atraumatic causes of childhood hip pain. Table 14.1 outlines the indications for hip arthroscopy in children and the procedures described for each diagnosis. Because children are changing so rapidly with growth and development, the differential diagnosis of their complaints changes with time. Hip maladies tend to cluster at several stages of childhood. In general, age can be used as a guideline to narrow a differential diagnosis of hip problems. In general, developmental dysplasia presents in infants and older children, Legg–Calvé–Perthes disease presents in children aged 4 to 10 years, slipped capital femoral epiphysis is seen in preteen or early teenage (generally obese) children, and labral injury may occur in older pediatric and adolescent patients following traumatic events.[5] All these common musculoskeletal conditions may manifest during athletic participation.[6] Although family members and children may associate a particular event with the onset of the hip pain, the underlying cause of the pain may actually be a more insidious process such as infection manifesting acutely. In some circumstances, the role of the traumatic event in the initiation of the hip pain is clear and unmistakable. However, when the trauma or athletic injury history is at all vague, sepsis should conclusively ruled out. This is especially true with the presentation of atraumatic hip pain in the young child (ages 0 to 6 years).[7–9]

Although it is clear that the role of hip arthroscopy in children remains limited, several conditions have been investigated and treated successfully using arthroscopic surgery of the hip. Since Burman's description of the use of an arthroscope to visualize joints in a cadaveric model, arthroscopy has risen in popularity to become the most commonly performed orthopedic procedure in this country today.[10,11] Despite the diverse applications of arthroscopy of the knee, shoulder, ankle, and wrist joints, arthroscopy of the hip has remained an infrequently performed procedure. The reasons for the delayed enthusiasm of surgeons for hip arthroscopy have been multifactorial: the relative technical difficulty of the procedure, the lack of well-documented clinical indications and proven results, and the potential risk of neurovascular injury. Surgeons have not previously had the opportunity to view the interior of the hip joint using a minimally invasive approach, thus limiting the understanding of occult sources of hip joint pain, especially in the active young patient. Finally, the majority of hip pathology in children occurs outside the actual joint space, further limiting the role of arthroscopy for this group of patients.

Hip pain that is persistent despite appropriate nonoperative treatment is a clinical entity that can be particularly difficult to manage when patients are young, and standard radiographic imaging is unrevealing. The advent of hip arthroscopy provides a minimally invasive avenue for diagnosis and treatment in these difficult cases. Thus, early reports on arthroscopy of the hip have centered on the utility of the procedure in providing a diagnosis in occult, intraarticular pathology. Enhanced understanding of the appropriate application of the procedure has led surgeons further into management and treatment of children's hip disorders. Nevertheless, refinement of the specific indications for arthroscopy of the hip and the efficacy of the procedure are only more recently becoming clearer in

TABLE 14.1. Indications for Hip Arthroscopy in Adolescence and Childhood.

Diagnosis	Therapy	Author
LCP disease: sequelae	Chondral debridement Loose body removal Osteochondral fragment excision	Bowen et al. 1986[29] Glick 1988 Kuklo et al. 1999[27] O'Leary et al. 2001[21] Berend and Vail 2001
Juvenile chronic arthritis JRA	Diagnostic Synovial biopsy Synovectomy	Holgersson et al. 1981[30] Kim et al. 1998[36]
Septic arthritis/pyogenic	Irrigation and debridement	Blitzer 1993[7] Chung et al. 1993[19] Kim et al. 1998[36]
SCFE	Diagnostic findings Evacuation of hematoma	Futami et al. 1992[33]
DDH	Labral debridement Diagnostic/chondral condition	Noguchi et al. 1999[35]
Labral tear	Diagnostic Partial limbectomy (labral excision)	Ikeda et al. 1988[2] Farjo et al. 1999[24]
Athletic injuries	Diagnostic Partial limbectomy Chondral debridement Loose body removal	O'Leary et al. 2001[21] Berend and Vail 2001[48]
Ligamentum teres avulsion	Avulsion fracture fragment excision Debridement of midsubstance tear	Kashiwagi et al. 2001
Diagnostic dilemma	Arthroscopic examination Treatment of findings	Kim et al. 1998[36]
Miscellaneous diagnoses (NOS)		Ide et al. 1991[22] Byrd and Jones 2000[44]

LCP, Legg–Calve–Perthes disease; JRA, juvenile rheumatoid arthritis; SCFE, slipped capital femoral epiphysis; DDH, developmental dysplasia of hip; NOS, age not otherwise specified in the article.

the literature and in practice. This chapter provides an overview of the role for arthroscopy of the hip in the pediatric and adolescent patient.

SAFETY OF HIP ARTHROSCOPY IN CHILDREN

The technique of hip arthroscopy is now well described and considered safe in most patients. Griffin and Villar reported a 1.6% incidence of complications in their review of 640 consecutive procedures. The most commonly reported complications involve nerve palsy injuries with three transient sciatic palsies and one femoral nerve palsy identified in Griffin's study.[12] Schindler et al. reported two transient pudendal nerve injuries, both with full recovery in their series.[13] All these adverse events are attributable to traction injury, for which the overall incidence is reported to be 0.8%.[12] Other less frequently described complications include injury to perineal structures, injury to the lateral femoral cutaneous nerve, extravasation of fluid causing abdominal pain, equipment failure, and inability to complete the procedure secondary to patient obesity.[12–18] No deep infections or serious major complications have been described in any study that includes pediatric or adolescent patients, and we have

not encountered any in our experience. We prefer to perform the procedure in the supine position on the fracture table with simple longitudinal traction. Using this technique and keeping operative times under an hour, we have avoided nerve injury, knee collateral ligament injury, and other complications reported with the use of traction. The possibility of manual traction in the very young child adds to the overall efficacy of this procedure in small children.[19]

Many believe that arthroscopy for the diagnosis and treatment of conditions about the hip in children decreases the need for open arthrotomy and possible dislocation of the hip. This less-invasive approach represents a distinct advantage for arthroscopy due to the potential complications of standard arthrotomy such as avascular necrosis. Children have a particularly vulnerable intracapsular blood supply to the femoral head.[20] Initial concerns that hip arthroscopy, which usually requires fluid distension of the joint capsule, might damage the blood supply has not borne out in clinical practice. No cases of avascular necrosis following hip arthroscopy in the young patient have been described to date. On the contrary, the physical size of the pediatric patient may add technical difficulty to the procedure because of limited size and space for instrumentation. Despite these challenges, careful portal placement and controlled traction techniques have made arthroscopy not only feasible but also often preferred in these patients. Hip arthroscopy in patients as young as 2.4 years has been reported, using only manual traction in these patients.[19] In a series of nine children aged 2.4 to 7.3 years, no intraoperative or postoperative complications related to arthroscopy were identified using this technique of manual traction and joint distension.[19]

INDICATIONS AND DIAGNOSTIC ACCURACY

Schindler et al. reviewed 21 children and adolescents undergoing 24 arthroscopies for varied diagnoses. In this study, arthroscopy supported the presumed diagnosis in 56%, concluding that hip arthroscopy may not be useful as a diagnostic tool.[13] This finding was corroborated in a large series, in which it was concluded that the diagnostic use of hip arthroscopy remains viable only in specific cases. Furthermore, Dorfmann and Boyer suggested that the improvements in imaging modalities have decreased and may continue to decrease the indications for diagnostic arthroscopy in the hip.[9]

Although hip scope for diagnosis alone may have limited applications, Schindler went on to conclude that arthroscopy in children is helpful in obtaining synovial biopsies and removing loose bodies and should decrease the need for open surgery with dislocation of the hip and its associated risk of avascular necrosis. The reported complication rate in Schindler's series was no higher than in the adult population, which has been reported to be 1% to 2%, with two patients having transient pudendal nerve dysesthesias and no infections or cases of residual stiffness being observed.[12,13]

More recent information has placed the surgeon in a more informed position when considering the role of hip arthroscopy. The surgeon can weigh the small risk of complications associated with hip arthroscopy, the merits of imaging alternatives such as magnetic resonance imaging, and the emerging data on accuracy of diagnosis and outcomes of treatment using hip arthroscopy. To properly take advantage of maximum benefit given the defined risk for hip arthroscopy, it is extremely important to consider which preoperative factors might portend a better outcome. Awareness of predictive factors such as mechanical symptoms is especially important in cases of occult pain in the young active patient who does not have an underlying developmental disorder, childhood aliment, or a revealing imaging study. In a review of patients treated at our institution, we concluded that regardless of the preoperative diagnosis, the presence of definite mechanical symptoms is an important prognostic indicator of symptomatic relief following operative hip arthroscopy. Removal of loose bodies, manage-

ment of labral tears, and debridement of focal chondral injury were found to be associated with better outcomes. Less-desirable results were achieved in patients with osteonecrosis and degenerative arthritis. However, mechanical symptoms in these patients, including pediatric and adolescent patients, may still signal potentially treatable pathology because treatment with arthroscopy may prevent or delay the need for open arthrotomy in children or arthroplasty in adults.[21]

HISTORY AND PHYSICAL EXAMINATION

Pediatric and adolescent patients do not frequently complain of hip pain. In fact, it is not uncommon for hip pathology to be discovered after complaints of knee pain in the young patient. This pattern of referred pain occurs frequently enough that the treating physician should have a high index of suspicion that hip pathology or hip injury may be the causative factor for knee pain in the patient with a normal examination of the knee. Another frequent presentation is limping in a child who has suffered no known injury. When this scenario occurs, a history of preceding illness, which is found in up to 40% of patients, directs the examiner toward a diagnosis of transient synovitis of the hip. In one study of 243 children seen in the emergency department, 39.5% subsequently had this diagnosis.[22]

In the pediatric or adolescent patient, as with any orthopedic patient, the history with careful attention to mechanism of injury can be revealing. Running, jumping, and kicking-based activities are frequently involved, especially in causing labral pathology. A patient with a labral tear often reports an acute twisting injury, but an axial load on a flexed hip can also result in trauma to the labrum. In our series of 86 hip arthroscopies, only 17% of patients gave a definite history of traumatic event preceding the onset of symptoms. Of the patients diagnosed at arthroscopy with labral tears, 36% had antecedent trauma, whereas 44% of patients with loose bodies attributed their pain to trauma.[21] McCarthy's analysis revealed a 44% incidence of traumatic injury in his patients with labral tears.[23] Again, it should be stressed that because hip injury is an infrequent occurrence in pediatric patients, underlying hip disorders should be investigated thoroughly.

In our experience and that of others, subjective complaints of catching, locking, popping, and giving way are helpful at defining those patients who may benefit from surgery.[9,21,23,24] We found the presence of mechanical symptoms to be suggestive of treatable intraarticular pathology in 100% of our patients who had labral tears, loose bodies, or chondral injury. However, in one study, only 64% of patients with a labral tear diagnosed at arthroscopy had mechanical symptoms.[24] McCarthy found a positive correlation between giving-way or locking episodes with labral tears and the presence of locking episodes correlated with chondral injury.[23] Selection bias toward these patients was undoubtedly present in our study because mechanical symptoms were considered an indication for surgery.[21] Locking or catching symptoms should be distinguished from popping or snapping symptoms because the latter may herald extraarticular pathology that is not amenable to arthroscopic surgery, such as anteromedial catching or psoas tendon bursitis.[9] Anecdotally, complaints of the hip feeling tired or weak have been helpful as an indicator of intraarticular pathology in our series.

Physical examination of the injured hip can be quite vexing, likely because of the complex anatomy both within and surrounding the hip joint. Examination frequently reveals pain in provocative positions, but this is individualized and entirely patient dependent. Reproducible pain with passive flexion and medial or internal rotation of the hip has been identified as predictors of intraarticular pathology.[24] This finding has been corroborated in young athletic patients.[2] The direction of these provocative maneuvers does not correlate well with the location of labral tears, according to Farjo et al.[24] McCarthy noted painful clicks in 56% of patients during a Thomas hip flexion-to-extension test and concluded that this finding had a significant positive correlation with acetabular labral tear on arthroscopic evaluation. He states that pertinent physical findings such as these represent the best predictors of treatable intraarticular pathology.[23]

We believe that decreased range of motion as compared with the contralateral unaffected hip is also a useful sign of significant hip pathology. Flexion and internal rotation appear to be affected most and earliest in these patients. These findings on physical examination are obviously nonspecific, as internal rotation of the hip is often lost early in degenerative conditions of the hip. Most would agree that limited abduction in flexion is a cardinal indication for treatment of LCP, and this examination should be performed on all pediatric patients with hip pain. Furthermore, a reduction in adduction of the flexed hip has been described as being the earliest physical sign of hip irritability, whether the underlying diagnosis is LCP or other causes.[25]

ROLE OF HIP ARTHROSCOPY IN SPECIFIC CONDITIONS OF CHILDREN AND ADOLESCENTS

Arthroscopy of any joint is less common in children than in adults because of the preponderance of peri-articular and growth plate-related injuries that are peculiar to skeletally immature patients. Likewise, when focusing the discussion to arthroscopy of the hip joint, the indications for and outcomes of the procedure are even less well defined than in the adult. In 1977, Gross noted, in his experience with 32 arthroscopic hip surgeries in children, that the procedure did not seem to more accurately delineate the diagnosis or add to the therapeutic outcome,[26] thus quelling early efforts in the application of this technique to young patients. However, since this early report, there have been renewed interest in and enthusiasm toward minimally invasive alternatives to open surgery on the hip in children with a multitude of diagnoses. The following discussion focuses on some of the more common childhood conditions in which hip arthroscopy does potentially play a beneficial role.

Legg–Calvé–Perthes Disease

Perhaps the most common indication for hip arthroscopy in the pediatric and adolescent population, and certainly the most common indication in our series, has been in cases of Legg–Calvé–Perthes disease (LCP), both for diagnosis of severity and the treatment of late sequelae including the removal of loose bodies.[27] Suzuki et al. reported on their series of 19 children undergoing diagnostic and operative hip arthroscopy for LCP disease. From this study a new breadth of knowledge has been gained on the gross and histologic pathology of this disease. Among their novel findings were the presence of synovial proliferation in both the acetabular fossa and the inner wall of the capsule. They postulate that this mass effect and the presence of hypervascularity add to the instability and femoral head coverage problems seen in this condition. Furthermore, the microscopic in vivo anatomy was shown to be that of proliferative hyperplasia and not inflammation. Although lavage was the only therapeutic modality applied at the time of arthroscopy, the authors reported that postoperative range of motion about the hip was significantly increased and pain was decreased.[28]

Four main sequelae of LCP disease are commonly seen (see Figure 14.1). These include, first, coxa magna, with an enlarged spherical or oval femoral head and relatively normal neck–shaft angles (Figure 14.1A,B). Second, coxa brevis can occur, with associated shortening of the femoral neck, overgrowth of the greater trochanter, and a shortened extremity (Figure 14.1C). Least commonly, osteochondritis dissecans (OCD) may be present, which involves an incomplete healing of the necrotic epiphysis (Figure 14.1D,E). Coxa irregularis is also described, which appears on radiographs as an irregular grooved and incongruent femoral head (Figure 14.1F,G). Bowen and his group described the arthroscopic treatment of OCD of the hip following Perthes' disease in a review of 14 patients with 15 hips involved. The standard treatment of this condition includes observation, bed rest, and activity modification with nonsteroidal antiinflammatory drugs. In this series, 5 patients underwent arthroscopic evaluation of the extent of degenerative disease; removal of the necrotic segment was attempted in 4, and successful in 3 patients. Femoral valgus osteotomy was performed in 2 patients based on arthroscopic findings, and both procedures were con-

sidered successful. This review has served to expand the indications and therapeutic validity for hip arthroscopy in LCP.[29]

Juvenile Rheumatoid Arthritis/ Juvenile Chronic Arthritis

As the field of minimally invasive surgery including arthroscopy has advanced, so has the enthusiasm for

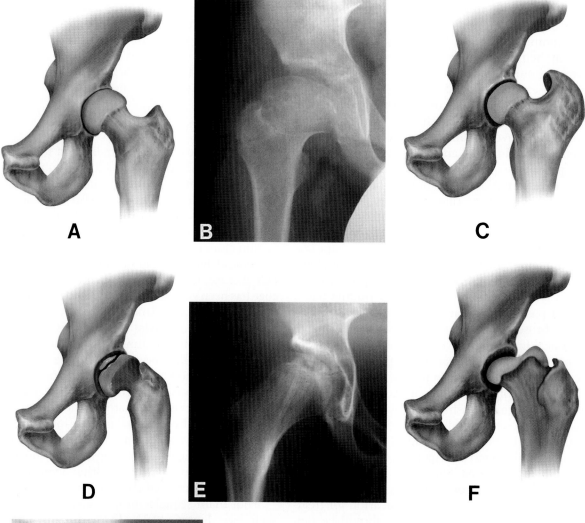

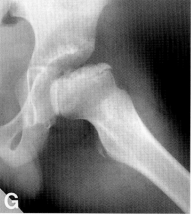

FIGURE 14.1. Late sequelae of Legg–Calvé–Perthes (LCP) disease. (A) Coxa magna: enlarged femoral head with lack of lateral acetabular coverage is shown. A relatively normal neck-shaft angle is preserved. (B) Coxa magna radiograph: anteroposterior (AP) radiograph of hip demonstrating the classic findings of coxa magna, enlarged oval femoral head. (C) Coxa breva: shortened femoral head and overgrowth of the greater trochanter are shown. (D) Osteochondritis dissecans (OCD): incomplete healing of the femoral epiphysis with entrapment of a fragment of necrotic bone within the femoral head. (E) OCD radiograph: clinical radiograph demonstrating a necrotic focus of bone entrapped in the femoral head, likely a result of incomplete healing of the necrotic epiphysis during LCP. (F) Coxa irregularis: an irregular and grooved femoral head is shown. Frequently this leads to advanced degenerative changes in the lateral and superior weight-bearing portions of the acetabulum. (G) Coxa irregularis radiograph: frog leg lateral radiograph demonstrates an irregular femoral head nearing the end of the healing phase of the disease; this is likely to result in coxa irregularis.

the application of arthroscopy to more unusual and less well understood joints such as the pediatric hip joint. Examples of this evolution include two more favorable series published in 1981 and 1986 reviewing the use of arthroscopy in juvenile chronic arthritis. Both reports tout hip arthroscopy as being valuable in diagnosing the extent of cartilage damage and the severity of synovitis, concluding that the procedure has value in the diagnosis of this condition.[30,31] Furthermore, Blitzer, in his series of patients treated with hip arthroscopy for septic arthritis, diagnosed one of his patients with JRA, adding to the diagnostic validity of this procedure.[7] Synovial biopsy of the hip joint, without the potential of avascular necrosis associated with open arthrotomy, is also a valuable and easily performed procedure in the workup of a patient with suspected JRA to evaluate the polyarticular nature of the disease. On a less positive note, the therapeutic efficacy of arthroscopic synovectomy for rheumatoid arthritis (RA) of the hip can be questioned based on a report by Ide et al. They performed arthroscopic synovectomy in three cases (six hips) and noted that there was no significant recovery of motion and that the pain relief was only temporary. However, all their patients were adults with stage III RA and severe cartilage damage. They concluded that the procedure would have been more helpful if it was performed earlier before the articular cartilage was destroyed.[32] It is likely that early in the course of JRA, when it affects the hip joint, arthroscopic synovectomy and debridement may provide improved results over those seen in the adult population.

Slipped Capital Femoral Epiphysis

Arthroscopy for slipped capital femoral epiphysis (SCFE) was reviewed in 1992 by Futami et al. Arthroscopy was performed to investigate the magnitude of articular cartilage and labral injury and to decompress the hematoma resulting from the fracture. In their review of five hips, they observed three associated labral injuries in the posterolateral portion of the labrum.[33] This finding was in contrast to the reports by Suzuki and Ikeda, who found labral tears in the posterosuperior position in young patients with occult hip pain. Arthroscopy also showed erosion of the acetabular cartilage anterosuperiorly, a transverse cleft on the anterior surface of the femoral head, and metaphyseal cartilage damage. They believed these findings corresponded to joint cartilage being crushed between the acetabulum and the femoral head and friction on the joint cartilage during joint motion after the slippage occurs.[2,28] From the information gained by preoperative diagnostic arthroscopy, Futami et al. concluded that this knowledge should be of great benefit in the therapy for and interpretation of the pathology in SCFE. They further added that evacuation of the resultant hematoma by arthroscopic lavage effectively reduces pain and may permit earlier postoperative motion and weight bearing.[33]

Developmental Dysplasia

Treatment of early symptomatic developmental dysplasia of the hip centers on obtaining adequate coverage for the femoral head. As the femoral head subluxates laterally, contact pressures on the acetabular and, subsequently, femoral side of the joint increase to critical levels, eventually resulting in degenerative arthritis. Multiple procedures in the child have been described and validated in the literature for obtaining this coverage, including both femoral and acetabular osteotomies. Most series support the use of pelvic or femoral osteotomy in the child both to prevent this end-stage disease and to encourage the normal development of the acetabulum and femoral head. However, when an older child or young adult presents with pain attributable to DDH, the indications for and results of hip osteotomies are less well defined. Even in the best of hands, thee procedures can have unpredictable results.

In the adolescent or young adult who presents with hip pain and a diagnosis of DDH, labral pathology has been shown to be the first stage of the development of degenerative arthritis. Klaue et al. confirmed that "acetabular rim syndrome" is a precursor to the development of secondary osteoarthritis in these patients.[34] It is not yet known if direct treatment of these labral injuries can change the natural history of the disease, but it has been shown that arthroscopic resection of the torn labrum in these patients provides symptomatic relief.[35] Noguchi et al. demonstrated the efficacy of using the arthroscope to determine the amount of degenerative changes in the hip joint before performing osteotomies. The results of osteotomy procedures are known to be worse in patients with degenerative changes, and these changes may not be easily visualized radiographically. However, arthroscopic examination can show the extent of acetabular and femoral head degenerative changes and could be used as a guide to determining appropriate candidates for osteotomy.[35]

Hip Arthroscopy in Pediatric Athletic Injuries

In the many series of athletic hip injuries reported in the current literature, seldom is the role of arthroscopy of the hip in pediatric and adolescent patients addressed. In Dorfmann's large series, the age range of patients was from 14 to 81 years. However, no specific mention of the mechanism of injury or pathology is noted for the younger patients.[9] Similarly, Schindler et al., in their comprehensive article, do not address the issue of the young athlete.[13]

In the last several years, only a few pediatric cases have been described specifically addressing the role of arthroscopy for hip pain associated with an injury during sporting activity. In a review by Ikeda et al., three patients, aged 15, 15, and 16 years, had acute onset of pain related to athletic participation. The first patient was injured during a sprinting event, the second was injured while competing in rugby football, and the last had sudden onset of pain while playing volleyball. All three patients were diagnosed arthroscopically as having tears of the acetabular labrum.[2] In this series, attempts at resection of the tear were not undertaken; however, multiple reports have described techniques for doing so.[21,23,24,36–38] The authors supported previous findings of a posterosuperior location of the tear, thought to be secondary to anatomic vulnerability to injury in that location.[11,23,39] It can be concluded that, similar to the glenoid labrum in the athlete, the acetabular labrum can be adequately examined and tears treated using arthroscopic techniques.

Hip Arthroscopy for Pediatric and Adolescent Pyarthrosis

One group of pediatric patients for which hip arthroscopy may provide effective treatment is those patients with a suspected diagnosis of pyarthrosis. This potentially catastrophic condition can be evaluated with laboratory studies including leukocyte count and erythrocyte sedimentation rate. Of these, the erythrocyte sedimentation rate appears to be the most sensitive and specific.[40] Although ultrasonic-guided aspiration of the hip joint may provide the definitive diagnosis, routine radiographs can rule out many of the possible etiologies, such as DDH, LCP, and SCFE, in children with normal laboratory results.[41] Arthroscopic washout of an infected hip has been reported in several studies in both the child and adult, and this procedure, which spares the child the possible iatrogenic problems associated with open washout, is becoming more routinely used.

Two series in the literature show a definite role for arthroscopic management of hip sepsis in the pediatric patient. Blitzer described the use of the arthroscope for the treatment of five patients with a presumed diagnosis of septic arthritis. The author cites the potential complications of open arthrotomy to be aseptic necrosis of the femoral head, subsequent dislocation of the hip, the cosmetic appearance of the standard open procedure, and prolongation of hospital stay. With the high index of suspicion necessary in cases of possible hip sepsis, and the extensive differential diagnoses, including transient synovitis, JRA, and periacetabular or pelvic abscesses or myositis, a certain number of pediatric patients would undergo unnecessary arthrotomy if arthroscopy is not used. Blitzer further concludes that, in a patient who is "old enough"

to be safely arthroscoped, the procedure is beneficial. This vague definition of age, however, does not provide the reader with a true definition of the appropriate candidate for arthroscopic lavage.[7] A more accurate age limit for arthroscopic treatment of hip pyarthrosis is provided by Chung et al., who in their series report the safe application of this procedure in patients as young as 2.4 years. They conclude that arthroscopic lavage and synovectomy are safe and effective in patients between the ages of 2 and 7 years, that the associated morbidity is low and the recovery of mobility rapid. The use of the arthroscope as a large-bore instrument to deliver a high-volume lavage has the added benefit of direct visualization of clot and infected joint debris.[19] Although arthroscopic debridement does not allow for direct identification of or treatment for foci of osteomyelitis, Chung et al. found that this did not influence the success of treatment. Two of their nine patients had focal metaphyseal radiodensities that resolved after arthroscopic treatment and routine antibiotics.[19] As mentioned, arthroscopic lavage and debridement also provide synovium for tissue diagnosis in equivocal cases in which JRA or transient synovitis may be the underlying cause of the hip pain and abnormal laboratory values.

Tumors About the Hip

Benign tumors about the hip are not uncommon in childhood, and some present in the intracapsular location, which may be amenable to arthroscopic management. Khapchik et al. reported on two cases of osteoid osteoma, a common benign tumor presenting in the first three decades of life, managed with arthroscopic excision. They noted that the procedure was relatively easy and had the added benefit of enabling the surgeon to obtain a biopsy specimen before treatment, something that is not available using percutaneous ablation techniques.[42] Thompson and Wooward described the use of the arthroscope in aiding the treatment of a chondroblastoma of the femoral head.[43] The obvious benefits of using minimally invasive techniques to treat intracapsular benign tumors in children and young adults are the ability to obtain a tissue diagnosis and the reduced morbidity and rapid functional recovery possible. Furthermore, arthroscopy would not complicate a subsequent open resection for the treatment of a recurrence, if it should occur. One can envision future endeavors to treat childhood benign tumors of the proximal femur such as unicameral bone cysts arthroscopically. Another tumor, of sorts, that has been successfully treated arthroscopically is synovial chondromatosis of the hip. In the prospective analysis by Byrd and Jones, they described treating a patient with synovial chondromatosis of the hip successfully with the arthroscope. Of particular interest is that at the time of a second procedure for the excision of heterotopic ossification of the soft tissues, no recurrent loose bodies were noted.[44]

AUTHORS' EXPERIENCE

We have treated 17 patients 18 years of age or younger over the past several years at our institution with arthroscopic surgery of the hip. Patient age ranged from 11 to 18 years. Diagnostic evaluation included plain radiographs of the pelvis and affected hip in each case. Supplemental imaging studies such as magnetic resonance imaging (MRI) or computed tomography (CT) scans were either obtained by the referring physician or performed at our institution. Physical examinations, including range of motion and the presence of reproducible mechanical symptoms, were also reviewed. Mechanical symptoms, in this group of patients, were defined as a subjective complaint of clicking, locking, popping, or giving way documented during routine history taking and the presence of reproducible pain with provocative maneuvers. In the routine treatment of LCP disease, which is a common diagnosis treated at our institution, we use arthroscopy only for those patients with mechanical symptoms and radiographic evidence of treatable intraarticular pathology. Findings of OCD, chondral injury, or labral pathology in these patients are thought to be good indications for surgical intervention. Most pediatric patients presenting with hip pathology are not offered arthroscopic surgery because their conditions are thought not to be amenable to this type of treatment. For example, a 14-year-old cheerleader with Ehlers–Danlos syndrome and recurrent painful popping in the hip, generalized ligamentous laxity, and a normal MRI arthrogram was excluded from operative treatment and is being followed to skeletal maturity.

Table 14.2 outlines the indications for arthroscopy and the treatments performed in our patients.

Hip arthroscopy was performed typically on an outpatient basis. The patient was positioned supine on a standard fracture table with a traction device and arthroscopy performed in a fashion similar to that described by Byrd and others.[1,9,15,17,45,46] Both regional and general anesthesia techniques were used, depending on patient and anesthesia preference. Paratrochanteric and anterior portals were created under direct fluoroscopic guidance. An 18-gauge angiocath needle was used to localize and distend the joint, with release of the vacuum pressure. Between 5 and 10 mm of joint distraction was then achieved through traction on the extremity and was confirmed by fluoroscopy.[9,14,17,38,46] Careful patient positioning and padding of the perineal post was used to avoid possible neurologic complications. Portals were then dilated over a guidewire, and either a 30- or 70-degree arthroscope was introduced into the joint (Figure 14.2). Standard arthroscopic instruments were then used as needed for chondral and labral debridement, synovectomy, and removal of loose bodies.[14]

All these patients had a diagnosis of hip pain persisting for more than 3 months that had not responded to appropriate nonoperative measures. Three patients had acetabular labral tears addressed at arthroscopy following motor vehicle accidents and dashboard-type injuries. One of these patients had underlying developmental dysplasia of the hip, a labral tear in the superoanterior location (as described for DDH), but no evidence of degenerative joint disease was noted. The second patient sustained a femoral neck fracture at the time of injury and had continued pain in the affected hip for 48 months before arthroscopy. An unstable chondral lesion and a labral tear were identified and treated arthroscopically with 24 months of relief of pain. This patient did require repeat arthroscopy of

TABLE 14.2. Indications for Hip Arthroscopy and Therapeutic Procedures Performed: The Author's Experience.

Diagnosis	Therapy	Number of cases
LCP: sequelae	Removal loose body Debridement chondral injury Partial limbectomy Removal OCD	6
MVA/trauma	Partial limbectomy Debridement chondral injury Removal loose body	3
AVN	Debridement chondral injury	1 (status post FVFG)
DDH	Partial limbectomy Evaluation of cartilage surfaces	2 (associated with trauma and athletics)
Athletics	Debridement chondral injury Partial limbectomy Removal of loose body Decompression of ganglion	7 (4 with antecedent hip pathology: LCP, DDH, SCD)

LCP, Legg–Calvé–Perthes disease; MVA, motor vehicle accident; AVN, avascular necrosis; FVFG, free vascularized fibular graft; DDH, developmental dysplasia of hip; SCD, sickle cell disease

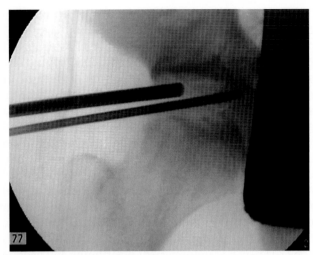

FIGURE 14.2. Intraoperative fluoroscopy image of instrument placement. Intraoperative fluoroscopy image shows the position of the 30-degree arthroscopic camera and an arthroscopic shaver instrument in place. Note the distension of the joint obtained with controlled traction and gravity-assisted inflow.

the hip for new onset of pain secondary to an extension of the chondral delamination and is now doing well. The third patient had continued mechanical symptoms and pain after a motor vehicle accident and underwent hip arthroscopy after 24 months of nonoperative therapy. The patient had loose bodies that were successfully resected arthroscopically (Figure 14.3). He remains symptom free at 2.5-year follow-up.

Seven of the patients presented with hip pain and mechanical symptoms after an injury sustained during athletic training or competition. These seven patients underwent eight arthroscopic procedures. Of these patients, four had a previous history of hip disease, likely placing them at increased risk of intraarticular hip injury. The first, an 11-year-old active boy, was diagnosed and treated for LCP disease as a younger child, but was pain free and was able to participate in sports. He presented with acute onset of pain after a twisting injury occurred during sporting activity. A chondral injury and a separate degenerative labral tear were identified arthroscopically, and a partial chondroplasty of the femoral head and resection of the unstable labral tear were performed. The second patient had a similar presentation, also with a known previous history of Perthes' disease. This 15-year-old boy presented after an injury that occurred while playing softball. Radiographic evaluation was remarkable only for findings of previous Perthes' disease, but no loose bodies or fractures were noted. At arthroscopy, a labral tear was identified and resected back to a stable base. An unstable chondral flap was also apparent and addressed arthroscopically. No significant synovitis or degenerative changes were noted. The patient had prompt resolution of symptoms and relief of pain after the procedure. Twenty-three months following the

initial arthroscopy, the patient had a more insidious onset of pain and decreasing range of motion in the same hip. Repeat arthroscopy was performed. A new femoral chondral lesion was noted, as was a small degenerative tear in the acetabular labrum. These were resected using standard arthroscopic instruments and the patient has remained symptom free for 26 months. More detailed case examples of the role of arthroscopy in LCP are given next.

The third of our patients who presented with hip pain following an injury in the setting of previous hip pathology sustained during sports had sickle cell disease, but she had not had complaints of hip pain before her injury. This 17-year-old girl presented with 6 months of pain and mechanical symptoms after an injury that occurred while running. At the time of arthroscopy, a loose body was identified and removed. The presumed donor site was identified on the femoral head and was also addressed arthroscopically with debridement back to a stable margin (Figure 14.4). She had complete resolution of symptoms and has been painfree for more than 4 years.

Athletic trauma was also identified in a 14-year-old girl who was treated with bracing for DDH as a child. She was asymptomatic until 6 months before her presentation when she fell while playing softball. She noted the acute onset of left hip pain that did not resolve despite treatment with nonsteroidal medications and physical therapy. Figure 14.5 shows the prearthroscopy radiographs. During her workup she underwent an MRI scan that demonstrated an acetabular labral tear. Because of her positive radiographic findings and her continued pain despite 6 months of conservative treatment, she underwent arthroscopic examination. At arthroscopy she was noted

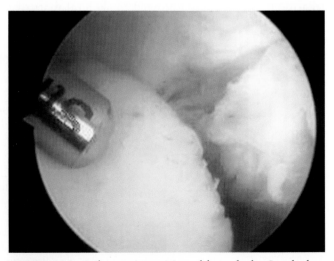

FIGURE 14.3. Arthroscopic excision of loose body. Standard arthroscopic instruments, including an aggressive shaver, are used routinely to excise loose bodies, as shown, from the hip joint. A large loose body is seen below the arthroscopic instrument. View is from the anterolateral portal.

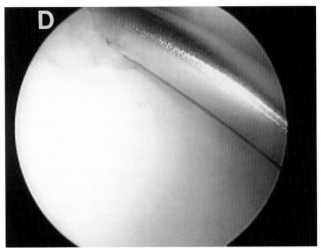

FIGURE 14.4. Loose body donor site (D) on femoral head. Friable, loose, and degenerative fibrocartilage, presumed to be a donor site for a loose body, which was extracted, is shown. Again, standard arthroscopic instrumentation can be used to perform chondral shaving or chondroplasty to these pathologic areas. View is from the anterolateral portal.

to have a large degenerative acetabular labral tear extending from the superior to the anterosuperior location (Figure 14.6). This finding is in agreement with those of Noguchi et al., who demonstrated that, in DDH, most prearthritic hips and all arthritic hips have labral tears in this location.[35] A partial limbectomy

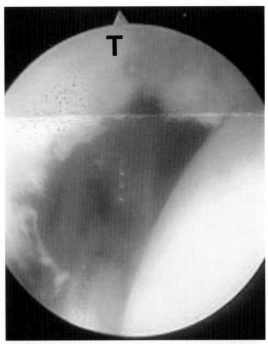

FIGURE 14.6. Degenerative tear (T) of the anterosuperior and posterosuperior labrum in DDH. At arthroscopy, the patient had a large degenerative tear of the acetabular labrum extending from anterior to posterior. This was resected to a stable base. View is from the anterolateral portal.

(labral excision) was performed. It was also noted that the articular cartilage of the hip was normal throughout, and no evidence of osteophyte formation was seen. The patient had 1 year of relief from her symptoms, but then presented with the onset of new, achy pain in the groin. She described her pain as being different from her previous pain at that time. She was also noted to have significant pain in the provocative position of adduction and internal rotation. Repeat MRI failed to demonstrate a recurrent labral tear. From the information gained at arthroscopy, normal cartilage without degenerative changes, it was thought that she was a candidate for a periacetabular osteotomy in an attempt to provide increased coverage and to prevent the eventual development of osteoarthritis. She underwent this procedure and is doing well at 4 months postoperatively (Figure 14.7).

The remaining three patients who sustained injury to the hip during athletics did not have an appreciable antecedent pathologic diagnosis of the hip. The first patient, a 13-year-old girl, sustained a posterior hip dislocation while snow skiing. She presented with popping and pain in the hip 4 months after the injury. MRI evaluation revealed a small ganglion in the posterior portion of the hip (Figure 14.8A). A possible labral tear was seen on MRI (Figure 14.8B), and the presence of the cyst and mechanical symptoms prompted arthroscopic evaluation. At arthroscopy, she was noted to have a tear of the posterior labrum in area of her cyst

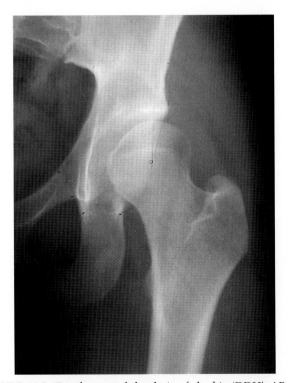

FIGURE 14.5. Developmental dysplasia of the hip (DDH). AP radiograph of the hip demonstrates poor superior acetabular coverage with a well preserved and congruous joint space. The patient had acute onset of mechanical hip pain following an injury while playing softball. Magnetic resonance imaging (MRI) revealed a torn acetabular labrum.

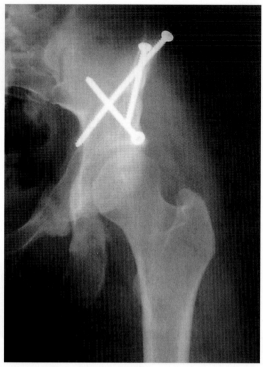

FIGURE 14.7. Ganz periacetabular osteotomy for DDH. After labral excision, the patient had 1 year of relief from symptoms. The information gained from arthroscopy, of normal articular cartilage, was used as an indication for periacetabular osteotomy. Arthroscopy before osteotomy can be beneficial to demonstrate cartilage wear and stratify patient outcomes from osteotomy.

(Figure 14.9A,B). This tear was resected via the arthroscope and she is now symptom free (Figure 14.10).

The second patient is a 15-year-old cheerleader who noted the insidious onset of hip pain after start-ing her cheerleading season. She gave a history of popping, clicking, and locking in the hip. After conservative management failed to provide relief, she underwent arthroscopic examination that, despite a normal MRI study, revealed a flaplike or bucket-handle labral tear, which was resected arthroscopically (Figure 14.11).

The third patient in the group who sustained a hip injury during athletics was 15 years old when he felt the sudden onset of anterolateral thigh pain while playing basketball. With continued complaints of radiating thigh pain, an MRI revealed a small acetabular labral tear (Figure 14.12), which was resected with the arthroscope (Figure 14.13A,B).

The remaining young patients in our series had no antecedent trauma or injury. Six patients had arthroscopy of the hip for late sequelae of LCP disease. As mentioned, it is common for patients with irregularly shaped femoral heads to present with new mechanical symptoms. Four of our patients had similar presentations of chronic hip pain accompanied by mechanical symptoms and either degenerative changes or loose bodies noted on radiographs. The other two patients had radiographic findings and MRI results of OCD consistent with incomplete healing of the femoral head.

Case examples of each indication are given. The first is a 12-year-old boy who was treated for LCP discovered at age 6 years. He complained of daily pain requiring home schooling and narcotic pain medications. He presented for a second opinion as to hip arthrodesis. His radiographs, including a recent arthrogram, revealed a relatively congruous joint surface,

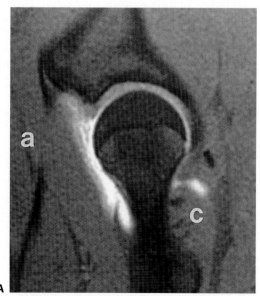

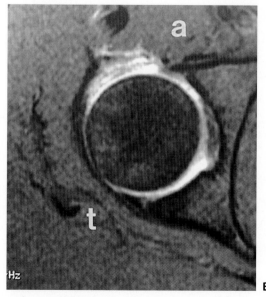

FIGURE 14.8. (A) MRI for preoperative diagnosis of hip pathology. Along with labral and chondral pathology, MRI is valuable for detecting other pathologic lesions in and around the hip joint. MRI revealed a posterior ganglion (c) that was thought to be associated with a small labral tear. (B) MRI with possible posterior labral tear (t). Given the findings of a posterior ganglion, suspicion for labral tear was heightened. A possible posterior tear was noted on the axial MRI image, and this was confirmed arthroscopically. a, anterior.

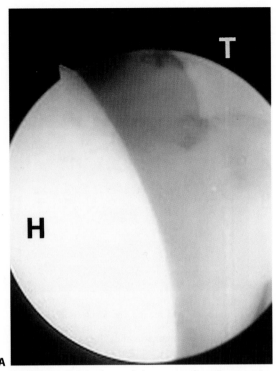

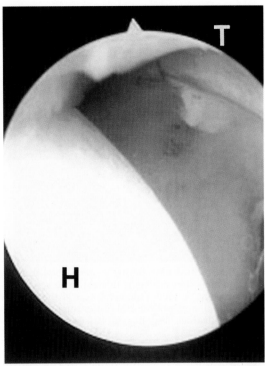

FIGURE 14.9. (A) Small labral tear (T) associated with posterior ganglion. A small tear at the margin of the articular cartilage and the labrum was seen arthroscopically in a position associated with the posterior ganglion. The tear is seen as a triangular flap in the 2 o'clock position. (B) Small labral tear. The tear was probed and found to be unstable, as shown herein. Both views are from the anterolateral portal. H, head.

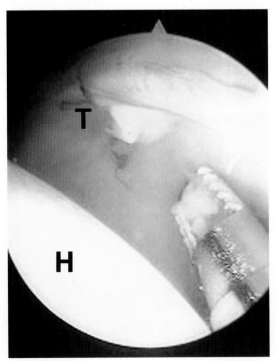

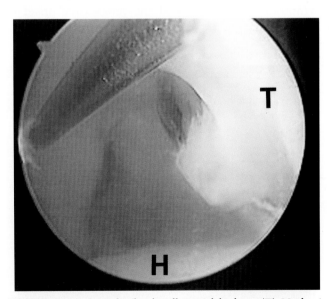

FIGURE 14.10. Labral tear (T) debridement. The flap was debrided back to the acetabular rim, preserving the overlying normal labrum. Standard arthroscopic instrumentation can be used for these procedures, such as this aggressive meniscal shaver. View is from the anterolateral portal. H, head.

FIGURE 14.11. Large bucket-handle-type labral tear (T). Mechanical symptoms can herald significant intraarticular pathology, such as this unstable tear of the acetabular labrum. The tear extends from the 11 o'clock position (under the tip of the instrument) to the 3 o'clock position, with a large flap extruding into the joint. View is from the anterolateral portal. H, head.

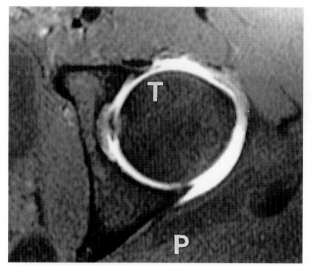

FIGURE 14.12. Axial MRI demonstrating a small labral tear (T). MRI with arthrogram, as shown here, is thought to be very sensitive for labral pathology. A small radial-type tear of the anterior labrum is denoted by thinning of the rim of the anterior acetabular labrum, losing its distinct black margin. P, posterior.

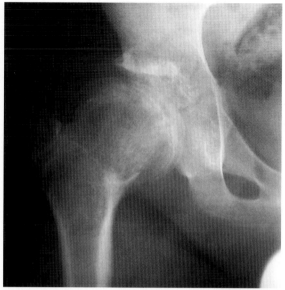

FIGURE 14.14. LCP disease. Preoperative radiograph of the hip reveals findings of coxa magna and a sclerotic nidus thought to be a loose body. With mechanical symptoms and pain requiring narcotic medications, the patient was thought to be a good candidate for arthroscopic surgery.

coxa magna, and with a possible defect in the center of the femoral head (Figure 14.14). He underwent arthroscopic resection of a frayed labrum and debridement of degenerative cartilage (Figure 14.15A,B). At follow-up, he has returned to school, no longer requires narcotic pain medication, and has resumed playing basketball, soccer, and baseball.

One of the two patients who presented with a definite OCD was a 12-year-old boy diagnosed with Perthes' as a 7 year old. After treatment with bracing, radiographic progression to an OCD was noted (Figure 14.16). He had a period of 4 years in which he was symptom free, then noted the progressive onset of

activity-related hip pain. MRI evaluation demonstrated a central OCD that was thought to be unstable (Figure 14.17A). He underwent arthroscopic surgery, at which time a large loose body was noted and removed (Figure 14.17B). The donor site was debrided with an arthroscopic bur. Six months postoperatively, he has returned to playing competitive basketball in a local league.

An additional patient underwent arthroscopic examination for an unstable chondral lesion following free vascularized fibula grafting for osteonecrosis

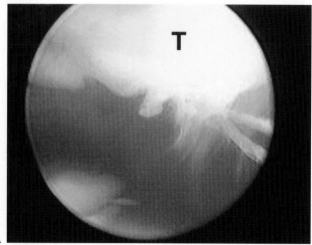

A

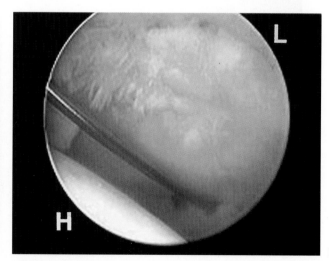

B

FIGURE 14.13. (A) Arthroscopic image of labral tear (T). Fraying and instability of the labrum to probing can indicate labral injury. The labrum, here, is noted to be degenerative and unstable, with friable tissue impinging into the joint. (B) Partial limbectomy (labral excision). Using standard arthroscopic instrumentation, the torn labrum (L) is resected back to a stable level. Before completing the excision, a probe is used (as shown) to test the stability of the remaining labral tissue. The free edge, where shaving will resume, is in the 10 o'clock position. Both views are from the anterolateral portal. H, head.

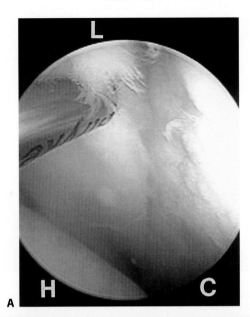

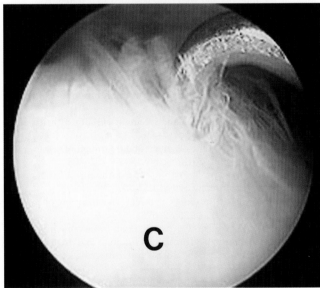

FIGURE 14.15. (A) Frayed labral tissue and early degenerative cartilage changes. At arthroscopy, the patient was found to have fraying of the labrum (L) and early degenerative changes of the acetabulum and the femoral head (H). Arthroscopic resection of the labral tear is shown. Chondromalacia (C) of the acetabulum is noted at the 3 o'clock position. (B) Grade 2 and 3 chondromalacia of the femoral head. Moderate degenerative changes including this area of chondromalacia were noted on the femoral head. These were addressed by gentle abrasion chondroplasty with an arthroscopic shaver. Despite kissing-type chondral injury, the patient has returned to full activity and no longer requires pain medication. Both views are from the anterolateral portal.

(Figure 14.18).[47] The results of this procedure were encouraging, with the patient remaining well at 4 years follow-up.

DISCUSSION

In the current literature, there are several convincing reports of the use of hip arthroscopy in the pediatric

patient. The role of this technique in the diagnosis and treatment of multiple childhood hip conditions including pyarthrosis, LCP disease, SCFE, coxa vara, juvenile chronic arthritis (JCA), chondrolysis, and avascular necrosis is well described.[7,18,19,28,30,31,33] The ability to examine and treat traumatic intraarticular pathology with minimal morbidity and prompt recovery is mandated by the young age of these patients and their demanding activity levels. Hip arthroscopists are now beginning to correlate preoperative physical examination findings and history with diagnosis and expectations for outcome. As our combined experience with this technique grows, the specific indications for its use in the young patient become increasingly better defined. In pediatric and adolescent patients, the new onset of hip pain should warrant a high level of suspicion for the more frequent causes of pain such as infection, LCP disease, SCFE, or DDH. When these have been evaluated, further differential diagnosis should include labral tears, loose bodies, synovitis, and chondral lesions. Many of these conditions appear to be amenable to arthroscopic evaluation and treatment. At this time, the presence of reproducible mechanical symptoms after a twisting or axial loading injury, persistent pain following trauma, or a diagnosis of avascular necrosis (AVN), JRA, or chronic juvenile arthritis (CJA) should prompt the orthopedic surgeon to consider arthroscopic examination of the hip if conservative therapy fails. Satisfying and reproducible results using this technique have been achieved when using hip arthroscopy within these parameters.

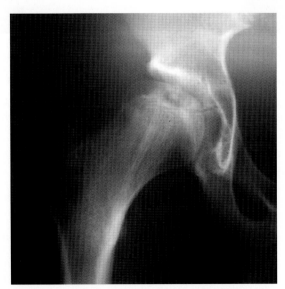

FIGURE 14.16. OCD of the femoral head following LCP disease. AP radiograph demonstrates a well-preserved femoral head with a focal area of sclerotic bone in the center surrounded by lucent fibrous tissue. The patient had progressive activity-related pain and mechanical symptoms.

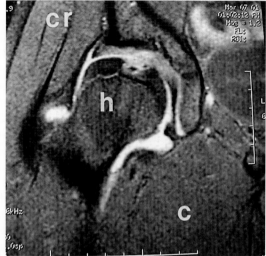
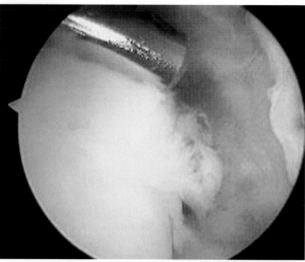

FIGURE 14.17. (A) Coronal MRI of the femoral head with unstable OCD. MRI arthrogram shows fluid (bright signal) surrounding the osteochondral lesion in the femoral head (h), suggesting the lesion is complete and loose. c, caudal; cr, cranial. (B) OCD of the femoral head. Arthroscopically, the patient was noted to have a large OCD, which was unstable to manipulation. The arthroscopic shaver is being used to debride the lesion. Fibrocartilage and friable tissue were noted at the margins and were also debrided to a stable base.

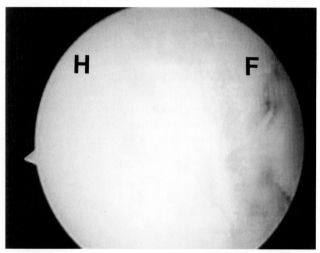

FIGURE 14.18. Chondromalacia associated with an unstable chondral fracture (F). Following free vascularized fibular grafting to the hip for osteonecrosis, the patient had mechanical symptoms and severe pain with activity. Arthroscopic examination revealed a delaminating chondral injury and associated chondromalacia. This tissue was debrided, and the patient has been symptom free for more than 4 years. View is from the anterolateral portal. H, head.

References

1. Byrd JW: Hip arthroscopy for posttraumatic loose fragments in the young active adult: three case reports. Clin J Sport Med 1996;6:129–133.
2. Ikeda T, Awaya G, Suzuki S, et al: Torn acetabular labrum in young patients. J Bone Joint Surg [Br] 1998;70:13–16.
3. Mehlmann CT, Hubbard GW, Crawford AH, et al: Traumatic hip dislocation in children: long-term follow-up of 42 patients. Clin Orthop 2000;376:68–79.
4. Quarrier NF, Wightman AB: A ballet dancer with chronic hip pain due to a lesser trochanter bony avulsion: the challenge of a differential diagnosis. J Orthop Sports Phys Ther 1998;28:168–173.
5. Skinner HB, Scherger JE: Identifying structural hip and knee problems. Patient age, history, and limited physical examination may be all that's needed. Postgrad Med 1999;106:51–52.
6. Boyd KT, Peirce NS, Batt ME: Common hip injuries in sport. Sports Med 1997;24:273–288.
7. Blitzer CM: Arthroscopic management of septic arthritis of the hip. Arthroscopy 1993;9:414–416.
8. Bould M: Arthroscopic diagnosis and treatment of septic arthritis of the hip joint. Arthroscopy 1993;9:707–708.
9. Dorfmann H, Boyer T: Arthroscopy of the hip: 12 years of experience. Arthroscopy 1999;15:67–72.
10. Burman MS: Arthroscopy or direct visualization of joints. J Bone Joint Surg 1931;13:669–695.
11. McCarthy JC, Aluisio F, Krebs V, et al: Intractable hip pain after occult trauma: arthroscopic findings and treatment (abstract). Presented at the 18th annual meeting of the AANA, Vancouver, BC, 1999.
12. Griffin DR, Villar RN: Complications in arthroscopy of the hip. J Bone Joint Surg [Br] 1999;81:604–606.
13. Schindler A, Lechevallier JJC, Rao NS, Bowen JR: Diagnostic and therapeutic arthroscopy of the hip in children and adolescents: evaluation of results. J Pediatr Orthop 1995;15:317–321.
14. Eriksson E, Arvidsson I, Arvidsson H: Diagnostic and operative arthroscopy of the hip. Orthopaedics 1986;9:169–176.
15. Frich LH, Lauritzen J, Juhl M: Arthroscopy in diagnosis and treatment of hip disorders. Orthopaedics 1989;12:389–392.
16. Funke EL, Munzinger U: Complications in hip arthroscopy. Arthroscopy 1996;12:156–159.
17. Glick JM: Hip arthroscopy. In: McGinty JB (ed). Arthroscopy. New York: Raven, 1991:663–676.
18. Rodeo S, Forster R, Weiland A: Neurological complications due to arthroscopy. J Bone Joint Surg 1993;75A:917–926.
19. Chung WK, Slater GL, Bates EH: Treatment of septic arthritis of the hip by arthroscopic lavage. J Pediatr Orthop 1993;13:444–446.
20. Gross RH. Arthroscopy in children. In: McGinty JB, Caspari RW, Jackson GG (eds). Operative Arthroscopy, 2nd ed. Philadelphia: Lippincott-Raven, 1996:83–90.
21. O'Leary AJ, Berend KR, Vail TP: The relationship between diagnosis and outcome in arthroscopy of the hip. Arthroscopy 2001;24:339–343.
22. Fischer SU, Beattie TF: The limping child: epidemiology, as-

sessment, and outcome. J Bone Joint Surg [Br] 1999;81:1029–1034.

23. McCarthy JC, Busconi B: The role of hip arthroscopy in the diagnosis and treatment of hip disease. Orthopaedics 1995;18:753–756.

24. Farjo LA, Glick JM, Sampson TG: Hip arthroscopy for labral tears. Arthroscopy 1999;15:132–137.

25. Manelaus MB: Lessons learned in the management of Legg-Calvé-Perthes disease. Clin Orthop 1986;209:42–48.

26. Gross RH: Arthroscopy in hip disorders in children. Orthop Rev 1977;6:43–49.

27. Kuklo TR, Mackenzie WG, Keeler KA: Hip arthroscopy in Legg-Calve-Perthes disease. Arthroscopy 1999;15:88–92.

28. Suzuki S, Kasahara Y, Seto Y, et al: Arthroscopy in 19 children with Perthes' disease: pathologic changes of the synovium and the joint surface. Acta Orthop Scand 1994;65:581–584.

29. Bowen JR, Kumar VP, Joyce JJ III, et al: Osteochondritis dissecans following Perthes disease. Clin Orthop 1986;209:49–56.

30. Holgersson S, Brattstrom H, Mogensen B, et al: Arthroscopy of the hip in juvenile chronic arthritis. J Pediatr Orthop 1981;1:273–278.

31. Rydhold U, Wingstrand H, Egund N, et al: Sonography, arthroscopy, and intracapsular pressure in juvenile chronic arthritis of the hip. Acta Orthop Scand 1986;57:295–298.

32. Ide T, Akamatsu N, Nakajima I: Arthroscopic surgery of the hip joint. Arthroscopy 1991;7:204–211.

33. Futami T, Kasahara Y, Suzuki S, et al: Arthroscopy for slipped capital femoral epiphysis. J Pediatr Orthop 1992;12:592–597.

34. Klaue K, Durnin CW, Ganz R: The acetabular rim syndrome. A clinical presentation of dysplasia of the hip. J Bone Joint Surg [Br] 1991;73:423–429.

35. Noguchi Y, Hiromasa M, Takasugi S, et al: Cartilage and labrum degeneration in the dysplastic hip generally originates in the anterosuperior weight-bearing area: an arthroscopic observation. Arthroscopy 1999;15:496–506.

36. Kim SJ, Choi NH, Kim HJ: Operative hip arthroscopy. Clin Orthop 1998;253:163–165.

37. McCarthy JC: Hip arthroscopy: applications and technique. J Am Acad Orthop Surg 1995;3:115–122.

38. Villar RN: Hip arthroscopy. Br J Hosp Med 1992;47:763–766.

39. Lage LA, Patel JV, Villar RN: The acetabular labral tear: an arthroscopic classification. Arthroscopy 1996;12:269–272.

40. Klein DM, Barbera C, Gray ST, et al: Sensitivity of objective parameters in the diagnosis of pediatric septic hips. Clin Orthop 1997;338:153–159.

41. Hollingworth P: Differential diagnosis and management of hip pain in childhood. Br J Rheumatol 1995;34:78–82.

42. Khapchik V, O'Donnell RJ, Glick JM: Arthroscopically assisted excision of osteoid osteoma Involving the hip. Arthroscopy 2001;17:56–61.

43. Thompson MS, Wooward JS: The use of the arthroscope as an adjunct in the resection of a chondroblastoma of the femoral head. Arthroscopy 1995;11:106–111.

44. Byrd JW, Jones KS: Prospective analysis of hip arthroscopy with 2-year follow-up. Arthroscopy 2000;16:578–587.

45. Byrd JW: Labral lesions: an elusive source of hip pain case reports and literature review. Arthroscopy 1996;12:603–612.

46. Glick JM, Sampson TG, Gordon RB, et al: Hip arthroscopy by the lateral approach. Arthroscopy 1987;3:4–12.

47. Urbaniak JR, Coogan PG, Gunneson EB, Nunley JA: Treatment of osteonecrosis of the femoral head with free-vascularized fibular grafting: a long term follow-up study of 103 hips. J Bone Joint Surg 1995;77A;681–694.

48. Berend KR, Vail TP. Hip arthroscopy in the adolescent and pediatric athlete. Clin Sports Med 2001;20(4):763–778.

15

Unique Populations: Dysplasia and the Elderly

J.W. Thomas Byrd

Two cohorts with common implications are developmental dysplasia and the elderly. A propensity for hip joint pathology exists in both populations, and both are generally considered to be a harbinger of poor results with arthroscopy. However, arthroscopy has a role in both of these groups and has been instrumental in gaining an appreciation for the pathomechanics associated with various lesions. Operative arthroscopy can meet with significant success when understanding the appropriate indications within these circumstances.

DEVELOPMENTAL DYSPLASIA

Developmental dysplasia of the hip (DDH) is not a cause of hip pain. It is simply a morphologic condition that makes the hip vulnerable to an intraarticular lesion that may then become symptomatic. The three most likely structures to be involved are the acetabular labrum, articular surface, and ligamentum teres.

Accompanying a shallow bony acetabulum, the labrum may be enlarged, assuming a more important role as a weight-bearing surface as well as added responsibility for joint stability. This hypertrophic labrum is thus exposed to greater joint reaction forces and may be at increased risk for developing symptomatic tearing.[1–3] Inversion of the acetabular labrum is also known to occur in association with dysplasia, being entrapped within the joint and again being a source of painful tearing.[4,5]

The reduced area of the acetabular articular surface results in increased contact forces,[6,7] which can result in early development of degenerative wear and may make the articular cartilage more vulnerable to acute fragmentation.[8–11]

Third, elongation or hypertrophy of the ligamentum teres accompanies lateral subluxation of the femoral head within the acetabulum.[12,13] Entrapment of this ligament can be a source of significant mechanical hip pain, whether from its redundant nature or partial degenerate rupture.

Thus, dysplasia is well recognized as an etiologic factor in the development of various painful intraarticular lesions that may be amenable to arthroscopic intervention. In fact, in our study, which is the only published report on outcomes of arthroscopy in a dysplastic population, the results were comparable with those previously published in a general population.[14] However, several caveats need to be fully appreciated.

It is important to assess patients carefully for the presence of dysplastic disease of the hip. Although arthroscopic debridement may result in significant symptomatic improvement, it may not seriously influence the long-term outlook. Especially for young individuals, arthroscopy should not be used solely for symptomatic improvement when long-term issues need to be addressed. Specifically, patients who are candidates for osteotomy to improve the joint mechanics and weight distribution must be carefully assessed.

As noted, the enlarged labrum accompanying a shallow acetabulum may carry greater weight-bearing responsibility as well as provide a buttress to superolateral subluxation of the femoral head. It is unlikely that simple debridement of the deteriorated portion of the labrum will accentuate this subluxation potential, but great care must be taken in the debridement procedure, especially avoiding an overly zealous resection.

Similarly, indiscriminate debridement of the ligamentum teres should be avoided. The vessel of the ligamentum teres remains patent and contributes to the blood supply of the femoral head in a significant percentage of adults. Arbitrary debridement could unnecessarily place the femoral head at risk for avascular necrosis. However, it seems unlikely that debridement of the ruptured portion should present a problem, and it has produced gratifying symptomatic results.

In summary, radiographic evidence of dysplasia is not a contraindication to arthroscopy, nor is it necessarily an indicator of poor outcome. Results are more dictated by the nature of the pathology. Nonetheless, it is prudent to view arthroscopy as but one tool in the complement of resources necessary in the assessment and management of patients with developmental dysplasia of the hip.

Case 1

A 14-year-old girl was referred with a 4-month history of painful locking and catching of her right hip. Symptoms first occurred when simply raising her leg to step over a railing. Her symptoms had since been unremitting. Her history was remarkable for dysplastic disease of both hips since birth. These were initially treated with closed reduction, but she had subsequently undergone multiple osteotomies of the proximal femur and pelvis. Most recently, she was being evaluated for an acetabular procedure to improve the coverage of her femoral head when she developed incapacitating mechanical right hip symptoms. Radiographs revealed changes consistent with her underlying disease and previous surgical procedures as well as slight lateral joint space loss on the right compared with the left (Figure 15.1A).

Based on her symptoms and examination findings, arthroscopy was recommended as a method to assess the extent of intraarticular damage that may be contributing to her symptoms and to see if this could be addressed. She was found to have an unstable inverted labrum (see Figure 15.1B). This was debrided in a cautious fashion (see Figure 15.1C). Care was taken to excise the entrapped portion contributing to her symptoms while preserving as much of the remaining labrum as possible to avoid potentially destabilizing the joint. Additionally, there was grade IV articular loss of the acetabulum. The unstable fragments were debrided, creating a stable edge of surrounding cartilage (see Figure 15.1D). Microfracture of the lesion was performed to stimulate a fibrocartilaginous healing response (see Figure 15.1E). Occluding the inflow confirmed vascular access through the perforations (see Figure 15.1F). Postoperatively, she was maintained on a strict protected weight-bearing status for 2 months, emphasizing range of motion. She was then able to resume normal light daily activities with resolution of her mechanical hip pain.

Case 2

A 16-year-old boy presented with a 9-month history of pain and locking of his left hip. This first occurred while playing football as a freshman in high school. He had received no previous specific treatment, but was known to have a developmental abnormality of his hip since early childhood. Radiographs revealed evidence of a separate bone fragment within the femoral head (Figure 15.2A), which was further substantiated by a computed tomography (CT) scan (Figure 15.2B).

With his mechanical symptoms and imaging evidence of a loose fragment, arthroscopy was recommended. The fragment was actually found to be fixed within the femoral head, but there was a grade IV unstable articular fragment over this area that was debrided (see Figure 15.2C–E). Postoperatively, he had resolution of his mechanical pain and catching.

Case 3

A 37-year-old woman presented with a 4-year history of progressively worsening right hip pain. There was no history of injury or precipitating event; she simply began experiencing discomfort that had worsened over recent months. Twisting maneuvers were especially painful. Her examination findings suggested that her hip joint was the source of pain. Radiographs revealed evidence of modest underlying dysplasia but were otherwise unremarkable (Figure 15.3A). Magnetic resonance imaging (MRI) was also unremarkable. She then underwent 6 months of continued activity restriction as well as various trials of oral antiinflammatory medications and physical therapy without improvement. She obtained pronounced temporary alleviation of her symptoms from a fluoroscopically guided intraarticular injection of anesthetic.

Based on her clinical circumstances, arthroscopy was offered as the next step in her management. She was found to have a hypertrophic ligamentum teres with an accompanying degenerate rupture that was debrided (see Figure 15.3B–D). Postoperatively, she demonstrated pronounced symptomatic improvement and was able to resume fitness exercises.

ELDERLY

Our population is aging, and the most rapid shift in this age distribution is set to occur as the baby boomers reach their senior years. In the United States alone, the Centers for Disease Control and Prevention estimate that approximately 70 million Americans suffer from arthritis or chronic joint ailments, and, according to the American Academy of Orthopaedic Surgeons, approximately 300,000 hip arthroplasties are performed annually.[15,16] Even in absence of arthritis, the hip joint is known to undergo senile changes. An MRI study has demonstrated an increasing incidence of labral pathology with age, even among asymptomatic volunteers.[17] An electron microscopy study had documented degenerative labral changes associated with the aging process, and this is consistent with two separate cadaveric studies that showed a 96% preva-

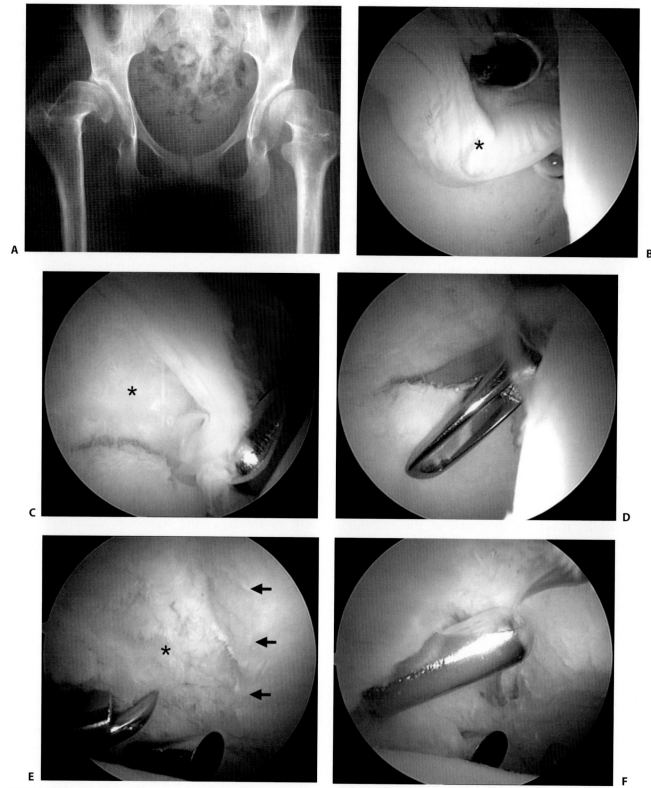

FIGURE 15.1. A 14-year-old girl with acute locking and catching of the right hip. (A) Anteroposterior radiograph demonstrates evidence of residual developmental dysplasia of the hip (DDH) of both hips and changes consistent with multiple previous osteotomies. Slight lateral joint space narrowing of the right hip is seen compared with the left. (B) Arthroscopic view from the anterolateral portal demonstrates an unstable entrapped anterior labrum (asterisk). (C) Debridement of the unstable portion of the labrum is begun, revealing extensive exposed subchondral bone (asterisk) with full-thickness articular loss. (D) Debridement of unstable articular fragments is performed with a basket. (E) Now viewing from the anterior portal, a stable articular edge has been achieved (arrows), and microfracture is begun through the subchondral surface (asterisk) that still has a thin covering of fibrous tissue. (F) With suction through the shaver, bleeding confirms vascular access through the areas of perforation.

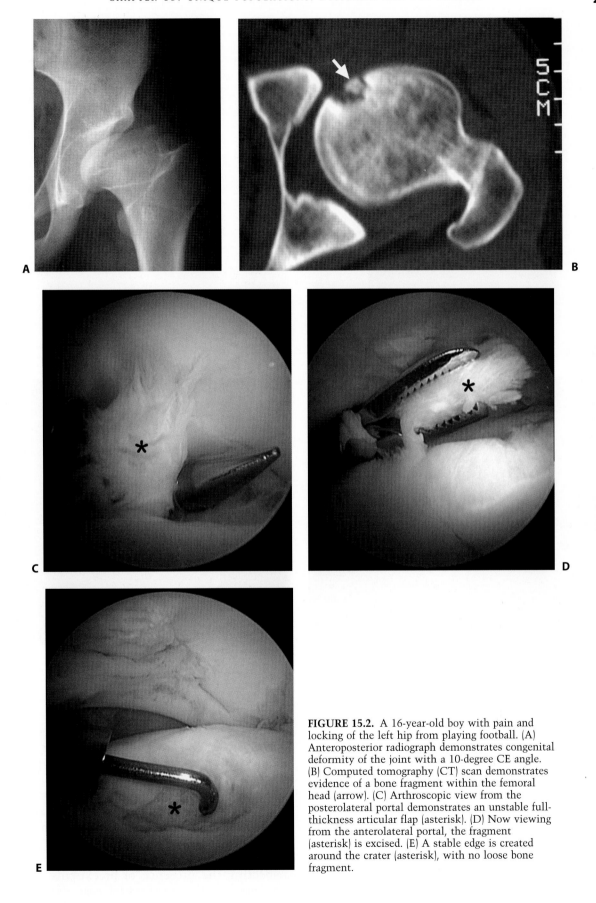

FIGURE 15.2. A 16-year-old boy with pain and locking of the left hip from playing football. (A) Anteroposterior radiograph demonstrates congenital deformity of the joint with a 10-degree CE angle. (B) Computed tomography (CT) scan demonstrates evidence of a bone fragment within the femoral head (arrow). (C) Arthroscopic view from the posterolateral portal demonstrates an unstable full-thickness articular flap (asterisk). (D) Now viewing from the anterolateral portal, the fragment (asterisk) is excised. (E) A stable edge is created around the crater (asterisk), with no loose bone fragment.

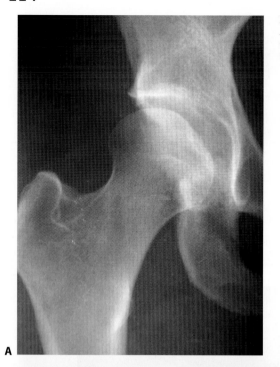

FIGURE 15.3. A 37-year-old woman with recalcitrant right hip pain. (A) Anteroposterior radiograph demonstrates moderate dysplasia with an 18-degree CE angle. (B) Arthroscopy reveals a hypertrophic ligamentum teres (arrows). (C) The degenerated hypertrophic portion of the ligament is debrided.

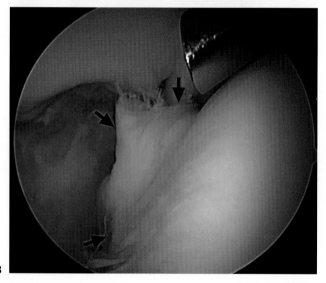

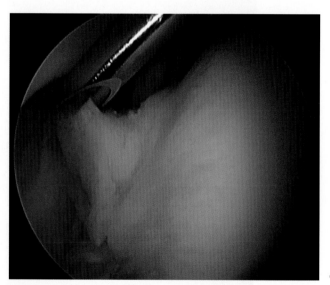

lence of labral lesions in specimens averaging 78 years of age.[18–20]

As our population ages, there remains an emphasis on maintaining an active lifestyle. Many individuals wish to maintain the physical prowess of their youth and, for the more reasonably oriented, there are fitness programs designed specifically for aging bodies. There is also greater interest in continuing to participate in competitive activities with advancing age at both the professional and recreational levels, which is reflected in the flourishing number of masters programs and senior events. Thus, the aging hip joint is subjected to many of the same forces (i.e., torsion, twisting, impact load-

ing) that are often a source of injury in younger joints. The mechanism of injury may be similar, but the propensity for injury may be greater because of underlying joint changes, and the recovery may be slower and less complete.

Arthroscopy has a role for many of the conditions that are encountered in older individuals, but expectations of success must be modified because of underlying senile changes or arthritis. Age is not a contraindication to arthroscopy, but is a factor in suspecting the presence of preexisting, subclinical degenerative disease. Several case examples illustrate the role and limitations of arthroscopy in an aging population.

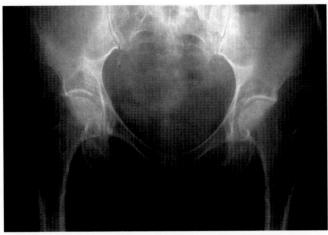

FIGURE 15.4. A 74-year-old woman with recalcitrant left hip pain. (A) Anteroposterior radiograph is remarkable only for subtle joint space loss of the left compared with the right hip. (B) Arthroscopy demonstrates severe grade IV articular fragmentation of both the acetabulum and femoral head, which is debrided.

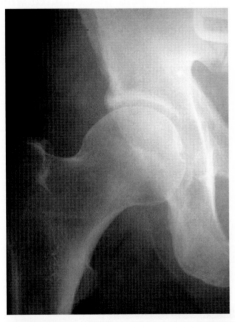

FIGURE 15.5. A 73-year-old man with acute-onset intractable hip pain. (A) Anteroposterior radiograph reveals modest degenerate changes, but good joint space preservation. (B) Viewing from the anterolateral portal, a large comminuted tear of the anterior labrum (asterisk) is excised. (C) Accompanying areas of grade IV articular fragmentation are debrided as well.

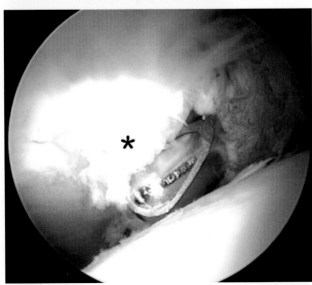

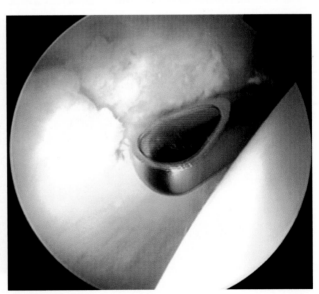

Case 4

A 74-year-old woman presented with a 16-month history of progressively incapacitating left hip pain. Radiographs were interpreted to show only mild degenerative changes (Figure 15.4A), insufficient to explain the magnitude of her symptoms. She had been managed under the auspices of four different physicians, having undergone an extensive evaluation of her lower back and a psychiatric consultation with recommendation for a pain management program. On examination, her hip seemed to be the principal origin of pain. This was further supported by a brief period of relief from an intraarticular injection.

Because of the intractable nature of her symptoms, arthroscopy was offered and revealed grade IV articular loss of both the acetabular and femoral surfaces (see Figure 15.4B). Debridement resulted in improvement for only a few months. However, with the documented severity of her disease, she was thought to be an appropriate candidate for total hip arthroplasty. This procedure was performed with gratifying results.

It has become evident that often subtle radiographic findings may have significant clinical implications. It has been our experience that advanced intraarticular damage may occur before there are any radiographic indicators of change. As in this case, for degenerative disease, when the symptoms are out of proportion to the radiographic findings, often arthroscopy will define more advanced damage in accordance with the patient's symptoms. Thus, we are beginning to learn how to interpret subtle radiographic features, especially the presence of any asymmetric joint space loss.

Case 5

A 73-year-old man presented with a 1-month history of incapacitating right hip pain that occurred while

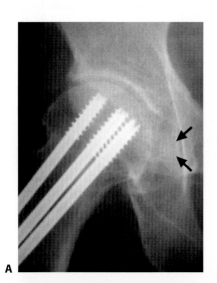

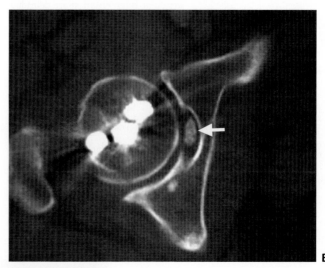

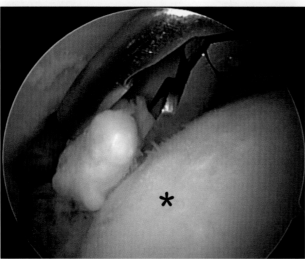

FIGURE 15.6. A 69-year-old woman with spontaneous onset of sharp stabbing right hip pain. (A) Anteroposterior radiograph reveals a well-healed femoral neck fracture with joint space narrowing and areas suggestive of a loose body (arrows). (B) CT scan further delineates the presence of an intraarticular fragment (arrow). (C) Arthroscopy reveals the loose bone fragment, which is retrieved, but there is also evidence of chronic grade IV articular loss, especially of the femoral head, with exposed eburnated bone (asterisk).

playing golf. Any movement of the hip was painful, and his symptoms were only partially alleviated by using crutches. Radiographs revealed mild degenerative changes but fairly good joint space preservation (Figure 15.5A). A bone scan and serologic testing were performed to rule out occult fracture, neoplasia, or infection. All results were unremarkable. Evaluation of the lumbar spine was also carried out to rule out a source of referred symptoms. An MRI of the hip was also unremarkable. Because of his recalcitrant symptoms, a fluoroscopically guided intraarticular injection of bupivacaine and corticosteroid was performed, which provided pronounced alleviation of his symptoms, but only for a few days. Arthroscopy was subsequently recommended. He was found to have extensive tearing of the anterolateral labrum as well as associated grade IV articular fragmentation of the acetabulum, which was excised (see Figure 15.5B,C). Postoperatively, he experienced pronounced symptomatic improvement and was able to return to his normal sports activities for the following 6 years.

Case 6

A 69-year-old woman was referred with a 6-week history of spontaneous onset incapacitating sharp, stabbing right hip pain. Her history was remarkable in that she had undergone multiple screw fixation of a femoral neck fracture 9 years previously. However, she had been asymptomatic and unrestricted in her activities until her recent onset of symptoms. Radiographs revealed her fracture to be fully healed. Evidence suggested an intraarticular loose body, but also modest joint space narrowing (Figure 15.6A). A CT scan further defined the extent of the intraarticular fragment (Figure 15.6B).

It was uncertain how much of her symptoms was simply due to the degenerative changes and how much might be attributable to the bone fragment. However, with her recent spontaneous onset of sharp stabbing pain and evidence of an intraarticular fragment, it was thought that arthroscopy to retrieve the fragment was the next step in her management to remove this as a potential contributing source. At arthroscopy, the large loose body was identified and retrieved. However, there was also noted to be severe articular damage with grade IV changes of the acetabulum and grade III damage to the femoral head (see Figure 15.6C). Postoperatively, the sharp stabbing symptoms were eliminated, but she continued to experience pain with daily activities. This was thought to be attributable to her underlying degenerative disease.

In this case, the patient experienced an acute episode of pain, mechanical symptoms, and clear evidence of an intraarticular loose body, all of which are normally good prognostic indicators of a potentially successful outcome of hip arthroscopy. However, radiographically, she had evidence of joint space loss reflecting underlying degenerative disease. In our experience, whenever there is radiographic evidence of degenerative disease, this is often the limiting factor in the response to arthroscopy and should be considered an overriding poor prognostic indicator, even in the presence of more favorable clinical findings. Degenerative disease is also often a great imitator. It may present with gradually worsening activity-related symptoms, but also may present with the acute onset of pain in absence of any prodromal findings.

References

1. Dorell JH, Catterall A: The torn acetabular labrum. J Bone Joint Surg 1986;68B(3):400–403.
2. Klaue K, Durnin CW, Ganz R: The acetabular rim syndrome. J Bone Joint Surg 1991;73B:423–429.
3. Nishina T, Saito S, Ohzono K, et al: Chiari pelvic osteotomy for osteoarthritis: the influence of the torn and detached acetabular labrum. J Bone Joint Surg 1990;72B(5):765–769.
4. Byrd JWT: Labral lesions: an elusive source of hip pain: case reports and review of the literature. Arthroscopy 1996;12(5): 603–612.
5. Byrd JWT, Jones KS: Inverted acetabular labrum and secondary osteoarthritis: radiographic diagnosis and arthroscopic treatment. Arthroscopy 2000;16(4):417.
6. Hadley NA, Brown TD, Weinstein SL: The effect of contact pressure elevations and aseptic necrosis on the long term outcome of congenital hip dislocation. J Orthop Rev 1990;8(4): 504–513.
7. Maxian TA, Brown TD, Weinstein SL: Chronic stress tolerance levels for human articular cartilage: two non-uniform contact models applied to long term follow up of CDH. J Biomech 1995;28:159–166.
8. Cooperman DR, Wallensten R, Stulberg SD: Acetabular dysplasia in the adult. Clin Orthop 1983;175:79–85.
9. Malvitz TA, Weinstein SL: Closed reduction for congenital dysplasia of the hip. Functional and radiographic results after an average of thirty years. J Bone Joint Surg 1994;76A:1777–1792.
10. Nishii T, Sugano N, Tanaka H, Nakanishi K, Ohzono K, Yoshikawa H: Articular cartilage abnormalities in dysplastic hips without joint space narrowing. Clin Orthop 2001;383: 183–190.
11. Noguchi Y, Miura H, Takasugi S, et al: Cartilage and labrum degeneration in the dysplastic hip generally originates in the anterosuperior weight bearing area: an arthroscopic observation. Arthroscopy 1999;15:496–506.
12. Michaels G, Matles AL: The role of the ligamentum teres in congenital dislocation of the hip. Clin Orthop 1970;71:199–201.
13. Ippolito E, Ishii Y, Ponseti IV: Histologic, histochemical, and ultrastructural studies of the hip joint capsule and ligamentum teres in congenital dislocation of the hip. Clin Orthop 1980;146:246–258.
14. Byrd JWT, Jones KS: Hip arthroscopy in the presence of dysplasia. Arthroscopy 19(10):1055–1060; 2003.

15. Centers for Disease Control and Prevention: Prevalence of self-reported arthritis or chronic joint symptoms among adults–United States, 2001. JAMA 2002;288(24):3103–3104.

16. AAOS Orthopaedic-Related Statistics. Rosemond, IL: American Academy of Orthopaedic Surgeons, 2000.

17. Lecouvet FE, VandeBerg BC, Melghem J, et al: MR imaging of the acetabular labrum: variations in 200 asymptomatic hips. AJR Am J Roentgenol 1996;167:1025–1028.

18. Tanabe H: Aging process of the acetabular labrum: an electron-microscopic study. J Jpn Orthop Assoc 1991;65:18–25.

19. Seldes RM, Tan V, Hunt J, Katz M, Winiarsky R, Fitzgerald RH Jr: Anatomy, histologic features, and vascularity of the adult acetabular labrum. Clin Orthop 2001;382:232–240.

20. McCarthy JC, Nobel PC, Schuck MR, Wright J, Lee J: The watershed labral lesion: its relationship to early arthritis of the hip. J Arthroplasty 2001;16(8 suppl 1):81–87.

16

Complications Associated with Hip Arthroscopy

J.W. Thomas Byrd

According to the Arthroscopy Association of North American's Committee on Complications, on reviewing almost 400,000 arthroscopic procedures, the overall incidence of complications was 0.56%.[1] However, this series represented predominantly knees, followed by shoulders, ankles, elbows, and wrists. There were no hips in the population.

In a previous review by this author of 1491 cases of hip arthroscopy from several of the world's leading centers, a total of 20 complications were defined for an overall incidence of 1.34% (Table 16.1).[2] The most common feature of these complications was that they usually occurred early in the surgeon's experience, which reflects the learning curve associated with the developmental phase experienced by these pioneers in hip arthroscopy.

In 1992, Glick was the first to report specifically on the complications associated with hip arthroscopy.[3] He described 9 complications among 60 cases for an overall incidence of 15%, including 8 neuropraxias (4 sciatic, 4 pudendal), of which 7 were transient and 1 was lost to follow-up, and 1 instrument breakage. Additionally, there was an unrecorded number of articular scuffings that the author thought were due to inadequate distraction. Most of their complications occurred in the early phases of their experience, and the author believed that the development of a custom distractor with better padding and positioning of the extremity and use of a tensiometer would reduce the likelihood of complications.

In 1996, Funke and Munzinger reported on 3 complications in 19 cases.[4] These included a transient neuropraxia of the pudendal nerve, a hematoma of the labia majora, and acute abdominal pain during a procedure performed under regional anesthesia. All problems occurred early in their experience. The first 2 were attributed to poor positioning and insufficient padding of the perineal post, and the latter was thought to be due to irritation of the peritoneum from extravasation of fluid. They believed these problems would be avoidable in the future by careful positioning and padding, use of general anesthesia for the procedure, and careful monitoring of the fluid pressure by use of a fluid management system.

In 1999, Griffin and Villar reported on the senior author's experience in a prospective study of 640 consecutive procedures.[5] They identified 10 complications with a 1.6% incidence, but none were major or long term; included were transient nerve palsies (3 sciatic; 1 femoral), 2 instrument breakages, and 1 each of a small vaginal tear, persistent bleeding from a portal, portal hematoma, and trochanteric bursitis. They found no correlation between the occurrence of complications and the stage of experience of the senior surgeon.

In 2001, Sampson reviewed the combined experience of himself and James Glick.[6] They reported on 530 cases with 34 complications for an incidence of 6.4%. Among these, only 3 (0.5%) were thought to be significant and the rest (27) were transient. The complications included 20 transient neuropraxias (10 perineal; 4 pudendal; 1 lateral femoral cutaneous; 1 femoral/sciatic; 4 sciatic), 9 fluid extravasations, 2 instrument breakages, 2 scuffings, and 1 avascular necrosis (AVN) of the femoral head.

Among 412 consecutive cases prospectively assessed by this author, 6 complications were identified, representing a 1.46% incidence: 3 partial neuropraxias of the lateral femoral cutaneous nerve (2 transient, 1 permanent), 1 transient obturator neuropraxia, 1 area of localized heterotopic ossification, and 1 possible deep vein thrombosis. Additionally, 1 patient felt that she simply was made worse as a consequence of the procedure. There was no identifiable cause or explanation, but this experience does reflect the potential deleterious effect of any operation.

NEUROVASCULAR TRACTION INJURY

Neuropraxia due to traction has been reported, most commonly involving the sciatic nerve. Glick was the first to report four such cases, which he attributed to his early technique for performing the procedure.[3] Later, Sampson reported on a larger series from this same center, observing that all neuropraxias were associated with prolonged traction times.[6] He advocates that the traction time should be kept under 2 hours

TABLE 16.1. Complications Associated with 1491 Arthroscopic Hip Procedures (Number in Parentheses).

Transient pudendal nerve neuropraxia (5)
Permanent pudendal nerve neuropraxia (1)
Transient sciatic nerve neuropraxia (4)
Intraabdominal fluid extravasation (3)
Partial lateral femoral cutaneous nerve neuropraxia (2)
Laceration of the lateral femoral cutaneous nerve (1)
Scrotal skin necrosis (1)
Femoral nerve palsy (1)
Instrument breakage (1)
Heterotopic ossification (1)

and, if more prolonged surgery is necessary, the traction should be intermittently released. Additionally, the amount of traction should be gauged to the laxity of the individual. Excessive traction on a loose joint can result in hyperelongation of the extremity and greater risk of neuropraxia. Villar has also reported three sciatic neuropraxias.[5] All three occurred on the same day, and he thought that this was probably due to a technical error in application of the traction. Villar and Sampson have each reported one femoral neuropraxia as well.

All reported traction neuropraxias were transient and the recovery was complete. However, this author is anecdotally aware of two cases by different surgeons in which the patients demonstrated evidence of sciatic nerve damage that only partially recovered. In both cases, the traction time was well under 2 hours, indicating that other factors may be involved in addition to the duration of traction. Sufficient traction force is necessary to ensure adequate joint space separation. Otherwise, there is greater risk of damage from the instruments entering the joint. However, care should be taken to use the least amount of traction force necessary to achieve adequate distraction.

This author has not experienced any traction neuropraxias. The greatest risk seems to be to the sciatic nerve. Some authors advocate hip flexion to relax the capsule, making distraction easier. However, this may place the sciatic nerve under greater stretch, increasing the risk of injury. We deliberately maintain the hip in extension or perhaps with only a few degrees (<10 degrees) of flexion. This practice may explain why we have not observed any sciatic neuropraxias.

It is worthy to note, when considering the amount of distraction of the hip (approximately 1 cm), that this proportionately represents a small change relative to the overall length of the sciatic and femoral nerves. Perhaps some nerves are simply more at risk for injury. However, currently there are no parameters by which to define this circumstance. Some patients with hip joint pathology may have coexistent radicular or neurologic-type pain. For these patients, it is especially prudent to offer counseling on the uncertain risk of exacerbating neurologic symptoms.

DIRECT TRAUMA TO NEUROVASCULAR STRUCTURES

Injury to the sciatic nerve or femoral nerve or vessels is a disastrous complication of hip arthroscopy. Evidence from anatomic studies suggests that the structures are at a safe distance when proper technique in portal placement is observed.[7] The reported clinical experiences also suggest that this is a relatively safe technique. However, one femoral nerve palsy has been reported.[2] This author is also aware of one anecdotal case of laceration of the femoral nerve associated with arthroscopy of the hip. This further emphasizes that those embarking on this technique should know the anatomy and landmarks and be versed in proper portal placement.

Although the femoral neurovascular structures and the sciatic nerve should be safely away from the operative field, the lateral femoral cutaneous nerve (LFCN) warrants special mention. The LFCN is always vulnerable to injury from the anterior portal.[7] One of its branches will invariably lie close to the portal. It cannot be predictably avoided by significantly altering the position of the anterior portal. Anatomic studies have shown that moving the portal more laterally does not avoid the nerve unless it is moved so far away as to encroach on the anterolateral portal. The nerve could actually be more readily avoided by moving the portal medially; however, this is ill advised for reasons of increasing proximity to the more important femoral nerve and vessels.

The LFCN can usually be avoided by using meticulous technique in portal placement. The nerve is especially vulnerable to laceration by a skin incision placed too deeply through the subcutaneous tissue. One case of laceration has been reported.[8]

Even with proper technique, neuropraxia of small branches of the LFCN can occur. This damage is most likely to occur when vigorous instrumentation of the joint from the anterior position is necessary, such as when removing loose bodies too large to be brought through a cannula. This author has observed three such cases (0.7% incidence); two were transient and one resulted in a permanent small patch of reduced sensation in the lateral thigh. The LFCN has arborized at the level of the anterior portal so, if injury occurs, it is to small branches involving only a limited portion of the area of distribution of the LFCN.

The anterior portal is important for optimal visualization and access to recesses of the hip joint. Thus, it is prudent to include as part of the preoperative discussion with the patient the small possibility of a partial neuropraxia of the LFCN.

COMPRESSION INJURY TO THE PERINEUM

Hip arthroscopy is unique in that the forces needed to distract the joint for arthroscopy necessitate counter-traction provided by a perineal post. This requirement introduces the potential for compression injury to the perineum and especially neuropraxia of the pudendal nerve.

Soft tissue pressure necrosis of the perineum has been reported by Eriksson et al.[8] This was an early experience and should be avoidable by proper padding and careful positioning. Nonetheless, it does emphasize the potential consequences of the magnitude of distraction forces generated for this procedure. Funke and Munzinger reported a hematoma of the labia majora that they attributed to poor positioning and insufficient padding of the perineal area.[4] Griffin and Villar have also reported a small vaginal tear that healed uneventfully, and they believed it was caused by excessive lateral force from the perineal bar.[5]

Transient neuropraxia of the pudendal nerve is the most common problem attributed to compression of the perineum. Glick reported this, especially in his early experience before switching to a custom distractor.[3] This author encountered two such cases when first beginning to perform hip arthroscopy on an antiquated fracture table with a poorly devised, poorly padded perineal post.[9] This problem has been observed once in more than 400 cases (0.2% incidence) performed on a newer table with a well-padded post. This case occurred after having performed more than 300 procedures without incident. The patient was loose jointed and did not require much distraction force. She had a simple labral tear that was debrided, and the procedure did not take very long. The patient was positioned by the senior author in the same manner used for more than 400 cases. Thus, there were no factors normally attributed to the development of a neuropraxia. Recovery, as in other cases, was complete within a few weeks.

This author has also observed one case of transient dysesthesias in the medial thigh that resolved uneventfully. It was thought that this likely represented a neuropraxia of the obturator nerve. This example illustrates that although moving the perineal post laterally reduces the risk of compression against the pudendal nerve, it does not eliminate all potential compression problems.

In general, proper padding and positioning are critical to the safety of the procedure. The minimal traction force necessary to achieve adequate distraction should be employed, and the traction duration should be kept as brief as possible. However, even when observing all these safety parameters, there is still a slight risk of some type of compression neuropraxia.

TRACTION FIXATION DEVICES

Most distraction systems use some type of device for capturing the distal lower leg including the foot and ankle. It is important that these areas be well padded before the application of traction. There have been no reports of major pressure injuries, although patients may occasionally describe aching in the foot or ankle for a short period of time following the procedure. Sampson described 10 cases of transient peroneal neuropraxia that was thought to be due to the early development and evolution of their hip distractors in addition to prolonged traction times. This author is also aware of one case of altered sensation in the saphenous nerve distribution of the foot from a case performed on a standard fracture table.

Skeletal traction is not necessary for routine hip arthroscopy, although this author has used a distal femoral traction pin in cases of ipsilateral total knee arthroplasty and ipsilateral tibial shaft fractures. The morbidity of a skeletal traction pin is minimal but unnecessary for most cases.

This author is familiar with one case of deep infection at the pin site following skeletal traction used for attempted arthroscopy. Interestingly, years later, this patient did undergo successful arthroscopy to address the hip lesion.

Occasionally, patients may present with ipsilateral cruciate ligament injury and hip joint pathology. Most commonly, these are the result of previous motor vehicle accidents. This author has performed hip arthroscopy using the standard distraction method in eight patients who have undergone previous ipsilateral cruciate ligament reconstruction without any untoward effects. However, it is recommended that the reconstructed knee ligament be fully matured before hip arthroscopy. Alternatively, a distal femoral traction pin may be appropriate in conjunction with a recent ipsilateral knee injury or reconstructive surgery.

FLUID EXTRAVASATION

Glick was the first to report on the potentially serious complications associated with excessive fluid extravasation, especially into the abdominal cavity.[2] All cases resolved without long-term sequelae, but one required paracentesis and ventilatory support overnight. Sampson subsequently reported nine cases of intraabdominal fluid extravasation.[6] Contributing factors included long operative times, fresh acetabular fractures, and extraarticular procedures such as iliopsoas tendon release. They believed that switching to an outflow-dependent pump reduced the incidence of extravasation and the total amount of fluid necessary for performing arthroscopy. They emphasized that it is important to pay attention to the amount of fluid that is being pumped in and how much is flowing out.

Bartlett et al. reported a case of cardiac arrest due to intraabdominal fluid extravasation through a central acetabular fracture.[10] The patient was successfully resuscitated, but this case further emphasizes the potential magnitude of this serious complication. Funke and Munzinger also noted a case that had to be terminated due to severe lower abdominal pain that they believed was caused by irritation of the peritoneum from fluid leakage when the procedure was performed under regional anesthesia.

It is this author's perspective that several points become imperative when performing arthroscopy in the presence of an acetabular fracture or when procedures are performed outside of the confines of the hip capsule (i.e., excision of extracapsular fragments or iliopsoas tendon release). First, the operation should be performed in an expeditious fashion. There is no need to rush, but steady progress should be made toward completion of the procedure. If difficulties are encountered and extravasation becomes a problem, it is appropriate, if necessary, to terminate the procedure rather than risk a potentially serious complication. Second, a high-flow fluid management system is especially helpful; this allows adequate flow without necessitating excessive pressure, which potentiates extravasation. Adequate flow is critical to maintaining good visualization, which is essential to completing the procedure in a timely and effective manner. A gravity fluid system is suboptimal for this purpose because flow and pressure are poorly modulated. Pumps, although much better suited, are not infallible and thus the surgeon must be cognizant of pump function and corresponding fluid egress. If fluid is being pumped in, but a corresponding amount is not coming out, then fluid extravasation should be suspected. Also of note: for acetabular fractures, it may be preferable to wait several weeks for the early healing response to develop a fluid seal.

Last, all the reported cases of intraabdominal fluid extravasation have been performed in the lateral position. It is unclear whether there is a predilection to this problem that is unique to the lateral position but, with this position, the intrapelvic and intraabdominal cavity becomes a sink into which fluid can pool simply by the dependent flow of gravity.

SCOPE TRAUMA

The single most common complication, which is probably underreported, is *scope trauma*. Glick alluded to this as a complication in an unrecorded number of cases.[3] He thought that this was most likely ascribed to inadequate traction, emphasizing the importance of proper joint distraction. Sampson reported two such cases as serious complications.[6] Realistically, iatrogenic intraarticular damage can occur to a varying degree in a number of cases.

The dense surrounding soft tissue envelope and the constrained architecture of the joint limit the maneuverability of instruments. The convex articular surface of the femoral head is especially vulnerable to injury, which may occur either during portal placement or during subsequent maneuvering of instruments in and out of the joint. Thus, a thoughtful approach is necessary with every aspect of carrying out operative arthroscopy of the hip.

The labrum is also susceptible to damage during portal placement. This is most likely to occur when trying to use a more cephalad position for penetrating the capsule to avoid the articular surface of the femoral head. The labrum may be inadvertently penetrated, potentially resulting in significant damage and uncertain long-term consequences.[10]

Minimizing joint damage begins with ensuring adequate joint surface separation for introduction of the instruments. Particular steps are necessary in placing the initial portal for the arthroscope, including precise positioning and liberal use of the C arm to avoid perforating the labrum or scuffing the femoral head.[11] Placement of subsequent portals is then facilitated by direct arthroscopic control as the cannulas enter the joint. Also, during the course of the procedure, it is prudent to directly visualize every entry and exit of the instruments.

It is this author's practice to tell patients that any surgery is a violation of the joint. Arthroscopic surgery is a much less invasive alternative to open procedures. However, any time the joint is violated, there is some risk of causing harm. Thus, the surgeon can only try to be as careful as possible and be certain that the procedure is being performed for the right reason, namely clinical circumstances that at least provide a good probability that there is some type of pathology that can potentially be addressed by the arthroscopic procedure.

INSTRUMENT BREAKAGE

The overall incidence of instrument failure in arthroscopy is reported as 0.1%. However, the risk of instrument breakage in the hip is greater than with other joints. As noted previously, the dense envelope and constrained joint architecture limit maneuverability of the instruments and this increases the potential for breakage. Additionally, the extra-length instruments used in the hip create a longer lever arm and greater potential for excess torque or bending. It is essential that the surgeon use only sturdy instruments that can withstand the rigors imposed by the anatomy of the hip. Extra-length instruments designed for other endoscopic procedures are often more delicate and would easily be broken if improperly employed for hip arthroscopy.

Villar and Sampson each reported two cases of instrument breakage, representing a 0.3% and 0.4% incidence, respectively.[5,6] In one case, the broken fragment could not be retrieved but there were no untoward problems encountered due to the broken instrument in any case. This author has not yet had an instrument break within the joint. However, it is not infrequent that a shaver blade becomes inoperable because of slight bending; this reflects the amount of torque that is delivered on the instruments in the hip because bent blades are rarely encountered during arthroscopy of other joints.

VASCULAR INSULT TO THE FEMORAL HEAD

It has been at least a theoretical concern that distraction of the joint and distension with fluid could compromise vascular flow to the femoral head. Anecdotal information is available regarding problems associated with AVN in patients undergoing hip arthroscopy.

However, these reports are sporadic and infrequent, and there is no pattern to suggest that there is a causal relationship.

Sampson reported the occurrence of AVN in one patient who had undergone uneventful arthroscopy for a labral tear incurred from a work-related injury.[6] This author has observed a case of previously documented AVN that progressed following arthroscopy.[2] A similar case has been observed by Villar as well.[12] With these sparse examples, it is uncertain whether these cases simply represent the natural course of the disease, or whether the progression could have been precipitated by the arthroscopic intervention.

HETEROTOPIC OSSIFICATION

This author has had experience with one case of heterotopic bone formation along the tract of the anterior portal following hip arthroscopy (Figure 16.1). This patient had multiple loose bodies associated with synovial osteochondromatosis. Most of the fragments were removed via the anterior portal.

The patient underwent successful excision of the heterotopic bone via a limited incision over the pal-

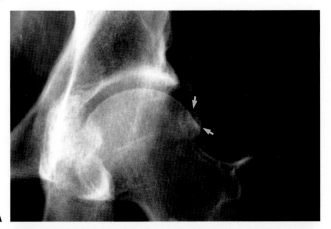

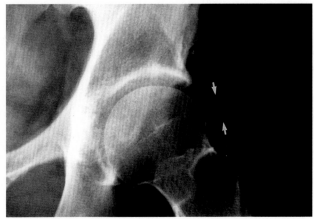

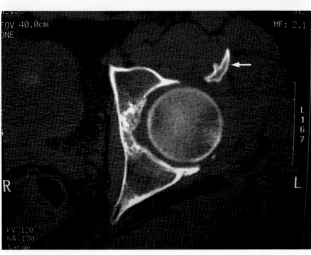

FIGURE 16.1. (A) Anteroposterior (AP) and (B) lateral radiographic view demonstrating the area of heterotopic bone formation (arrows). (C) Computed tomography (CT) scan further defines the characteristic features of heterotopic ossification (arrow).

pable area of involvement. The radiographic appearance and histology were both consistent with a localized area of heterotopic ossification.

Heterotopic ossification is a well-recognized complication associated with open hip surgery such as total hip arthroplasty.[13] As with many complications, while the risk associated with arthroscopy may be small, the procedure is not immune.

INFECTION

Infection is an exceedingly rare (overall incidence, 0.07%) but potentially devastating complication of any arthroscopic procedure.[1] Although it has not been reported in the hip, it is still a concern. It is known that joints with thin subcutaneous coverage, such as the ankle and elbow, carry the highest risks of infection. Conversely, the hip is protected by a very dense soft tissue envelope, but this protective feature may be offset by the close proximity to the groin and perineum, a highly contaminated area.

Overall, there is always a small but finite risk of infection with arthroscopy. One must always adhere to meticulous technique in prepping and draping and in the surgical procedure. Also, routine use of preoperative broad-spectrum intravenous antibiotics for prophylaxis is well accepted. Under these circumstances, if or when infection occurs, one is assured that all appropriate precautionary measures have been observed. The key then simply becomes prompt recognition and treatment of infection when it occurs.

THROMBOPHLEBITIS

Deep vein thrombosis (DVT) is an infrequent, but recognized, complication of lower extremity arthroscopic surgery. The incidence of subclinical DVT is greater when investigated with more sensitive tools such as duplex ultrasonography.[14,15] However, the clinical significance of these silent cases is unclear. There have been no previous published reports of thrombophlebitis as a complication of hip arthroscopy, but it is a potential concern as with any lower extremity surgery. This author has had one possible case of DVT. A professional athlete began to experience gastrocnemius discomfort during the course of his conditioning 2 months following arthroscopic hip surgery. He had no clinical findings suggesting DVT. Magnetic resonance imaging (MRI) was performed to see if he had sustained any injury to the gastrocnemius muscle, and this image noted evidence of thrombus in the deep calf system. A venous Doppler study revealed no evidence of occlusion or flow obstruction, but as a precautionary measure, he was placed on oral Coumadin for 1 month. His calf soreness resolved with modifica-

tion of his conditioning program and there were no further ramifications. The principal prophylaxis against DVT is early mobilization. Additional maneuvers may also be appropriate as advocated for other types of lower extremity arthroscopy.

SOFT TISSUE DISORDERS

It is this author's experience that trochanteric bursitis and other lateral soft tissue symptoms sometimes coexist with intraarticular pathology and may obscure the diagnosis. These soft tissue disorders may be incompletely resolved before arthroscopy and may still need management afterward. Tenderness around the portals may also occur, and Villar has reported trochanteric bursitis following arthroscopy that responded to a corticosteroid injection.[5] It is likely that this is more common than has been reported, but does not seem to represent a causally related long-term problem. Rare incidents of bleeding around a portal site or local hematoma (0.3%) have also been reported, but with spontaneous and uneventful resolution.[5]

CONCLUSION

Glick summarized complications of hip arthroscopy as being caused by either excessive or inadequate traction.[3] Too much traction or traction improperly applied results in traction neuropraxia or compression injury to the perineum. Inadequate traction leads to iatrogenic joint damage from instrumentation when the surfaces are not properly distracted.

Overall, reported complications associated with hip arthroscopy are infrequent, but not insignificant. It is hoped that many of the problems encountered by the pioneers in this field do not have to be relearned by others. There is a learning curve associated with hip arthroscopy. However, knowledge of many of the potential complications can be gained through education and instruction and not necessarily through personal experience.

It is especially important to note that complications are usually reported by those most experienced in arthroscopic techniques. These are the surgeons who should have the best opportunity to have the lowest complication rate. Many serious problems, and the frequency with which they are encountered by inexperienced surgeons, may never be reported.

References

1. Committee on Complications of the Arthroscopy Association of North America: Complications in arthroscopy, the knee and other joints. Arthroscopy 1986;2:253–258.

2. Byrd JWT: Complications associated with hip arthroscopy. In: Byrd JWT (ed). Operative Hip Arthroscopy. New York: Thieme, 1998:171–176.

3. Glick JM: Complications of hip arthroscopy by the lateral approach. In: Sherman OH, Minkoff J (eds). Current Management of Complications in Orthopaedics: Arthroscopic Surgery. Baltimore: Williams & Wilkins 1990:193–201.

4. Funke EL, Munzinger U: Complications in hip arthroscopy. Arthroscopy 1996;12:156–159.

5. Griffin DR, Villar RN: Complications of arthroscopy of the hip. J Bone Joint Surg [Br] 1999;81:604–606.

6. Sampson TG: Complications of hip arthroscopy. Clin Sports Med 2001;20:831–835.

7. Byrd JWT, Pappas JN, Pedley MJ: Hip arthroscopy: an anatomic study of portal placement and relationship to the extraarticular structures. Arthroscopy 1995;11:418–423.

8. Eriksson E, Arvidsson I, Arvidsson H: Diagnostic and operative arthroscopy of the hip. Orthopaedics 1986;9:169–176.

9. Byrd JWT: Hip arthroscopy utilizing the supine position. Arthroscopy 1994;10:275–280.

10. Bartlett CS, DiFelice GS, Buly RL, et al: Cardiac arrest as a result of intraabdominal extravasation of fluid during arthroscopic removal of a loose body from the hip joint of a patient with an acetabular fracture. J Orthop Trauma 1998;12:294–299.

11. Byrd JWT: Avoiding the labrum in hip arthroscopy. Arthroscopy 2000;16:770–773.

12. Villar RN: Hip Arthroscopy. Oxford: Butterworth-Heinemann, 1992.

13. Lewallen DG: Heterotopic ossification following total hip arthroplasty. Instr Course Lect 1995;44:287–292.

14. Jaureguito JW, Greenwald AE, Wilcox JF, Paulos LE, Rosenberg TD: The incidence of deep venous thrombosis after arthroscopic knee surgery. Am J Sports Med 1999;27:707–710.

15. Williams JS Jr, Hulstyn MJ, Fadale PD, et al: Incidence of deep vein thrombosis after arthroscopic knee surgery: a prospective study. Arthroscopy 1995;11:701–705.

17

Rehabilitation

T. Kevin Robinson and Karen M. Griffin

The evolution of hip arthroscopy has necessitated a progression in hip rehabilitation to ensure optimal postsurgical results. Rehabilitative methodology and techniques commonly employed after minimally invasive surgical techniques for other joints, such as the knee, shoulder, elbow, and ankle, have found application in the management of hip disorders. Understanding and respecting basic principles is always key to maintaining successful outcomes with any technique.

Traditional issues in hip management focused on three areas: (1) maintaining protective weight-bearing status through gait training with hip fractures; (2) instruction in routine postoperative hip precautions following hip arthroplasty; and (3) instruction in modification of their environment and activities of daily living for arthritic patients attempting to live with their symptoms.

Hip pain is a common orthopedic complaint. Injuries of the hip and pelvis represent 5% to 6% of all injuries incurred by adult athletes and 10% to 24% of those in child athletes.[1] Certain activities have been found to have a higher incidence of hip pain. The occurrence of hip and pelvic injuries is especially common in ballet dancers (44%), soccer players (13%), and runners (11%).[1]

Arthroscopic assessment defines the presence of symptomatic hip pathology. Operative arthroscopy provides a less-invasive alternative to arthrotomy for some disorders and may offer definitive treatment for certain lesions of the labrum or articular surface.[2] Although the mechanical disorder can often be corrected through surgery; the functional deficit must be corrected through rehabilitation.[3]

The goal of the rehabilitation plan is to reduce symptoms (modulate pain and inflammation) and improve function (restore mobility, strength, proprioception, and endurance). This goal is approached through a systematic progression dependent on the patient's status (pathology present) and functional needs. During the assessment process, it is important to determine the patient's level of understanding regarding the pathology and expectations of goals and the time frame for achieving them. Patient education is the foundation of the rehabilitation plan. The patient must comprehend the related precautions and recommended progression per his or her individual situation. Through collaborative consultation with the physician concerning the specific patient cases, reasonable goals and expectations can be formulated for favorable outcomes.

ASSESSMENT

The physician's history, examination, and diagnostic studies determine the patient's diagnosis and prognosis of surgical or nonsurgical treatment. The patient's history and the clinical evaluation assist in determining how the symptoms will respond to treatment. A course of presurgical treatment (*prehab*) may be indicated in some hip cases to regain neuromotor control and decrease stresses to the joint. An appropriate exercise program can, at times, help restore normal mechanics and minimize joint stresses to facilitate healing. In other circumstances, it can *buy time* when a patient desires and the physician thinks it is beneficial to delay operative intervention. Rehabilitation of a patient preoperatively when the need for surgery has been confirmed better prepares patients psychologically and physically for postsurgical recovery.

Pathomechanics of the hip and pelvis are viewed as primarily reflecting the joint pathology and secondarily reflecting joint compensation. For example, for a patient with degenerative changes within the joint, the primary disorder is the antalgic gait caused by joint pain. Secondary dysfunction may ensue due to weakness of the gluteus medius, presenting as an abductor lurch (Trendelenburg's gait). Disorders of the sacroiliac joint (S-I joint) and lumbar spine also become considerations with chronic hip dysfunction because of altered gait and weight-bearing mechanics (Figures 17.1, 17.2).

The hip allows multidirectional mobility (Figure 17.3). Most activities do not occur in a specific plane but require combinations of movement. Activities of daily living such as sitting, walking, stair climbing, running, and squatting all require different functional ranges of motion. Common functional deficits include pain with prolonged sitting; difficulty donning socks or shoes; inability to squat or sit on low surfaces; and altered gait with a shortened stance phase, protraction

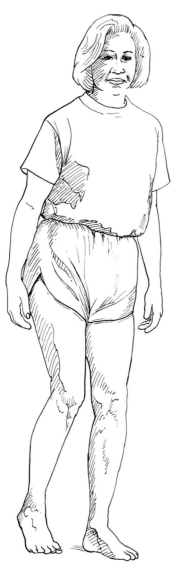

FIGURE 17.1. With a painful hip, the stance phase of gait is shortened. Hip extension is avoided by keeping the joint in a slightly flexed position. This slight flexion creates a functional leg length discrepancy with shortening on the involved side and may partially create a lurch.

of the hip, and decreased hip extension on the involved side. Normal gait uses multiplanar hip motion of 15 degrees of extension, 37 degrees of flexion, 7 degrees of abduction, 5 degrees of adduction, 4 degrees of internal rotation, and 9 degrees of external rotation[4] (Figure 17.4). Ascending stairs requires the motion of a normal walking pattern with additional 67 degrees of flexion and creates a force of three times body weight. Standing on one leg creates a force of two and one-half times, while loads approaching eight times body weight occur in the hip joint during jogging, with potentially greater loads resulting from vigorous athletic competition[5] (Figure 17.5).

These parameters must be considered when assessing sports injuries and the sport-specific demands on return to competition. It is estimated that a healthy hip joint can tolerate a force of approximately 12 to 15 times body weight.[6]

The clinical assessment includes observation of gait and basic functional transitional movements such as sitting to standing to sitting, ascending and descending stairs, and balance activities. It also includes understanding the patient's specific movement patterns and what elicits the pain symptoms; balance testing; assessment of involvement of the lumbar spine, pelvis, sacroiliac joint, and knee; range of motion and muscle testing; palpation; and special hip tests that may be indicated for flexibility and differentiation.

Primary problems of symptomatic hip pathology may involve the soft tissue encasing the joint, the surrounding capsule, or the joint structure. The irritation and inflammation of the musculotendinous structures, bursae, or joint capsule can result in concomitant tendonitis, bursitis, or capsulitis. The ligaments of the hip joint are susceptible to acute tearing and chronic degeneration. Within the joint, labral or chondral injury can be responsible for protracted hip symptoms. Loose bodies and labral lesions are well-recognized indications for arthroscopic surgery, which tends to produce gratifying results for properly selected patients.[7]

The acetabular labrum is a fibrocartilaginous rim around the perimeter of the acetabulum and is triangular in cross section. The labrum is thicker postero-superiorly and thinner anteroinferiorly.[8–11] The labrum is attached to the osseous rim of the acetabulum and blends with the transverse ligament at the margins of the acetabular notch. The labrum deepens the acetabulum and is thought to assist in the constraint of the femoral head within the bony socket.[12] Several studies have described a thickening or hyperplasia of the acetabular labrum in diseased states, expecially developmental dysplasia of the hip.[13–15] This finding supports the theory of the functional importance in restraint of the femoral head within the acetabulum.[12]

Free nerve endings and sensory organs have been found in the superficial layers of the acetabular labrum. It is believed that these free nerve endings contribute to nociceptive and proprioceptive mechanisms.[16] The acetabular labrum may also improve the stability of the hip joint by maintaining a negative intraarticular pressure.[17]

The clinical presentation of a patient with an acetabular labral tear is similar to the patient presentation with a meniscal tear. The patient can complain of a sharp *catching* pain that is often associated with a popping and a sensation of locking or giving way of the joint.[15,18,19] Patients can have pain in the anterior groin, anterior thigh, buttock, greater trochanter, and medial knee. The reason for the variety in location of complaints of pain is that the sensory supply to the hip joint is 65% from the obturator nerve, so pain in this area is referred to the groin and the medial aspect of the knee. Approximately 30% of the sensory dis-

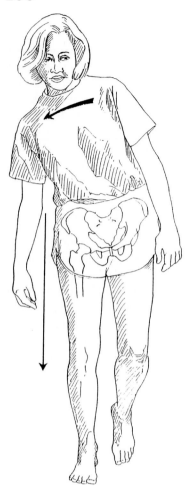

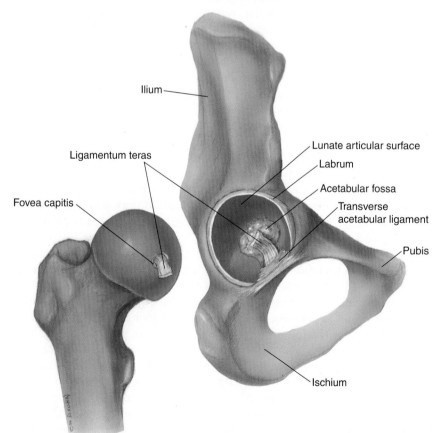

FIGURE 17.2. An abductor lurch may occur as a compensatory mechanism to reduce the forces across the joint. By shifting the torso over the involved hip, the center of gravity is moved closer to the axis of the hip, shortening the lever arm moment and reducing compressive joint forces.

Ilium

Ligamentum teras

Fovea capitis

Lunate articular surface

Labrum

Acetabular fossa

Transverse acetabular ligament

Pubis

Ischium

FIGURE 17.3. The ball-and-socket configuration of the hip allows multiplanar motion.

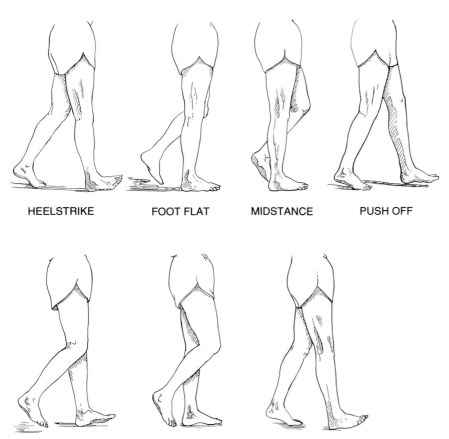

HEELSTRIKE FOOT FLAT MIDSTANCE PUSH OFF

ACCELERATION MIDSWING DECELERATION

FIGURE 17.4. Normal gait uses multiplanar hip motion.

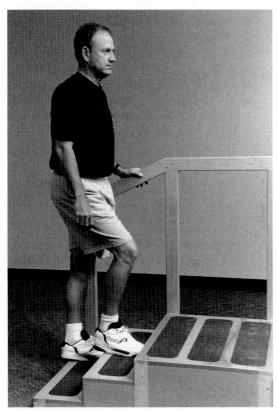

FIGURE 17.5. Ascending stairs, in a reciprocal fashion, requires a greater degree of hip flexion.

tribution is from the femoral nerve, which refers to the anterior portion of the thigh. The remaining sensory distribution is from a branch of the sciatic nerve; therefore, the pain is referred to the buttock[20] (Figure 17.6). In a retrospective study, McCarthy and associates reviewed 94 consecutive patients with intractable hip pain who underwent hip arthroscopy. They found statistically significant associations between the preoperative clinical presentation and arthroscopic operative findings. Acetabular labral tears detected arthroscopically correlated significantly with symptoms of anterior inquinal pain ($r = 1$), painful clicking episodes ($r = 0.809$), transient locking ($r = 0.307$), and giving way ($r = 0.320$). Byrd found the most common injury mechanism was hip hyperextension combined with external rotation causing an anterior acetabular labral tear. Axial loading of the hip in a flexed position was the most common mechanism for a posterior acetabular labral tear.[7]

Secondary problems can occur, such as joint mobility limitations analogous to adhesive capsulitis of the shoulder. Over time, limited joint motion and postural alterations can transfer into faulty mechanics and compensatory stress of joints above or below the hip. Additional musculoskeletal pain syndromes and functional limitation can develop. Secondary knee irritation or lumbopelvic problems are common and

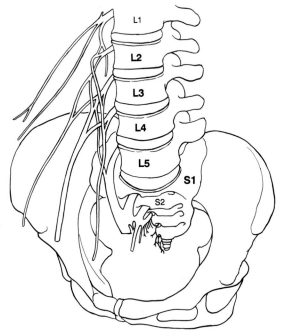

FIGURE 17.6. The hip receives innervation predominately from the L2–S1 nerve roots of the lumbosacral plexus.

may need to be addressed in the rehabilitation of the total kinetic chain and integrated functional unit.

Because of the mobile ball-and-socket configuration of the hip joint, few functional movements are uniplanar. However, for examination purposes, the six principal directions of movement are flexion, extension, abduction, adduction, internal rotation, and external rotation (Figure 17.7). The typical capsular pattern of restriction is characterized by a gross limitation of flexion, abduction, and internal rotation with minimal loss of extension and external rotation.[21–23] The capsular pattern indicates the capsule of the joint is affected. This is a common finding following an arthroscopic procedure. The joint is distended with saline during the procedure, and any bleeding that occurs from arthroscopic debridement within the joint can cause inflammation of the synovial lining of the joint.

Normal parameters of range of motion can vary greatly. Goniometric measurements of passive range of motion (PROM) are taken bilaterally of the patient's hip and knee joints. Typically, in the prone position, the hip can be extended 30 degrees (Figure 17.8). In the supine position, hip flexion requires that the contralateral extremity be flat on the table to eliminate accessory or compensatory movement that can occur due to pelvic tilt.

Recording abduction and adduction requires that the pelvis again be stabilized to eliminate accessory movement that may falsely indicate greater range of motion. Abduction averages 45 to 50 degrees and adduction 20 to 30 degrees (Figure 17.9). With the hip

flexed 90 degrees, internal rotation averages 35 degrees and external rotation averages 45 degrees (Figure 17.10).[24]

A succinct abbreviated examination can be used to quickly determine if there is any gross restriction in range of motion of the hip:

- To test for abduction, have the patient stand and spread his or her legs as far apart as possible. One should be able to abduct approximately 45 degrees from the midline (Figure 17.11).
- For adduction, instruct the patient to alternately cross his or her legs while standing. One should be able to achieve approximately 20 degrees of adduction (Figure 17.12).
- For flexion, have the patient draw each knee to the chest as far as possible without bending the back (Figure 17.13).
- For combined flexion and adduction, have the patient sit in a chair and alternately cross one thigh over the other (Figure 17.14).
- For extension, have the patient sit in a chair with the arms folded across the chest and then rise to a standing position (Figure 17.15).

The Thomas test can alternately be used to quantitate hip flexion or the presence of a hip flexion contracture (Figures 17.16, 17.17). For measuring flexion, the knee is brought toward the chest. The contralateral hip is maintained in extension and the degree of flexion of the hip being examined is recorded. Conversely, for assessing a flexion contracture, the knee of the contralateral extremity is brought maximally to the chest. The hip being examined is then brought toward extension. Inability to lay the leg flat on the table reflects a hip flexion contracture. Inordinate tightness of the iliotibial band can most easily be detected using the Ober test. The patient is positioned on his or her side with the suspect hip placed up. With the hip extended and knee flexed, limitation of passive adduction is indicative of a tight iliotibial band (Figure 17.18).

Strength of the hip muscles is assessed using manual muscle tests as described by Hislop and Montgomery.[25] Intrarater reliability of manual muscle testing grades has been found to be reliable by several authors.[26,27]

Common physical findings include (1) pain elicited by internal rotation of the hip joint flexed at 90 degrees[19]; (2) pain elicited by axial compression of the hip joint flexed at 90 degrees; (3) pain and/or a popping sensation with a Thomas test[15,28]; and (4) a positive hip extension test. This test is performed with the patient in a prone position.[15,29] The patient's affected lower extremity is passively taken into combined extension and external rotation. A positive test result is replication of the patient's pain and/or a popping sensation.[21] In a retrospective study comparing

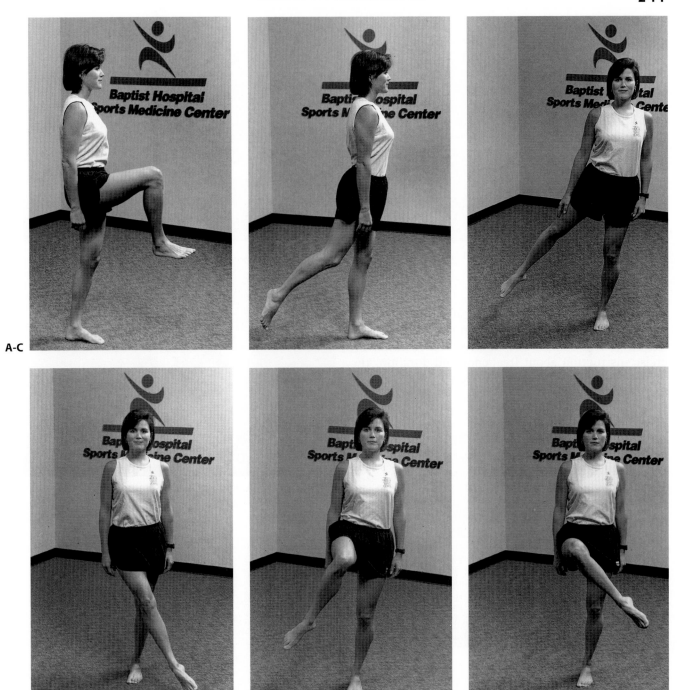

A-C

D-F

FIGURE 17.7. The six principal directions of movement are demonstrated for the right hip: (A) flexion; (B) extension; (C) abduction; (D) adduction; (E) internal rotation; and (F) external rotation.

preoperative clinical findings with arthroscopic findings, McCarthy et al. found that a positive hip extension test was correlated with an arthroscopic finding of an acetabular labral tear ($r = 0.676$).[20]

TREATMENT AND REHABILITATION PROGRESSION

From the clinician's subjective and objective assessment and the information provided by the physician,

specific areas of concern and needs will be identified. The rehabilitative treatment plan after arthroscopic hip surgery depends on the pathology recognized and the arthroscopic methods used. To achieve the overall goals for an individual patient, the clinician must assess what instruction, monitoring, and equipment are necessary and must gauge the intensiveness or aggressiveness of the patients's functional progression. For example, a patient with significant degenerative changes will have a slower recovery, dictated prima-

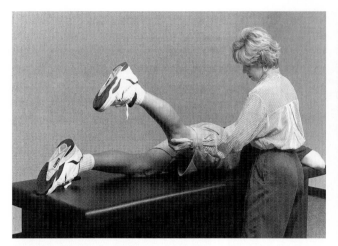

FIGURE 17.8. With the patient positioned prone, the hip is maximally extended 30 degrees.

rily by the symptoms. For this patient, a primarily home-based rehabilitation program may suffice. It relies on patient compliance, however. After initial exercise instruction about frequency and duration, the program can often be accomplished with the simplest

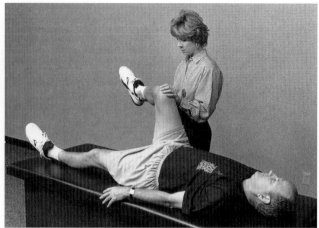

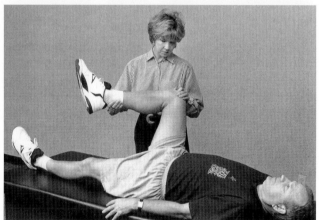

FIGURE 17.10. (A, B) With the hip flexed 90 degrees, maximal internal and external rotation are recorded.

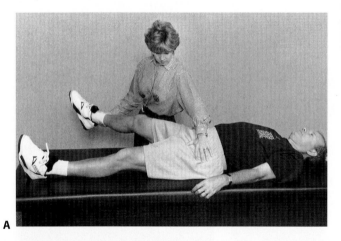

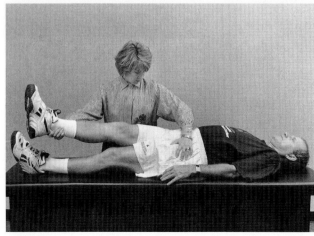

FIGURE 17.9. (A, B) Abduction and adduction are measured. Care is taken to avoid accessory movement by keeping the pelvis stable.

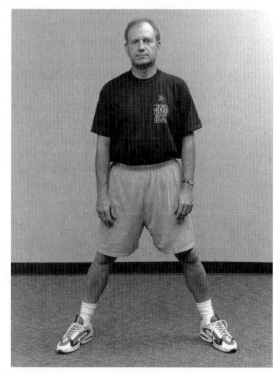

FIGURE 17.11. A quick test of abduction is performed by asking the patient to stand and spread his or her legs as far apart as possible.

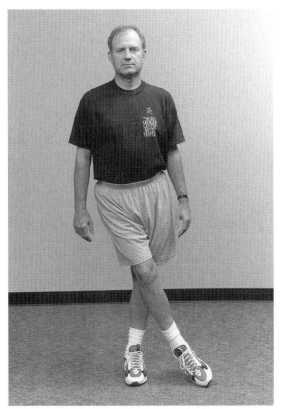

FIGURE 17.12. Adduction is checked by asking the patient to alternately cross his or her legs.

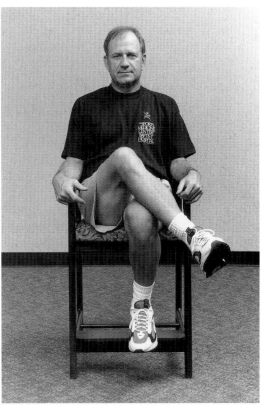

FIGURE 17.14. Combined flexion and adduction are checked by alternately crossing one thigh over the other in a seated position.

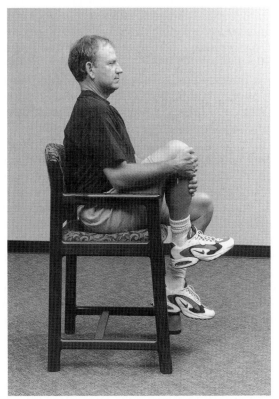

FIGURE 17.13. Flexion can be estimated by having the patient draw the knee toward the chest as far as possible without bending the back.

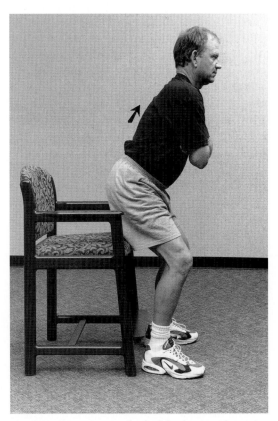

FIGURE 17.15. Extension is checked by having the patient rise from a seated position with arms folded across the chest.

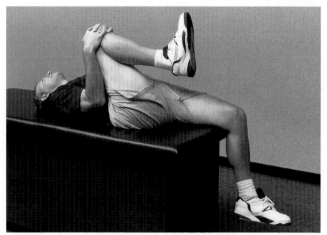

FIGURE 17.16. The Thomas test allows more accurate quantification of hip flexion. Accessory movement via pelvic tilt is eliminated by maintaining the contralateral hip in maximal extension. Flexion of the examined hip is then recorded.

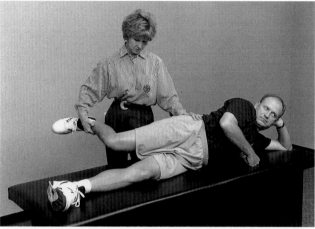

FIGURE 17.18. The Ober test assesses tightness of the iliotibial band. With the patient positioned on his or her side, the hip is extended and the knee flexed. Limitation of passive adduction is then indicative of a tight iliotibial band.

home equipment. For a patient undergoing abrasion arthroplasty, the rehabilitation process is much more deliberate, with a prolonged interval of protected weight bearing. During this time, the intensity of rehabilitation is conservative and often may be accomplished easily with an independent program and only occasional supervision. Conversely, an athlete with a labral tear and otherwise healthy joint may be expected to progress much more aggressively through the protocol phases with the anticipation of regaining full function and return to sports. In this case, the clinical environment, or at least access to a well-equipped workout facility, is preferred. More clinical attention is necessary to gauge the patient's response and ensure safe progression.

Postoperative recovery actually begins with the preoperative educational process. This may be a struc-

tured prehabilitation program that addresses impairments such as pain, swelling, postural deviations, compensated mobility, muscle length and muscle strength, decreased proprioception, and muscular and cardiovascular endurance. Hip pain may alter lumbopelvic hip movement patterns that lead to impairments of muscular balances and faulty mechanics. In other cases, a single comprehensive preoperative visit for instruction, explanation, and demonstration of the expected postoperative rehabilitation protocol is all that is needed. The patient should be aware that the rehabilitation responsibilities begin even before leaving the outpatient area. Many of the initial exercises can be performed independently, but the patient should understand the importance of beginning isometric contractions at the hip and ankle plantarflexion and dorsiflexion pumps to facilitate lower extremity circulation (Appendix A).

The patient's weight-bearing status can vary depending on the surgeon's findings and procedure performed. Typically, weight bearing is allowed as tolerated, and crutches are discontinued within the first week. Although the discomfort associated with arthroscopy might be surprisingly little, there can still be a significant amount of reflex inhibition and poor muscle firing as a result of the combination of penetration with the arthroscopic portals and the traction applied during the procedure. The gluteus medius muscle is a prime example of this. In a typical arthroscopic procedure the anterolateral and posterolateral portals pass through this muscle. Clinically, it is common for the patient to have a difficult time regaining muscle tone and appropriate firing of this muscle after surgery. This problem is analogous to the effects of an arthroscopic knee surgery on the vastus medialis muscle. Functionally, this muscle is needed to maintain a level pelvis during ambulation. Addi-

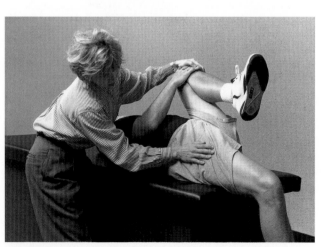

FIGURE 17.17. Conversely, the Thomas test can be used to check for a flexion contracture. The contralateral extremity is drawn maximally toward the chest. The examined hip is then extended. Inability to lay the leg flat on the table reflects a hip flexion contracture.

tionally, due to the short moment arm of the gluteus medius, this muscle causes a large joint compression force when it contracts during the single limb stance phase of gait.[5] In a patient with hip articular pathology it is common to find inhibition of the gluteus medius muscle as a result of pain. Consequently, assistive devices are helpful to reestablish a normal gait pattern and synchronous muscle activity. The most effective method of neutralizing compressive forces across the hip is to allow the patient to apply the equivalent weight of the leg on the ground (Figure 17.19). Maintaining a true nonweight-bearing status requires significant muscle force to suspend the extremity off the ground, thus generating considerable dynamic compression across the joint as a result of muscle contraction. Resting the weight of the leg on the ground neutralizes this dynamic compressive effect of the muscles. Additionally, simple devices such as insoles may help to relieve compressive stress for some patients.

Muscle-toning exercises are performed within the first week after surgery. These exercises require progression dependent on the patient's tolerance but should not be overly aggressive. Isometric exercises are the simplest and least likely to aggravate underlying joint symptoms: these include isometric sets for the gluteals, quadriceps, hamstrings, adductor and abductor muscle groups, and lower abdominals. Addi-

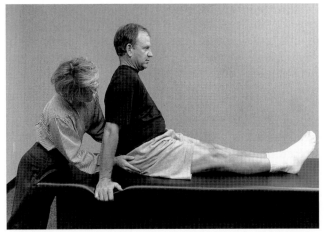

FIGURE 17.20. Gluteal isometrics may decrease overactivity of the iliopsoas and provide a decrease in anterior hip pain.

tionally, isometric contraction of the antagonistic muscle group may inhibit spasms and promote pain relief. Gluteal isometrics may decrease overactivity of the iliopsoas and provide a decrease in anterior hip pain (Figure 17.20) (Appendix B).

An aquatic program is often beneficial for allowing early return to exercise and can begin as soon as the portal sites have healed and the sutures have been removed. A pool program allows for earlier joint mobilization and gentle strengthening in a reduced-weight environment. The water buoyancy can provide assistance to movement in all planes as safer resistance with increased active exercises (Figure 17.21). Gait activities can be progressed in waist-deep water with minimized compression of the surgical site (Appendix C).

Active assisted range-of-motion exercises are begun early. These are then progressed to active range of motion, gravity-assisted, and then to gravity-resisted exercises during the postoperative recovery. Exercises

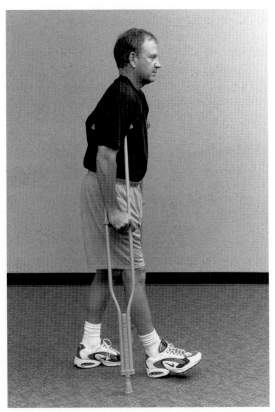

FIGURE 17.19. Protected weight bearing allows gradual transference of weight to the affected extremity.

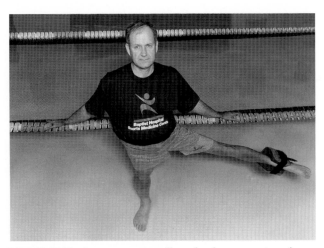

FIGURE 17.21. A water program allows for the progression of many exercises in a reduced-weight environment.

are directed in all planes of hip motion, and the end ranges of motion are determined by the patient's level of discomfort (Appendix D). Stretching is typically pushed only to tolerance, and the patient is educated as to these parameters. Pushing the extremes of range of motion does little to enhance function and may exacerbate discomfort. An exception to this is after excision of large bony osteophytes that had created a prominent bony block to motion. Aggressive early stretching under these circumstances can regain the previously blocked motion and might indeed improve function when there was a significant mechanical block. Manual mobilization techniques can assist in the reduction of compressive forces across the articular surfaces. This reduction may lessen discomfort, and over time enhance cartilage healing.[30] Small accessory oscillation movements stimulate joint mechanoreceptors, assisting in pain modulation. Graded mobilization with flexion and adduction movement or internal rotation is gently implemented with the moderately painful joint.[21]

Distraction techniques (longitudinal movement) are most useful when hip movements are painful. Oscillatory longitudinal movements are produced by pulling gently on the femur (Figure 17.22). This technique can be assisted by a rolling or sliding motion by the clinician with support under the patient's thigh in the direction of the treatment movement and can be performed in varying degrees of hip flexion (Figure 17.23). Oscillatory movements in a compression mode, stopping short of the pain position, can be helpful, especially for patients with pain on weight bearing.

Very little posteroanterior movement of the femoral head takes place within the acetabulum, but anterior and posterior glides can also be beneficial for the painful hip joint (Figure 17.24). It can also be used as an accessory movement at the limit of physiologic range when a goal of treatment is to increase the range of motion of the joint.[21] The presence of a capsular pattern of the hip as described by Cyriax is often found secondary to the postoperative effusion. Characteristic of that pattern is a gross limitation of flexion, abduction, and internal rotation, with minimal loss of extension and external rotation.[31]

Joint range of motion is normalized by restoring capsular extensibility. Limitation of hip flexion and internal rotation commonly occurs because of posterior capsular restrictions. In cases with painful restricted motion, the clinician must assess carefully whether mobilization techniques are a viable treatment option, depending on the physical status of the hip joint and the psychologic status of the patient. Because of apprehension or other psychomotor factors, some patients may not be good candidates for application of these techniques.

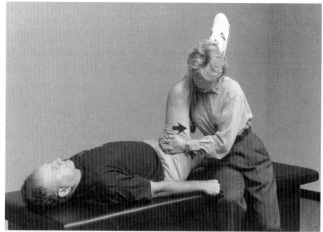

FIGURE 17.23. To perform inferior glides, the patient's lower leg rests on the therapist's shoulder. The therapist then manually applies a distraction force on the anterior proximal thigh.

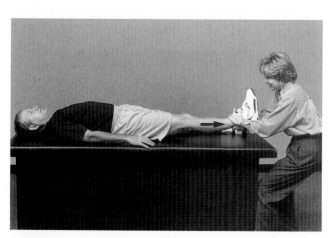

FIGURE 17.22. Straight plane distraction is demonstrated by applying an axial traction force on the extremity.

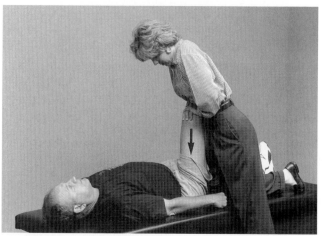

FIGURE 17.24. For posterior glides, the therapist applies pressure downward on the knee, creating posterior translation of the femoral head relative to the acetabulum.

NEUROMOTOR CONTROL

Proprioceptive deficits routinely occur in conjunction with articular injuries. The acetabular labrum contains free nerve endings and sensory organs. It is believed that these free nerve endings contribute in nociceptive and proprioceptive mechanisms.[16] The acetabular labrum also improves the stability of the hip joint by maintaining a negative intraarticular pressure.[17] With injury to the labrum, this negative pressure is lost and stability of the hip is adversely affected, inhibiting normal motor response and decreasing neuromuscular stabilization of the joint. The aim of proprioceptive retraining is to restore these deficits and assist in reestablishing neuromotor control. The elements necessary for reestablishing neuromuscular control are proprioception, dynamic joint stability, reactive neuromuscular control, and functional motor pathways. Joint positioning tasks early in the rehabilitative process can enhance proprioceptive and kinesthetic awareness.[32] More advanced proprioceptive neuromuscular techniques incorporated in functional patterns of movement or modified ranges may be acceptable transition exercises, depending on the symptoms and status of the hip.

Dynamic stabilization exercises encourage muscular cocontractions to balance joint forces. Closed-chain methods allow progressive weight-bearing trans-

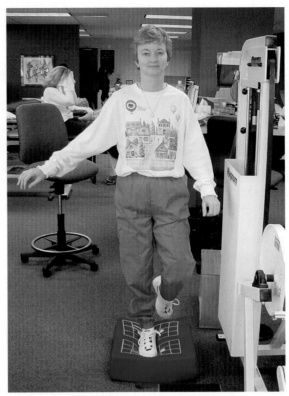

FIGURE 17.26. Reestablishing neuromuscular control may begin with simple static balance maneuvers evolving to single stance with balance devices with or without visual input.

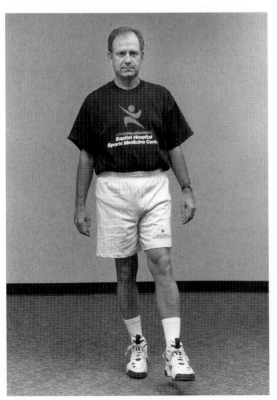

FIGURE 17.25. Controlled single-leg stance exercises facilitate pelvic toning and stimulate proprioceptive and balance functions in a closed-chain fashion.

ference to the lower extremity in a manner that lessens the shear and translational forces across the joint surface.[33,34] This begins with simple static balance maneuvers, starting with full stance, and evolving to single stance, with and without visual input (Figure 17.25). Progression is then made to a combination of balance and strength activities. Bilateral heel raises and mini-squats are progressed to unilateral heel raises and mini-squats. More advanced closed kinetic exercises such as increased partial squats, lunges, and dynamic weight shifts are encouraged initially in the pool. Low-force, slow-speed, and controlled activities may be transitioned to high progressive force, fast-speed, and uncontrolled activities if the joint allows without becoming overstressed. For example, balance devices, mini-trampolines, and unlimited creative upper extremity activities while balancing can further challenge the neuromuscular system (Figure 17.26).

Core stability is an exceedingly important, yet often overlooked, aspect of hip rehabilitation after both injury and surgery and may be especially critical in optimizing performance and minimizing the risk of reinjury. Core stabilization/strengthening emphasizes training of the trunk musculature to develop better pelvic stability and abdominal control (Figure 17.27). Often, patients develop the strength, power, and endurance of specific extremity musculature to perform required activities but are deficient in muscular

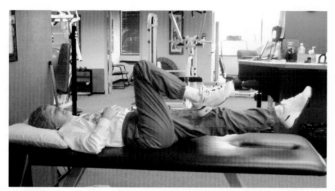

FIGURE 17.27. Beginning core stabilization emphasizes training of the trunk musculature to develop better stability and abdominal control.

strength of the lumbopelvic–hip complex. The core stabilization system must be specifically checked as part of the assessment and challenged as part of the rehabilitation program (Appendix E). An effective core stabilization system and strong lumbopelvic–hip musculature complex as an integrated functional unit is important for efficient weight distribution, absorption, and transfer of compressive forces.

Static stabilization, transitional stabilization, and dynamic stabilization are phases of progression from closed-chain loading and unloading, to conscious controlled motion with high joint tolerance, and ultimately to unconscious control and loading of the joint. Thus, depending on the patient's tolerance, the exer-

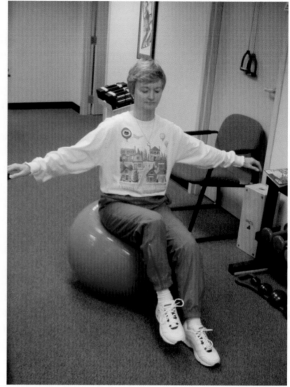

FIGURE 17.29. Depending on the patient's tolerance, the stabilization program may progress to complex on an unstable surface without visual input.

cise program may progress from slow to fast, simple to complex, stable to unstable, low force to high force, and general to specific[34,35] (Figures 17.28, 17.29).

Pilates exercises can be an adjunct to progression during the dynamic stability phase of rehabilitation, facilitating improved flexibility, joint mobility, and strength. The Pilates Reformer, an apparatus with cables, pulleys, springs, and sliding boards, is the foundation equipment of Pilates. This low-impact pro-

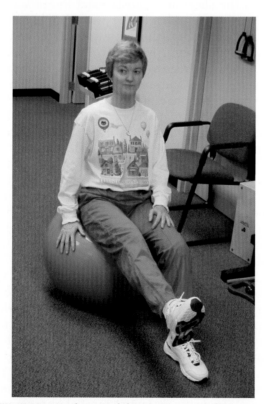

FIGURE 17.28. Initial core stabilization on gym ball may progress with hip flexion and knee extension.

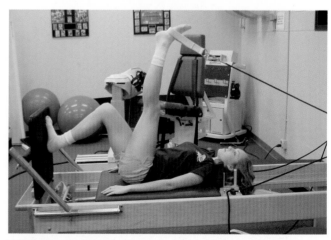

FIGURE 17.30. Pilates exercises with use of a Pilates Reformer can be an adjunct to progression during the dynamic stability phase of rehabilitation, facilitating improved flexibility, joint mobility, and strength.

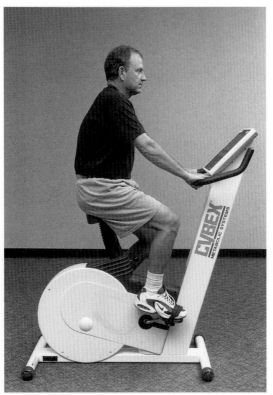

FIGURE 17.31. Used properly, a stationary bicycle can be useful to enhance smooth, fluid joint motion. The resistance is kept low. Initially, the seat is raised high, and then lowered as mobility improves.

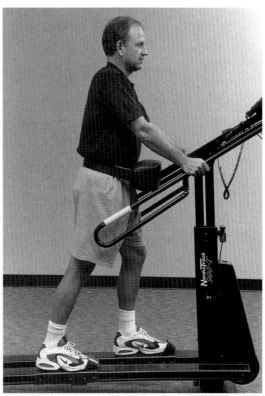

FIGURE 17.32. Performance on a NordicTrack or Elliptical Crosstrainer is better tolerated by some than others. Both are excellent devices for gradually enhancing endurance and strength, maintaining low impact.

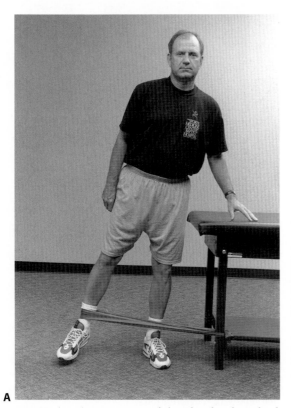

A

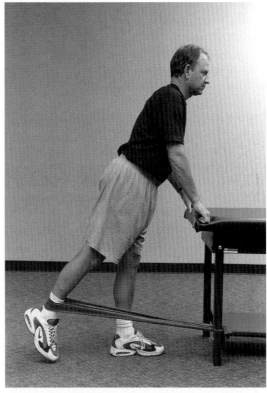

B

FIGURE 17.33. (A, B) Various uses of the Theraband can be devised for gentle hip abductor and extensor muscle strengthening.

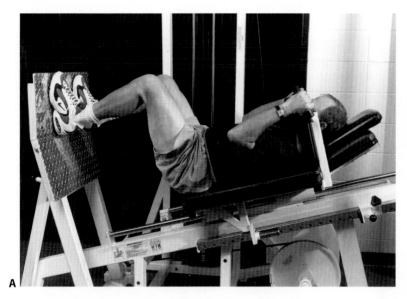

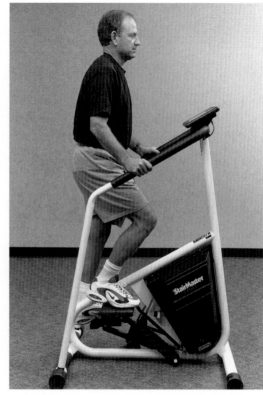

FIGURE 17.34. (A, B) Closed-chain activity on the leg press or StairMaster can generate high compressive forces across the joint and should be judiciously introduced.

gression uses the patient's body weight as resistance with the specialized equipment or mat exercises with a series emphasizing core stabilization and strengthening (Figure 17.30).

Functional progression during the rehabilitation program depends on the type of hip pathology present and the specific demands of the patient's anticipated activities. During the recovery phase, equipment may be used in a low-impact mode, such as a stationary bicycle, elliptical crosstrainer, cross-country ski machine, or water treadmill (Figures 17.31, 17.32). These devices may enhance mobility and encourage dynamic eccentric and concentric strengthening and endurance. Closed-chain activity on the stair machine or leg press and open-chain activities can generate high compressive and shear forces across the joint; these should be judiciously introduced (Figures 17.33, 17.34, 17.35).

Functional exercises simulating the patient's daily activities or sport-specific program must be individualized to meet the patient's goals. These exercises must be kept within the constraints as dictated by the type of hip pathology that has been addressed. Improving quality of life is certainly a goal of arthroscopic procedures, but this must be kept within the framework of a realistic outlook.

One unique feature of the hip compared with many other joints is that limitation of motion often does not represent a significant functional problem. Certainly

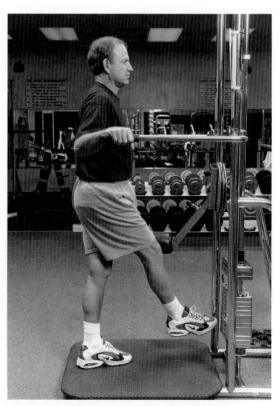

FIGURE 17.35. A multi-hip weight machine may be used in the final phases of rehabilitation.

optimizing motion is an integral part of rehabilitation management, but this must be kept in perspective. Remember that the common goals of hip rehabilitation are to reduce discomfort and improve function. Motion should not be pushed to the point of inordinately accentuating symptoms.

For some cases, depending on the extent of pathology and the extent of surgical debridement, the explosive character of compressive forces generated by certain specific physical and sports activities may need to be curtailed or modified with substitutions that the joint can tolerate during healing. In fact, some patients or athletes may need to change the sport position or the sport altogether. Last, the clinician must ensure that the patient's expectations and the goals of rehabilitation coincide by emphasizing education for current and future hip management. The patient's compliance with a continued management program should include maintaining muscle balance (strength, flexibility, proprioception) and improving overall function.

References

1. Boyd KT, Peirce NS, Batt ME: Common hip injuries in sport. Sports Med 1997;24:273–280.
2. Byrd JWT: Hip arthroscopy utilizing the supine position. Arthroscopy 1994;10(3):275–280.
3. Henry C, Middleton K, Byrd JWT: Hip rehabilitation following arthroscopy. IOI Theater (videotape). Presented at AAOS annual meeting, Orlando, FL, February 1995.
4. Norkin C, Levangie PK: Joint Structure and Function: A Comprehensive Analysis, 2nd ed. Philadelphia: Davis, 1992: 300–332.
5. Crowninsheild RD, Johnston RC, Andrews JG, et al: A biomechanical investigation of the human hip. J Biomech 1978;11: 75–85.
6. Byrd JW: Labral lesions: an elusive source of hip pain: case reports and literature review. Arthroscopy 1996;12:603–612.
7. Edwards DJ, Lomas D, Villar RN: Diagnosis of the painful hip by magnetic resonance imaging and arthroscopy. Radiology 1996;200:225–230.
8. Petersilge CA, Hague MA, Petersilge WJ, et al: Acetabular labral tears: evaluation with MR arthrography. Radiology 1996; 200:231–235.
9. Keene GS, Villar RN: Arthroscopic anatomy of the hip: an in vivo study. Arthroscopy 1994;10:392–399.
10. Cotton A, Boutry N, Demondion X, et al: Acetabular labrum: MRI in asymptomatic volunteers. J Comput Assist Tomogr 1998;22:1–7.
11. Mason JB: Acetabular labral tears in the athlete. Clin Sports Med 2000;20:779–790.
12. Ikeda T, Awaya G, Suzuki S, et al: Torn acetabular labrum in young patients. J Bone Joint Surg 1988;70:13–16.
13. McCarthy JC, Mason JB, Wardell SR: Hip arthroscopy for acetabular dysplasia: a pipe dream? Orthopedics 1998;21:997–999.
14. McCarthy JC, Busconi B: The role of hip arthroscopy in the diagnosis and treatment of hip disease. Orthopedics 1995;18: 753–756.
15. Kim YT, Azusa H: The nerve endings of the acetabular labrum. Clin Orthop 1995;320:176–181.
16. Takechi H, Nagashima H, Ito S: Intra-articular pressure of the hip joint outside and inside the limbus. J Jpn Orthop Assoc 1982;56:529–536.
17. Farjo LA, Glick JM, Sampson TG: Hip arthroscopy for acetabular labral tears. Arthroscopy 1999;15:132–137.
18. Hase T, Ueo T: Acetabular labral tear: arthroscopic diagnosis and treatment. Arthroscopy 1999;15:138–141.
19. Johnson EW: Location of hip pain. JAMA 1979;242:1849.
20. McCarthy J, Day B, Busconi B: Hip arthroscopy: applications and technique. J Am Acad Orthop Surg 1995;3:115–122.
21. Maitland GD: Peripheral Manipulation. Boston: Butterworth, 1977:207–229.
22. Magee DJ: Orthopedic Physical Assessment, 3rd ed. Philadelphia: Saunders, 1997:20–26.
23. Norkin CC, White DJ: Measurement of Joint Motion: A Guide to Goniometry. Philadelphia: Davis, 1985.
24. American Academy of Orthopaedic Surgeons: Joint Motion: Method of Measuring and Recording. Chicago: American Academy of Orthopaedic Surgeons, 1965.
25. Hislop HJ, Montgomery J: Daniels and Worthingham's Muscle Testing: Techniques of Manual Examination, 6th ed. Philadelphia: Saunders, 1995.
26. Frese E, Brown M, Norton BJ: Clinical reliability of manual muscle testing: middle trapezius and gluteus medius muscles. Phys Ther 1987;67:1072–1076.
27. Wadsworth CT, Krishnan R, Sear M, et al: Intrarater reliability of manual muscle testing and handheld dynamometric muscle testing. Phys Ther 1987;67:1342–1347.
28. Fitzgerald RH: Acetabular labrum tears: diagnosis and treatment. Clin Orthop 1995;311:60–68.
29. Santori N, Villar RN: Acetabular labral tears: result of arthroscopic partial limbectomy. Arthroscopy 2000;16:11–15.
30. Salter RB, Simmonds DF, Malcolm BW, et al: The biological effect of continuous passive motion on the healing of full-thickness defects in articular cartilage. J Bone Joint Surg 1980; 62A:1232–1251.
31. Cyriax J: Textbook of Orthopaedic Medicine: Diagnosis of Soft Tissue Lesions, 7th ed. London: Bailliere Tindall, 1978:78–84.
32. Voight M: Reactive neuromuscular training. Presented at Tennessee Athletic Trainers Society (TATS) annual meeting, Nashville, TN, January 2000.
33. Clark M: Core stabilization training. Advanced track seminar. Presented at National Athletic Trainers Association (NATA) annual conference, Nashville, TN, June 2000.
34. Sahrmann S: Diagnosis and treatment of muscle imbalances and musculoskeletal pain syndrome. Advanced track seminar. Presented at NATA annual conference, Nashville, TN, June 2000.

18

Clinical Nursing Care

Kay S. Jones

In hip arthroscopy, the physician places great emphasis on patient selection, the surgical procedure, and the rehabilitation process after surgery. It is also important to provide the necessary nursing care to the patient during this time of disability and altered functional state. The role of the clinical nurse is multifaceted and is an integral part of the patient's perioperative experience. The nurse's role commences when the decision for surgery is made and continues until recuperation and rehabilitation are complete and the surgeon releases the patient. Many of the clinical nurse's efforts are spent preparing the patient and the patient's family for the postoperative period, ensuring that their expectations are reasonable and appropriate and that they can adequately handle what is to come.

The clinical nurse provides comprehensive care, education, continuity, and support to patients undergoing hip arthroscopy. The nurse serves as a resource person, not only for the patients, but also for the surgeon, outpatient personnel, physical therapists, and other ancillary agencies. This role includes consulting and collaborating with others to help increase the effectiveness, efficiency, and safety of the care rendered to the patient. The clinical nurse also serves as the primary facilitator of communication among members of the health care team.

As health care resources and patient needs become more sophisticated, so must the skills of the person to whom the patients and staff turn for assistance and direction. To function most effectively in these multiple roles, the clinical nurse must be knowledgeable of all aspects of hip arthroscopy including anatomy and physical examination of the hip, the surgical procedure and its indications, expected outcomes, possible complications, and the postoperative rehabilitation process. This knowledge equips the nurse to provide the necessary nursing care and enables the implementation of the nurse's roles of educator, practitioner, consultant, and collaborator.

PREOPERATIVE CARE

Outpatient surgery is routine for many surgical procedures. It is advantageous because it reduces costs and allows patients to recuperate in their own environments. This approach requires that the patient and caregivers become actively involved in and responsible for the perioperative care.1 The clinical nurse's preparation of the patient starts with the first visit to the orthopedic surgeon's office. This visit may be for diagnostic purposes, or conservative measures for reducing the patient's discomfort may be rendered. The decision for surgery may be made at this time. It is important for the clinical nurse to establish an open and trusting relationship with the patient and other caregivers from the first encounter. It is through this special relationship and unique interaction that the foundation for the perioperative course is laid.

The clinical nurse also provides continuity of care through direct patient contact. Thus, there is one person in the surgeon's office with whom the patient can feel comfortable conversing and asking questions. The clinical nurse is there to help the patient and their caregivers manage their anxiety and to provide information regarding diagnoses, testing, surgery, and postoperative recovery.

It is important that the clinical nurse take a comprehensive systematic approach to the nursing care of the patient undergoing hip arthroscopy. The nurse must demonstrate an aptitude to foresee and discuss care options including potential short-term and long-term consequences. The clinical nurse continually assesses, diagnoses, plans, intervenes, and evaluates the patient's plan of care.

NURSING HEALTH HISTORY

The clinical nurse must spend enough time with the patient to obtain an adequate nursing health history. This step is done on the patient's first visit to the surgeon's office. This history is a composition of subjective and objective data that will assist the nurse in identifying nursing diagnoses and collaborative health problems. Patients are often referred for this procedure by their primary care physicians or other orthopedic surgeons. They may already have received advice on the role of hip arthroscopy that may or may not be entirely accurate. Perhaps of even greater significance, many patients are taking a more active role in their health management and present to the physician's office with extensive information, usually obtained from the Internet. The accuracy of this information can be highly variable. The clinical nurse's role is to assess how much information the patient has and help the patient decipher the information.

SUBJECTIVE DATA

The nursing interview is a communication process that focuses on the patient's developmental, psychologic, sociocultural, and spiritual responses that can be treated and supported with nursing and collaborative interventions. It is important for the nurse to be cognizant of the patient's comfort and anxiety levels, age, and current health status. These factors can influence the patient's ability to fully participate in the interview.

The interview process has three phases. During the introductory phase, the nurse and patient get to know each other. At this time, the nurse gives the patient a brief overview of the interview process and explains its purpose. The second phase is the working phase, in which the nurse begins to take the history. It is important that the nurse take cues from the patient, listen, and use critical thinking skills in interpreting and validating the information received from the patient. The final phase of the interview process is the summary phase, in which the nurse verbally summarizes the information obtained to ensure accuracy and to validate the problems and goals. Possible plans for problem resolution are discussed with the patient during the summary phase.[2]

A few specific communication techniques can be employed to facilitate the interview and ensure its efficiency. It is important for the nurse to ask open-ended questions to obtain patient perceptions. These questions begin with "What," "Where," and "How," and are important because they encourage the patient to use more than a one-word response. Close-ended questions are also important to help obtain facts and elicit specific information. This may help keep the patient from rambling. Offering the patient a list of words to choose from may help obtain specific answers while reducing the chance that patients will perceive and try to provide an expected answer. For example, in reference to the quality of pain, the nurse might ask, "Is the pain dull, sharp, mild, or stabbing?" In reference to the frequency, one might ask, "Does the pain occur daily, with or without activity?"

When the nurse obtains data that digress from normal, further exploration is necessary. These questions are useful: "What alleviates or aggravates the problem?" "How long has it occurred?" "When does it occur?" "Was the onset gradual or sudden?" Throughout the interview, it is important for the nurse to

rephrase the patient's responses to clarify information obtained.[2]

Several key points are important when interviewing a patient. The first is to avoid being judgmental. This attitude puts the patient at ease and encourages more specific information. It is important to use silence to help patients organize their thoughts. It is also helpful to provide answers to questions as they arise during the interview. Avoid leading questions, rushing the patient, and performing other tasks while taking the history.[2] By employing these principles during the interview, the clinical nurse obtains information used in developing a plan of care and assists the surgeon by providing information necessary for making a diagnosis.

While obtaining the patient's history, the clinical nurse must be aware that many disorders can present as a painful hip, including problems of the lower back as well as visceral disorders, and that the patient may describe *hip pain* that actually represents referred symptoms. Once the problem has been localized to the hip area, a distinction must be made between intraarticular and extraarticular symptoms.

A few characteristic features may clue the examiner to suspect an intraarticular hip problem. These hallmarks include complaints of anterior, inguinal, or medial thigh pain. Complaints of lateral hip pain or posterior or buttock symptoms are more commonly caused by extraarticular sources such as trochanteric bursitis, abductor muscle injury, or sciatica. A history of catching or popping of the hip may be related to intraarticular pathology, but these symptoms can also occur with disorders outside the joint.

Patients with intraarticular hip pathology commonly complain of pain in their groin with activities. Twisting maneuvers, such as turning to change direction, are often more problematic than straight-ahead walking. Inclines and ascending or descending stairs are more likely to exacerbate symptoms. Characteristically, getting in and out of an automobile can be difficult as it loads the hip in a flexed position while also twisting. Painful hip symptoms with intercourse is often a problem and is often more likely to be spontaneously mentioned when the patient and interviewer are of the same gender. There may be difficulty putting on shoes and socks, which often indicates restriction in rotational motion.

Objective Data and Physical Examination

After the subjective information has been obtained, the nurse can begin to explore the objective aspects of the patient's complaints. The surgeon may obtain this information, but it is important for the clinical nurse to understand the physical assessment process. This procedure is discussed in detail in Chapter 3 and summarized here.

Examination of the patient with a complaint of hip pain is straightforward but inclusive of the lumbar spine and pelvis. Many patients present with a chief complaint of *hip pain* but do not have an intraarticular hip problem. Therefore, the examiner must first consider extraarticular sources that could cause the patient's hip pain. Once the extraarticular sources are ruled out, intraarticular sources of the patient's pain can be considered.

Extraarticular sources of hip pain can be the lumbar spine, sacroiliac joint, or sciatic nerve. Strains of certain muscles, such as the hip adductors or flexors, can also imitate hip joint symptoms. When deep tendinous involvement occurs, such as from the piriformis or iliopsoas tendon, it may be difficult to differentiate these symptoms from mechanical hip symptoms. Although uncommon, a femoral hernia also produces groin pain.

Observation of the patient's gait pattern is meaningful. The gait may be antalgic or possibly reveal an abductor lurch, which reduces the forces generated across the hip. The patient may use an assistive device such as a cane or crutches. It is important to note the patient's base of support. While standing, the patient may assume a slightly flexed position of the affected hip. When seated the patient may slouch to avoid excessive hip flexion or lean to the uninvolved side with the hip in a slightly abducted, externally rotated position.

It is important to inspect the patient's hips and lower extremities for any asymmetry, gross atrophy, spinal malalignment, or pelvic obliquity that may be fixed or associated with a gross leg length discrepancy. Leg lengths are measured as a routine part of the examination. Thigh circumference is recorded as this may reflect the chronicity of the disease and may be a rough indicator of the response to therapy. It is also important to document range of motion of the affected hip compared with the unaffected hip.

It is helpful to ask the patient to use one finger to point to the area of most discomfort. This is a useful way of determining the area of maximal involvement. Intraarticular hip pathology usually has a component of anterior hip pain. The patient may also relate a sensation of deep, lateral discomfort or posterior pain, but this is usually in conjunction with a significant anterior component. Often, the patient demonstrates the *C-sign* in describing deep hip pain. This sign is characterized by placing the index finger and thumb around the hip, forming a C-shaped pattern over the area of involvement. The index finger rests in the groin area and the thumb rests over the posterior aspect of the trochanter.

Palpation is rarely helpful in determining intraarticular pathology, but it is important in the overall assessment of other sources of pain in the hip region, such as trochanteric bursitis. The examiner palpates the lumbar spine, sacroiliac joints, ischium, iliac crest, and the lateral hip around the greater trochanter, always comparing the unaffected to the affected side and examining the unaffected hip first.

Crepitus may be felt as the hips are put through range of motion. Manual muscle testing is a crude measure of hip function but may elicit symptoms localized to a specific muscle injury. Resisted active range of motion may also reproduce joint symptoms. The affected hip may have restricted range of motion because of pain or a mechanical block such as a loose body.

The most specific indicator for hip joint pain is log rolling of the patient's leg. This action moves only the femoral head in relation to the acetabulum and the surrounding capsule. The absence of pain on log rolling does not preclude the hip as the source of symptoms, but the presence of pain with this maneuver greatly raises the suspicion of mechanical joint pathology.

Two maneuvers elicit pain with even subtle hip pathology. These are the combination of forced flexion with internal rotation or abduction with external rotation. The Patrick or Faber (flexion, abduction, external rotation) test has been used to educe symptoms from both the hip and sacroiliac joint. The distinction is usually based on the origin of the pain. An active straight leg raise often elicits symptoms. This maneuver creates a force of several times body weight across the articular surfaces and actually generates more force than walking.

POSTOPERATIVE CARE

By the time the patient arrives in the operating suite, the educational process should be complete and the patient prepared to handle the events that will follow. As discussed earlier, this educational process is best accomplished before the patient arrives at the hospital. Three salient features are important in the postoperative care of the patient: pain control, wound care, and activity level. It is important that these three aspects are understood by the patient and the caregivers. These concepts may be difficult to comprehend preoperatively but should be discussed.

It is helpful to provide written postoperative instructions for the patient and caregiver (see Appendix). The instructions reiterate much of the information that has been verbalized preoperatively and immediately postoperatively. Providing written discharge instructions helps increase retention and understanding of the information provided.[3] The 1994 study by Oberle et al.[4] showed that timing of preoperative teaching is critical to retention and patient satisfaction. Approximately 25% of the patients in the study reported being given little or no information about their surgery, even through nurses had provided information during the perioperative period. This report suggests that patients and their caregivers do not always hear and understand the information being conveyed. Written postoperative discharge instructions can serve as a reference once the patient has returned home.

PAIN CONTROL

Postoperative pain is one of the greatest fears patients have about surgery and is often poorly addressed by physicians.[5] This concern should be discussed preoperatively to allay apprehension. Patients expect some postoperative pain or discomfort, but many are surprised at the low intensity of pain they actually experience. Most patients describe postoperative pain as a burning ache in the hip, but the severity depends on the pathology addressed. For example, a patient with loose bodies may find that the postoperative pain is less than the discomfort experienced preoperatively. Conversely, a patient undergoing an abrasion arthroplasty for chondral damage may experience considerably more discomfort immediately after surgery.

It should be explained to the patient that there will be pain from the surgical procedure, but also some muscular soreness in the operative leg. This soreness is related to manipulation of the hip, the traction, and distractive forces used during the arthroscopic procedure. Usually, there is soreness in the hip joint after the acute surgical pain has abated. Soreness due to the use of the perineal post for distraction is common with some patients. They typically describe it as feeling like they have ridden a horse and have soreness in their saddle area. Ankle soreness in the operative leg is related to the traction boot. It is reassuring for the patient to know that these various aches normally resolve in 5 to 7 days.

Narcotics or oral centrally acting medications, such as hydrocodone (5 mg) or oxycodone (5 mg) with acetaminophen (500 mg) are prescribed for pain control. Prescription pain medicine is generally used for the first 4 to 5 days after surgery. By the end of the first postoperative week, most patients no longer need narcotics to control pain. Patients should be reminded to take medications with food to prevent gastrointestinal discomfort. They should also be instructed to refrain from driving or operating heavy machinery while medicated.

After narcotics are discontinued, alternative nonprescription medications such as acetaminophen, ibuprofen, or other nonsteroidal antiinflammatories may be useful to ameliorate discomfort. It is important to note that analgesics, possibly narcotics, may be needed when physical therapy is initiated or when performing exercises. Some patients may experience prolonged discomfort or more intense pain. The reasons for this should be explored by the clinician.

The use of ice (cryotherapy) has several beneficial effects for tissues that have been injured, whether from trauma or by surgery. When ice is applied immediately after surgery, the body attempts to preserve core heat by constricting superficial cutaneous vessels, causing decreased capillary permeability and hemorrhaging. This reaction therapeutically alters the physiologic response of the tissues to injury by reducing inflammation, swelling, and pain.[6]

Ice may be most effective when used immediately after surgery. The ice bag can first be applied by the recovery room nurse. The patient should be instructed to apply ice for 15 to 20 minutes every 3 hours for the first 24 hours and even for 2 to 3 days after surgery if it helps alleviate discomfort.

Cryotherapy is not without hazards. Cold should not be used for longer than 30 minutes with conventional methods (ice bags/packs) because of the potential for freezing the skin; this could result in frostnip or frostbite. Nerve palsies can result from the application of cold to an extremity for longer than 30 minutes, or when cold is improperly applied to vulnerable areas.[7]

Contraindications to cryotherapy include patients recovering from an epidural infusion or spinal block. Ice should not be used until full sensation has returned in both lower extremities. Cryotherapy should not be used at all in the patient with a suspected neuropathy, such as with diabetes, or on patients with a true hypersensitivity or allergy to cold.[7]

WOUND CARE

A bulky dressing is applied to the surgical site (Figure 18.1). This dressing is left in place until the first postoperative day, allowing time for extravasated fluid from surgery to be absorbed into the dressing. Usually, this has subsided enough to remove the dressing within the first 24 hours. The patient should be reassured that it is normal for the dressing to feel wet from the irrigation fluid and that it may be blood tinged.

The patient should be aware that the surgeon will make three or four arthroscopy portals. Each of these portals will be closed with a single suture. Patients, and even allied health professionals, are often surprised at the anatomic location of the portals. They envision them being located more cephalad (Figure 18.2).

The portals are cleaned daily with hydrogen peroxide and water. An adhesive bandage can then be applied until the sutures are removed. The patient may shower on the first postoperative day, taking care to keep water from running directly over the portals. If the portals show signs of adequate healing, the sutures

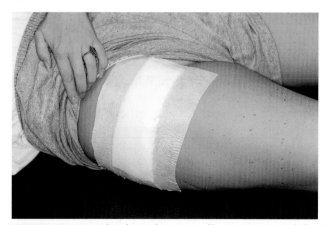

FIGURE 18.1. An absorbent dressing collects extravasated fluid that leaks out through the portals.

may be removed 3 to 5 days postoperatively and steri-strips applied.

It takes approximately 7 to 10 days for the portals to heal completely. During this time, showering is allowed, but the patient should avoid submersing the operative hip in a bathtub, hot tub, or swimming pool.

It is important to educate patients regarding the signs and symptoms of infection. They should be advised to contact the nurse if they develop any redness or drainage at the portal sites or if they develop a high fever.

ACTIVITY LEVEL

The activity level prescribed after hip arthroscopy is variable, depending on the pathology found at the time of surgery and the surgeon's preference. Generally, an assistive device such as crutches or a walker is recommended during the first week, with the patient bearing weight as tolerated. A normal gait pattern usually returns within this time frame, but patients should be encouraged to use their assistive devices until they see the physical therapist or return to the surgeon's office. Weight-bearing status may be more restricted in certain cases such as abrasion arthroplasty of the weight-bearing surface of the hip joint.

The patient will be most comfortable immediately after surgery in a reclining or sitting position. The most comfortable sleeping positions are usually supine or on the nonoperative side with a pillow between the legs. Sleeping on the operative side does not cause harm, but usually this is not comfortable until 4 or 5 days postoperatively.

Patients need to be reminded that it is easy for them to overdo activities in the first few days after surgery, and patients should be encouraged to limit their activities. Once they feel like being up and around, daily activities can be performed to tolerance, but they should be respectful of any discomfort felt in

the hip. Often patients experience a *honeymoon phase* during the first 3 to 4 weeks following surgery. They are enthused by the way their hip feels, but they have not yet resumed most of their normal daily activities. As patients resume more normal activities, there will always be some transiently increased soreness. If the patient is not prepared for this, it can be an abrupt and disheartening experience, shaking the patient's confidence in the eventual recovery process. The nurse can explain that it really takes a month to get over the actual surgical procedure. After that initial month, it can take 3 to 4 months before patients may actually appreciate the benefits of the surgery.

Fatigue is one of the biggest considerations after surgery.[4] This can be related to several factors including the anesthetic, analgesics, pain, or sleep disruption. The nurse should inform the patient that this effect generally dissipates after postoperative day 3 but can last as long as several weeks.

Physical therapy is usually initiated 2 days after surgery. The rehabilitation program for the postoperative patient is individualized to the pathology addressed and the procedure performed. The primary focus of the rehabilitation process is to reduce discomfort and improve function. A successful result after surgery is often dependent on a properly constructed rehabilitation program. This is an important concept to be relayed to the patient because there may often be a reluctance to go to physical therapy. When the hip hurts, the idea of exercise may not be appealing.

The most frequently asked question regarding activity is "When can I drive?" General guidelines include the following two parameters: the patient must have discontinued the use of narcotic analgesics and have regained adequate leg control to operate the accelerator and brake pedals or clutch.

It is important for the clinical nurse to remember several things pertinent to the postoperative recuperation. Patients want and need to hear that they are do-

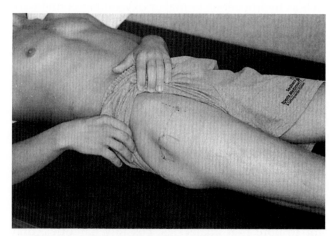

FIGURE 18.2. Inspection of the wound demonstrates the position of the standard portals. These are placed lower than many patients expect when conceptualizing the location of their hip joint.

ing well and are on schedule in their recovery. Patients are often impatient and may expect to recover more quickly than they actually do. Many prefer to have guidelines by which to gauge their progress. They want to know how other patients normally respond under the same circumstances.[4] Remember that patients often latch on to misinformation and often revert to this misinformation, despite the clinician's best effort at education. Patients and their caregivers may simply exhibit selective hearing or may forget to read postoperative instructions; therefore, frequent contact by telephone is one of the keys to the successful recovery of the hip arthroscopy patient.[8] The frequent contact between the clinical nurse and the patient can have a positive effect on patient satisfaction and also provides a mechanism for feedback from the patient and caregivers.[3]

CONCLUSIONS

Appropriate patient selection and education, skillful implementation of the surgical procedure, and a properly constructed rehabilitation program are all important factors in the success of hip arthroscopy. It is also important that the patient's expectations are properly matched with the results anticipated by the surgeon.

An optimal outcome is dependent on coordination of the perioperative care, from preoperative assessment through postoperative rehabilitation. The clinical nurse helps facilitate the patient's smooth transition through this experience and serves as a vital resource person for other members of the health care team. The nurse is an educator, practitioner, consultant, and collaborator. By serving in this multifaceted role, the nurse helps ensure appropriate and efficient use of resources through close patient follow-up and timely response to changes in the clinical circumstance. Thus, the other members of the health care team, whether it is as the patient, caregiver, surgeon, operating room personnel, or physical therapist, can better fulfill their respective roles.

References

1. Sutherland E: Day surgery: all in a day's work. Nurse Times 1991;87(11):26–30.
2. Weber J: Nurses' Handbook of Health Assessment. Philadelphia: Lippincott, 1988:1–7.
3. Dougherty J: Same-day surgery: the nurse's role. Orthop Nurs 1996;15(4):15–18.
4. Oberle K, Allen M, Lynkowski P: Follow-up of same day surgery patients. AORN J 1994;59(5):1016–1025.
5. Stephenson ME: Discharge criteria in day surgery. J Adv Nurs 1990;15(5):601–613.
6. Knight KL: Cryotherapy. Am Fam Physician 1990;23(3):141–144.
7. McDowell JH, McFarland EG, Nalli BJ: Cryotherapy in the orthopaedic patient. Orthop Nurs 1994;13(5):21–30.
8. Burden N: Telephone follow-up of ambulatory surgery patients following discharge is a nursing responsibility. J Post Anesth Nurs 1992;7(4):256–261.

APPENDIX: POSTOPERATIVE INSTRUCTIONS FOR ARTHROSCOPIC SURGERY OF THE HIP

The following information is designed to answer some frequently asked questions regarding what to expect and do after arthroscopic surgery. These are general guidelines; if you have any questions or concerns, please call.

Dressing and Wound Care

During arthroscopic surgery, the joint is irrigated with water. There are typically three small incisions closed with sutures. Your hip will be covered with a bulky dressing. Water may gradually leak through these incisions, saturating the bandage. This blood-tinged drainage may persist for 24 to 36 hours. If it has not significantly decreased by this time, call our office.

The bandage may be removed the day after surgery. The incisions should be cleaned with hydrogen peroxide and water and then covered with an adhesive bandage. As soon as the incisions are dry, you may leave them uncovered. Do not use ointments such as Neosporin on the incisions. You may shower the day after surgery, but avoid water running directly over the incisions. The incisions should not be soaked (e.g., bathtub, hot tub, swimming pool).

If the incisions show any signs of infection, contact our office. Specifically, if there is increased redness, persistent drainage, if you have fever, or if the pain does not progressively decrease, call the office.

Ice

During the first 48 hours, ice can be helpful to decrease pain and swelling and is especially important during the first 24 hours. Ice bags/packs should never be applied directly to the skin. They should be wrapped in a towel and applied for only 15 minutes at a time every 2 to 3 hours. If the skin becomes very cold or burns, discontinue the ice application immediately.

Ambulation and Movement

Unless you have been otherwise instructed, you will be allowed to bear as much weight on your leg as is comfortable immediately after surgery. Crutches may be used as necessary to help decrease discomfort while walking for the first few days after surgery. Please use crutches at least until your first physical therapy appointment.

Your level of discomfort will most often be your best guide in determining how much activity is allowed. Remember that it is easy to overdo the amount of activity in the first few days after surgery, and any increase in pain or swelling usually indicates that you need to decrease your activities. Please be careful on slippery surfaces, steps, or anywhere you might fall and injure yourself.

Medications

You will be given a prescription for pain medication. If you have any known drug allergies, check with the nurse before taking any medication. Please note that we are unable to call in prescriptions for narcotics after office hours. If you need a refill, please call early in the day so the nurse can call in your prescription. This is especially important if the weekend is approaching.

Some medications have side effects. If you have any difficulty with itching, nausea, or other side effects, discontinue the medication immediately and call our office. Pain medication often causes drowsiness, and we advise that you do not drive, operate machinery, or make important decisions while taking medication.

Aspirin serves as a mild blood thinner and may decrease the chance of blood clots forming in the leg. Although this is uncommon, it can be a difficult problem. If you are able to take aspirin, you should take one aspirin (325 mg) twice daily for 2 weeks following your surgery. It is best to take one in the morning and one in the evening and to avoid taking them on an empty stomach. If you are under the age of 16 or have any unusual medical problems, please check with the nurse about whether you should take aspirin.

Exercise and Physical Therapy

Physical therapy usually begins within a few days after your surgery. The therapist will outline an exercise program specific to your type of surgery. The purpose of physical therapy is to help you regain the use of your hip in a safe and progressive fashion. If you have any questions regarding your exercise program, please contact the physical therapist. If you are unaware of when or where your therapy is, please call the nurse and she can help you determine this.

First Postoperative Visit

Your first postoperative appointment will be within 1 week of your surgery. The findings at surgery, long-term prognosis, and plans for rehabilitation will be discussed at this appointment. If you are unsure of when your first postoperative visit is, please call the office and someone will help get one scheduled.

Communications

If you are having any problems, contact us right away. If it is after office hours, the answering service will contact the nurse or doctor on call.

Remember, if your pain increases, check for signs of infection (redness, fever, and so forth), decrease your activities, use ice, and take your pain medication as prescribed. If the pain persists, or if there are signs of infection, call our office.

A. PROTOCOL FOR ARTHROSCOPIC HIP DEBRIDEMENT

All patients are different and should be treated according to their tolerance in therapy. It is important that these patients <u>listen to their pain symptoms</u> and adjust their program as needed.

Immediate Post-Op: Work on ROM within tolerance

- ▸ Active assisted ROM allowed to all planes without pain

- ▸ Educate patient on importance of avoiding pain with stretch

- ▸ Crutches are used for comfort – weight bearing as tolerated. Patient can wean off crutches as tolerated over first two weeks if not instructed by the physician to remain on them longer. Patient may also stop crutches in the house, but continue use outside of the home until fully confident on involved leg.

- ▸ Some patients may benefit from some gentle hip mobilization and distraction techniques (perform these only if patient is able to tolerate and clinician feels comfortable in proper technique).

These include:
1. Straight plane distraction, force applied at distal lower leg.

2. Inferior glide with patient supine and hip and knee bent to 90°, force applied at superior aspect of anterior thigh with movement inferiorly.

3. Gentle posterior glide with patient supine (hip and knee bent to 90°) with force applied down through knee for posterior hip movement.

4. Oscillation mobilization in internal/external rotation (log-rolling).

AVOID EARLY STRAIGHT LEG RAISES (especially with patients suffering from articular surface damage)

As early as week one - if patient is able to tolerate - gentle toning exercises can begin - patient must be pain free and remain pain free throughout exercises.

These include: Progress down the list as tolerated, avoiding pain.

1. Isometrics	• **Quad Sets** • **Glut Sets**	• **Ham Sets** • **Adductor Sets**	• **Abductor Sets**

2. Initial core positioning/strengthening	• **Pelvic Toning Exercises**
	   anterior/posterior tilt
	   core hip flexion/extension
	• **Double and single leg bridging**
	• **4 pt hip flexion/extension**
		• **Balancing Drills, to single leg drills**
		   mini squats
		• **Standing core position**	

3. Pool Exercises	• **Water resisted toning exercises** • **Swimming and walking drills**		
4. Intermediate Exercises (some patients never reach this stage)	• **Theraband** • **Weight machines** • **Bike**	• **Elliptical Crosstrainer** • **Other Cardiovascular Exercises**	

B. HIP EXERCISES—PHASE I

1. HIP AND KNEE FLEXION/HEEL SLIDES - Bend the knee
of your involved leg by sliding your heel towards you as far as
possible. When you have reached the maximum bend, pause for a
few seconds, and then allow your leg to straighten back to the
starting position. Use your hands for assistance if needed. Repeat
____ times, ____ times a day.

2. HIP ABDUCTION - With your legs straight out in front of
you, slide your involved leg out to the side as flat as is
comfortable, then bring it back to the starting position. Repeat ____
times, ____ times a day.

3. INTERNAL ROTATION/EXTERNAL ROTATION - "Log
Roll" your involved leg with an inward and outward stretch as
comfort allows. Repeat ____ times, ____ times a day.

4. GLUT SETS - With your legs straight out in front of you,
contract and tighten your buttocks, holding for ____ seconds,
then relax.Repeat ____ times, ____ times a day.

* 5. QUAD SET - Tighten muscle in front of knee and hold 5
counts, then relax. Repeat ____ times, ____ times a day.

* 6. HAM SET - Press the heel of your foot down to the floor so
the muscle on the bottom of your thigh tightens. Hold 5 counts,
then relax. Repeat ____ times, ____ times a day.

** multi-angled co-contractions: exercises 5 and 6 can be
performed at various degrees of knee flexion (30°, 60°, and 90°).

7. HIP ADDUCTION (ISOMETRIC) - Lie on your back with your knees slightly bent. Place a pillow between your knees and squeeze for a count of _____, then relax. Repeat ____ times, ____ times a day.

8. HIP ABDUCTION (ISOMETRIC) - Lie on your back with your knees slightly bent. Now, wrap a strong, non-elastic strap (i.e. belt) around your legs just above your knee. Now, try to pull the legs apart against the resistance of the strap and hold for _____ seconds, then relax. Repeat ____ times, ____ times a day.

9. TERMINAL KNEE EXTENSION - Place a towel roll beneath your knee on the involved side. The roll should be approximately 4"-6" in diameter. Straighten your involved knee but keep your thigh in contact with the roll. Hold your leg straight for 5 seconds, then slowly lower your leg. Repeat _____ times, _____ times a day.

10. DOUBLE LEG BRIDGING - Lying on your back with your knees bent and your feet resting on the floor, raise your hips into the air. Hold for a count of _____, then lower. Repeat ____ times, ____ times a day.

11. SINGLE LEG BRIDGING - Lying on your back with your _____ knee bent and your _____ leg flat on the floor, raise your hips into the air. Hold for a count of _____ , then lower. Repeat ____ times, ____ times a day.

C. WATER EXERCISES—LOWER EXTREMITY

1. SQUATS - In the pool with water at chest level, place your feet shoulder width apart and slowly perform a mini-squat , bending your knees approximately 30° to 45°. From this position, straighten your legs, rise up on the balls of your feet, then return to the starting position. Repeat ____ times.

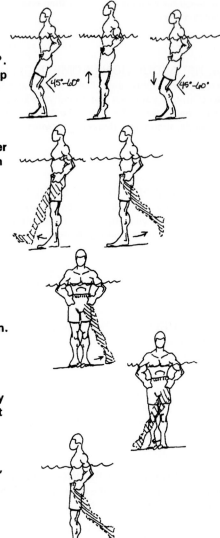

2. HIP SWINGS - (a) In the pool with water at chest level, shift your body weight on to your uninvolved leg. Keeping your knee straight, move your involved leg forward and back, being careful to maintain your balance. Repeat ____ times.

   (b) In the same position as above, shift your body weight on to the uninvolved leg. Keeping your knee straight, move your involved leg out to the side and back to the starting position. Repeat ____ times.

   (c) Again in the same position, move your involved leg across your body and back to the starting position. Repeat ____ times.

   (d) Finally, from the same position, move your involved leg behind you, keeping your knee straight, then return your leg to the starting position. Repeat ____ times.

D. THERABAND EXERCISES

1. HIP FLEXION - Secure one end of the band to an immovable object and the other just above the ankle of your involved leg. With your back to the object and keeping your knee straight, lift your leg straight out in front of you, then slowly lower. Repeat _____ times, _____ times a day.

2. HIP EXTENSION - Secure one end of the band to an immovable object and the other end just above the ankle of your involved leg. Facing the object and keeping your knee straight, pull your leg back, then return slowly. Repeat _____ times, _____ times a day.

3. HIP ABDUCTION - Secure one end of the band to an immovable object and the other end just above the ankle of your involved leg. With your uninvolved leg next to the object, push your other leg away from the object, then slowly lower. Repeat _____ times, _____ times a day.

4. HIP ADDUCTION - Secure one end of the band to an immovable object and the other end just above the ankle of the involved leg. With your involved leg next to the object, pull your leg straight across the other, then return slowly (as in A.). Or, if your therapist so instructs, begin with the involved leg out to the side and then pull it in next to the other (as in B.) Repeat _____ times, _____ times a day.

   * All the exercises listed above can be performed above the knee, if necessary.

HIP EXERCISES—PHASE II

1. SUPINE HIP INTERNAL/EXTERNAL ROTATION – Lie on back with knees straight and legs apart. Slowly roll toes and knees outward and then back inward. Gradually increase the amount of turn in both positions.
Repeat _____ times, _____ times a day.

2. SUPINE PELVIC FLEXION/EXTENSION – Lie on back with knees bent. Tighten lower abdominal muscles. Tighten buttock muscles and flatten back. Rotate pelvis upward and arch back. Find and position in your neutral (balanced) mid-position between flat and arched. Hold with lower abdominals.
Repeat _____ times, _____ times a day.

3. SUPINE PELVIC CORE STABILIZATION/MARCHING – Lie on back. Find and position in your neutral mid-position. Hold with lower abdominals while lifting bent knee up in "marching" position 3-4" off floor. Alternate legs.
Repeat _____ times, _____ times a day.

4. SUPINE PELVIC CORE STABILIZATION/LEG EXTENSION – Lie on back with knees bent. Find and hold neutral mid-position. Slowly straighten one leg and then return to bent position. Alternate legs. Repeat _____ times, _____ times a day.

5. SIDELYING HIP ABDUCTION (Gluteus Medius) – Lie on your _____ side on the floor or on a flat surface. Gently rotate and lift top leg outward (in clamshell position).
Repeat _____ times, _____ times a day.

6. <u>SEATED HIP INTERNAL/EXTERNAL ROTATION</u> – Sit and gradually turn your leg outward and then back inward.
Repeat _____ times, _____ times a day.

7. <u>SEATED HIP FLEXION STRETCH</u> – Sit and gradually lean forward /downward for an "easy" stretch.
Repeat _____ times, _____ times a day.

8. <u>SEATED HIP FLEXION</u> – Sit and raise legs in bent position (as if you were marching).
Repeat _____ times, _____ times a day.

9. <u>HANDS/KNEES POSITION HIP FLEXION/EXTENSION</u> – Position on hands and knees and find pelvic neutral mid-position. Hold with lower abdominals while moving hip in alternate flexion (knees toward chest) and extension (straightening hip backward) position.
Repeat _____ times, _____ times a day.

10. <u>**GYMBALL CORE STABILIZATION (Beginning Positions)**</u> –
Find mid-pelvic position while sitting on gymball. Hold with
abdominal muscles.
Repeat _____ times, _____ times a day.

11. <u>**GYMBALL CORE STABILIZATION/KNEE EXTENSION**</u>-
Find mid-pelvic position while sitting on gymball. While
holding neutral mid-position, slowly control lifting leg straight
into extension.   Alternate legs.
Repeat _____ times, _____ times a day.

12. <u>**GYMBALL CORE STABILIZATION/HIP FLEXION**</u> –
Find mid-pelvic position while sitting on gymball. While
holding neutral mid-position with abdominals, slowly control
lifting leg in a "marching" position. Alternate legs.
Repeat _____ times, _____ times a day.

Index